How to
Eat, Move *and*
Be Healthy!

How to
Eat, Move *and* Be Healthy!

Your personalized 4-step guide to
looking and feeling great from the inside out

by
Paul Chek

A C.H.E.K Institute Publication
San Diego, CA

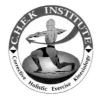

How to Eat, Move and Be Healthy!

First printing, February 2004
Second printing, September 2004

Cover design: Peri Poloni, Knockout Design
Book design: Cara Burke
Editors: Cara Burke, Ed Mann, Penthea Crozier
Proof readers: Paul McNeese, Marc Hertzberg
Illustrators: Charlie Aligaen, Joling Lee

C.H.E.K Institute
San Diego, CA, U.S.A.

800.552.8789
info@chekinstitute.com
www.chekinstitute.com

Printed in the U.S.A.

ISBN: 1-58387-006-7
Chek, Paul W.

Warning – Disclaimer

The workouts and other health-related activities described in this book were developed by the author and are to be used as an adjunct to improved strengthening, conditioning, health and fitness. These programs may not be appropriate for everyone. All individuals, especially those who suffer from any disease or are recovering from any injury, should consult their physicians regarding the advisability of undertaking any of the activities suggested in these programs. The author has been painstaking in his research. However, he is neither responsible nor liable for any harm or injury resulting from this program or the use of the exercises or exercise devices described herein.

As I sit here writing this preface, I am a happy, healthy, fit and strong 42-year-old man. Over 20 years of my life has been spent assisting others in achieving physical, emotional, mental and spiritual health, fitness and high-level athletic performance. This pursuit has helped me grow tremendously as a person. Through my experiences as an athlete, therapist, conditioning specialist and consultant to professional athletes, sports teams and corporations, it became evident that I could do more. It became clear that while I was growing as a person and my clients were growing through their experiences with their bodies and their lives, I could beneficially influence a greater number of people by designing educational programs for healthcare professionals, which I have now done successfully since 1988.

In the natural evolution from a person who thinks only of himself, feeding the *I* (ego), to one who thinks of those around him (*we* or *us*), I was destined to share the methods that have helped keep myself and my students healthy and vital with everyone, with *all*. This book provides *everyone* the opportunity to *choose* health and vitality. While many people think movement or exercise, eating correctly and being healthy is a lot of work, the fact of the matter is that moving too little, eating incorrectly and being devitalized are simply choices with ramifications. The ramifications I am speaking of are laid out clearly in Bill Wolcott's foreword as well as being discussed throughout this book; they include physical, emotional, mental and spiritual degeneration!

What society at large has lost touch with is the fact that for thousands of years, ancient enlightened men have been telling us that we are miniature models of the cosmos, that all in the Universe can be found within us. We are both *star people* and *people of the earth.* The current condition of the human race mirrors our management of Mother Earth. We breathe the air that is her lungs, we drink the water that is her blood; we eat the foods that are the product of her great and beautiful body. How can we be any healthier than *She*, for we are *She* and *She* is we!

In our pursuit for material gain and to better understand ourselves, we have focused on the sense world, the world of what we can see, touch, hear, feel and taste. We have become industrialized and institutionalized. Our science and medicine have become ever more complex and specialized, to the point that today we are surrounded by experts who have studied tirelessly to learn more and more about less and less, only to end up knowing *absolutely everything about nothing!* We have studied disease looking for health. We have made plastics, processed foods and medical drugs in an attempt to *make things easier*…yet we have not only made things harder for ourselves and our children, we have become the greatest parasite Mother Earth has ever known. In fact, we have even become a parasite to the Moon and made a garbage dump out of Space in the process!

The famous Naturalist, Edward O. Wilson, informs us that today we are killing more living species of all types than ever in history! The escalating rates of disease among plants, animals and human beings was forecasted in the pioneering works of great people such as Sir Albert Howard, Sir Robert McCarrison, William Albrecht, Rudolph Steiner, Ehrenfried Pfeiffer, Lady Eve Balfour, Weston A. Price and Francis Marion Pottenger Sr. and Jr. While these great pioneers studied plants, animals and man, and how to keep them healthy, they warned of the impending dangers we faced through chemical and industrialized management of plants and animals. We have come *a long way down the road they tried desperately to steer human- ity away from many years ago*. While they all warned of the danger in managing Mother Earth, her crops, animals and ourselves with such shortsightedness, they also stated that we could, with a concerted effort, turn things around and head back toward a healthy existence—a healthy existence for both the ecosystem of Mother Earth and the inner ecosystem of the human being.

I was fortunate to have a mother who was both health-minded and respectful of Mother Earth. We lived off the land when I was young. Produce and animals were our life bread, and on a farm you quickly learn that you only get what you give, you reap what you sow. We knew exactly where our food came from, and if there was anything wrong with it, it was our fault—*simple!* Today, hardly anyone ever sees their produce or the animals they eat in the field. Nor do they see what is done to the land in the process of growing produce and raising animals under the influence of the food processing industry, commercial farming in- dustry, chemical corporations and the pharmaceutical industry, which reap billions and billions each year from the drugs sold to patch both man and animal alike! We are living like an ostrich with its head in the sand, falsely believing that what is "out of sight" is "out of mind".

This book comes with a bit of tough love. It is truly *time to pull our heads out, be they in the sand or some other dark place.* Clearly the "experts" have not made us healthy, they have only allowed us to ignore the head, neck, back, heart and stomach aches that were intended to warn us of foul play. To change the world for the better, we must start with ourselves, IMMEDIATELY! It will be your children who are left with the mess we've either created or allowed to be created because our bad diets and lifestyles left us too lifeless to get involved, to care, to stand up to those with purely *I* or selfish motives.

To restore our health is to restore health to our ecosystem and Mother Earth, for the two are inextricably linked. To get healthy we must begin to think right, and as I always tell my clients and students, you have to:

- Drink right to think right
- Eat right to think right
- Move right to think right

And to drink right and eat right means that we will have to pay a lot more attention to what we put in our oceans, lakes, rivers and streams. To eat right, we will have to pay a lot more attention to what is being done to our food and the land it is grown upon! When we begin to move right, you won't see lazy or obese people driving around the parking lot for half an hour trying to get a parking spot right next to the entrance of the local shopping mall! When we are moving right, we will be much more respectful of the air we are polluting unnecessarily, *because we will be more conscious of the fact that we are breathing it!*

If the thought of eating correctly, moving your body and becoming healthy seems daunting and like a lot of work to you, don't worry. It's no more work than you are doing to manage a life of illness and fatigue right now! This book teaches you how to eat right so you can enjoy food and the vitality it gives you—right now. You may not realize how your food choices are directly linked to your aches, pains and sagging vital- ity. Many people today have lost sight of the fact that *life is movement and movement is life!*

The world is getting fat while it is getting sick, and you are the only one who can change that! How many people do you think realize that the human body is about 80% water as they pour coffee, tea, soda pop, alcohol and sugar drinks of neon blue and fluorescent green down their gullets? This book teaches you that to have a healthy body, a healthy mind and a productive life, you need to drink good clean water. Please don't wait to get involved until it is completely toxic with industrial waste! Your body manufactures 2,000,000 red blood cells every second; just look at what you ate and drank in the past 24 hours to see what your new red blood cells are made of! That observation alone may shed some light on the number of drugs being consumed by the population at large today. Clearly, you can't achieve the look or feel you want using your stomach as a garbage can, can you?

No, it's not hard to be healthy, to be vital, to be productive and to have a beautiful body, *it's just a choice*. All you have to do is change your mind, to change your thinking and allocate your energy to achieving what you *want*, not what you *don't want*. Famous Australian business consultant Brad Sugar says, "*The formula for change is when the desire for change is greater than the resistance to change.*" If you are ready to make that change, to become healthy, vital, productive, beautiful and happy with who you are, to make Mother Earth better by making yourself better, *this book is for you!* If you want to continue to be fat, tired, diseased, unhealthy, destructive to Mother Earth and keep drug lords rich, the formula is easy and you don't need a genius like Albert Einstein to give it to you – it's simple: *more of the same = more of the same!*

I invite you to follow the simple life changing principles in this book so that we can all set a good example for the next generation. We owe it to ourselves and to our children to be healthy and vital. If you've even read this far, chances are very good you are ready. Let's do it!

Your Personal Health and Vitality Consultant,

Paul Chek

Great speakers have always found violent opposition from mediocrities. The latter cannot understand it when a man does not thoughtlessly submit to hereditary prejudices but honestly and courageously uses his intelligence.

Albert Einstein

Anyone who has written a book can attest to the fact that in some ways the process is much like giving birth. A book begins as an idea—often an idea intended to serve a purpose, to fill a need. From there, we water this mental seed—this *idea*—with progressively more action in the form of further thought and discussion. Finally, we commit ourselves (and others!) to this idea and make it a reality. Once you evolve beyond the *idea* stage, others have to get involved, again, like creating and giving birth to a human being.

My idea to give birth to this book began as a mental seed that was first shared with my wife, Penny Crozier. While some people are easy to convince of an idea, *Penny is not.* Penny's mind immediately begins to think, "What should he be doing with his mental energy…article deadlines…course manual revisions…videos to be made…he has a new client coming in tomorrow"—she runs the business! When I explained my deep desire to write this book, she could see the importance of it and committed to helping me get the job done. Thank you, Penny, for your patience with me! I know that I am the father of this idea, which makes you the mother—complete with the pains of birthing. Once I get the idea on paper, I hand it off to Penny, the Institute staff and, finally, to the many reviewers, so that when it comes into the world it has more of my strengths, fewer of my weaknesses. There have been many *guardian angels* who have put their strengths and love into this book so that it may best serve you and Mother Earth. These people include:

Cara Burke: If Penny is the mother of this book, *Cara is the midwife!* There are few people in the world who could handle the many tasks of researching, editing, layout, graphics, schedule coordination for photo shoots, and the many details of book production without cracking up! While Cara would agree that performing the work of 10 people is a challenge, she would most likely tell you that trying to get me to write shorter chapters is *the mother of all challenges!* While my Golf Biomechanic's book took a year to write and produce, this book has been like the child that preferred the womb, tasking Cara with what is now three years of work.

Cara has carted reports, chapters and files of all sorts all over the world as we've progressively refined the book to what it is here. This book would not exist if not for Cara! Thank you, Cara, for your unselfish support and constant efforts to help me become a better writer and for your constant love and care for this project! This book is proof that an idea can have one father and two mothers, for it is *very much Cara Burke!*

Charlie Aligaen: For several years, Charlie worked as the C.H.E.K Institute artist. After having completed most of the diagrams and drawings for this book, Charlie went on to other pursuits in life. For over four years, his artwork allowed me to express my thoughts multi-dimensionally. Charlie's artwork contributes greatly to this book, improving the reader's ability to comprehend the message I am trying to convey. Charlie, you are an amazing talent and your work will serve humanity through all the books you and I have done together for a long time after we are both in another world. I love you and you will forever be dear to me, my friend!

Joling Lee: Joling took over where Charlie left off as company artist. Joling has done an amazing job, not only by maintaining the style developed by Charlie, but also by adding her own unique feel to the images. Thank you so much, Joling, for enhancing my ability to communicate to the world artistically through you. It is a great pleasure to see your smile every day at work! Joling, I appreciated your contributions to my work, this book, the Institute and its many students.

C.H.E.K Institute Staff: *How to Eat, Move, and Be Healthy!*, more than any other project I've completed, has involved the entire C.H.E.K Institute staff. They all have been involved in reading manuscript drafts, giving feedback and supporting the entire process. Their feedback has often been valuable for determining when my writing and message has been too complex for the general public. Because they are like family to me, they are reliably candid!

C.H.E.K Institute Students: My many consultations with students of the C.H.E.K Institute have not only offered me a chance to practice, but also to learn and grow as a practitioner faster than I could as a practitioner dealing only with a private clientele. Working with the students, I have become better and better at simplifying my explanations of physiological, emotional, mental and spiritual processes so that they may better convey information to their clients. I have always been challenged to find the point at which distilling technical information best serves the public without losing necessary dimension, depth or value. This process helped me learn what Cara and Penny have tried so hard to teach me for many years. Students, thank you for the opportunity to learn through you each day! You have helped make this a better book for the layperson.

Mentors: While there have been many mentors in my life who have served me in the development of a holistic approach to both life and the body, the following are most relevant to this book:

Bill Timmins has taught me an immense amount about the hormonal systems of the body. He has also served as a major contributor to my understanding of digestion, elimination, stress physiology and the importance of *lifestyle factors.* Dr. Timmins gave me valuable support and encouragement for the system I developed and teach today, and his training further motivated me to focus my efforts on what *causes* people's problems, not just the application of quick fix technologies, as so many in the health and exercise fields do today. Thank you for your wonderful influences, Dr. Timmins!

Cliff Oliver has been like a guardian angel, sent to look over me as I serve humanity as best I can. With his extensive background in the fields of nutrition, chiropractic, natural and holistic medicine, he has been an invaluable source of knowledge for me. Dr. Oliver has helped all instructors of the C.H.E.K Institute (Chris Maund, Janet Alexander and Suzi Nevell) with challenging clients, teaching us along the way. Dr. Oliver serves me each time I see, hear or think of him by showing me what kind of man I can grow up to be! Dr. Oliver, thank you for all your love and ongoing support, and for your direct and indirect contributions to this book.

Fong Ha taught me, by being a living example, that one could achieve an incredible amount through stillness. Fong gave me many great ideas for cultivating Chi, ideas that have been useful with my clients and now will be of use to all the readers of this book. Equally important, Fong Ha has served to show me that I can age into a splendid combination of graceful movement, beauty, intelligence, wisdom and natural power. Through his instruction and my application of that training, the seed of Fong Ha's mastery is offered to you through this book, too!

Bill Wolcott and Dodie Anderson mentored me through my training as a Metabolic Typing Advisor. Thank you, Dodie and Bill, for being incredibly patient with me and my students as we have learned to effectively apply metabolic typing. Bill, your work has served to change untold thousands of lives for the better, both through your own work and through mine and that of C.H.E.K Institute students! For anyone ready to take responsibility for their own health, the practice of metabolic typing presented here and expanded upon in your book, *The Metabolic Typing Diet*, is a necessary first step! Thank you for your many valuable contributions to this book.

Reviewers: One of the most challenging things a writer can do is expose his/her ideas to those with the knowledge and skill to critically analyze them. It is natural to nurture and protect your ideas, much like you would your own children, and it takes strength to accept critical feedback, particularly when it could mean that you may have been wrong, possibly even wrong for many years! The kind of people that have the knowledge and skill to provide feedback for a book such as this are highly-skilled, industrious and busy people; therefore, I must thank them not just for their feedback, but for their time and willingness to share their knowledge by improving the message contained in this book. Special thanks to reviewers Susan Oliver, Eric Soranno, M.D., Jay Smith, M.D., C.H.E.K Practitioner Level 3, CHEK NLC Level 2, Matthew Wallden, N.D., D.O., C.H.E.K Practitioner Level 3, CHEK NLC Level 2, Nigel Brooke, N.D., D.O., C.H.E.K Practitioner Level 3, Dr. Cliff Oliver, Bill Wolcott, Alun Biggart, CHEK NLC Level 2 and Emma Lane, C.H.E.K Practitioner Level 3, CHEK NLC Level 3. If I have missed any of you, please forgive me and know that I sincerely appreciate your support and efforts.

I would also like to thank Sue Chek and Paul Chek, Jr. for the love and support that fueled me through much of my professional career. The love and energy you gave me, and give me today are a part of everything I do!

Thank you all,

Paul Chek

It was the best of times, it was the worst of times, it was the age of wisdom, it was the age of foolishness, it was the epoch of belief, it was the epoch of incredulity . Charles Dickens, *A Tale of Two Cities.*

Dickens' assessment of human affairs is as true today as it was in 1859. In fact, it would be fair to say that it's even more true today because of the extraordinary nature of our times.

The belief in the importance of diet and nutrition to health is pervasive, more so today than ever before, yet the rates of chronic degenerative diseases in the U.S. continue to sky-rocket. One out of every two people die from (easily-prevented and easily-treated) heart disease, yet it was virtually unknown less than 100 years ago. One out of every three dies from cancer. Diabetes, relatively rare until recently, is becoming a raging epidemic. Alzheimer's Disease currently impacts about five million people a year, but that number is expected to triple, affecting nearly 40% of the U.S. population over age 65.

Incredulously, the number three cause of death in the U.S., as reported in the Journal of the American Medical Association (JAMA), is found at the hands of our doctors, the very ones we turn to for help. Is it any wonder that people are leaving doctors' offices in droves searching for alternatives and answers that make sense?

Although health expenditures are now out-pacing the growth of the U.S. economy, the U.S. ranked only 17th on the list of Health of Nations. Diseases that only a short time ago were thought to be relegated to the aged are appearing in younger and younger children each year. Twenty years ago, about 2% of all cases of new onset diabetes (type II) were in people between nine and 19 years old. Today, it's about 30% to 50%. Heart disease, arthritis and cancer are no longer for just the aged.

In spite of the thousands of books that have been written on diet and fitness, and regardless of the booming $40 billion a year supplement industry, one in 50 adults are more than 100 pounds overweight; two out of every 3 adults and 1 out of every 5 children are overweight. Today, schools are forced to obtain new weight scales that can measure 350 pounds and higher to monitor the weight *of our children.*

As health consumers, we encounter information overload at every turn. More information is available today than ever before, yet there is so little understanding. Bookstores across the land offer wall-to-wall books, each touting the one diet right for everyone or the latest and greatest supplement to make us well and keep us young. The TV airways are jam-packed with exercise gimmicks and "wondrous" machines "guaranteed" to make us fit and lean. The Internet, easily accessible to virtually anyone, contains vast amounts of invaluable information, but the sheer enormity of it only brings greater confusion instead of clarity, leading to even more questions than the answers we so desperately seek.

Whether you're a casual reader interested in learning about nutrition, a student consumed with the desire to understand the subject, a practitioner trying to stay abreast of the latest developments in the field, an athlete looking for that edge over the competition, a housewife looking for ways to keep her family healthy, or someone facing a dire health challenge desperately seeking solutions, the same questions are at the forefront of your quest: Whom can you trust? Where can you find accurate information? How do you distinguish right from wrong? *How do you find out what's right for you?*

Of the tens of thousands of books that have been written on the subject, most are flawed and not to be trusted. Either they are purely based in theory with no real world relevance, or they are based upon lab research that does not bear out in clinical application. Many tout one protocol for all people, which, due to the reality of biochemical individuality, has no logical or scientific basis and is doomed to failure. And often a book is written by someone who found something that worked and for some irrational reason made the fallacious leap in logic that if it worked for him/her it will work for everyone.

The best course of action is to follow the recommendations of someone who has had both many years of experience and a track record of proven results. Rarer than needles in haystacks, such books are few and far between and difficult to find. But they are treasures to those fortunate enough to find them.

How to Eat, Move and Be Healthy! is just such a book. Paul Chek has spent many years traveling the globe, seeking out the best of the best in their respective fields of expertise. He has studied with them. He has learned from them. In many cases he has worked with them. And, like a brilliant conductor who seeks out only the most gifted musicians, Paul has orchestrated a unique and masterful system of healing, regeneration and rejuvenation. Most importantly, over the past 20 years Paul has successfully helped thousands of people from all over the world achieve the optimum health that is their birthright. He has identified the steps required in this process and has made them readily available and easily accessible to anyone through this book.

At the root of Paul's success is his deep understanding of metabolic individuality. Each of us is unique. This is true in obvious ways such as our height, weight, color of skin, hair and eyes, strength, endurance, digestion, and so on. But in reality, our uniqueness extends to every part of ourselves. In every sense, like no two snowflakes are the same, we are as unique metabolically in terms of rates of cellular metabolism and how we metabolize food as we are in our fingerprints. This little known and even less understood secret of biochemical individuality permeates every aspect of Paul's approach.

It is not enough to eat only high quality, organic food. It is absolutely critical to customize your diet to your body's unique and ever-changing needs. It is not enough simply to exercise. Exercise must be done properly and, like diet, must be customized to the unique dictates of your individual metabolism, temperament and physiology. There is no one else in the world who has a better grasp of these principles or who is more capable of guiding you in their application than Paul Chek.

In order to achieve your goal you must take action, and in order to take action you must have faith in something. But it is absolutely necessary that you place your faith in the right thing. The right faith in the wrong thing can only produce disappointment. The right faith in the right thing will assuredly lead you to your goal.

How to Eat, Move and Be Healthy! will help you discover what is right for *you*. Follow the practical, easy steps Paul has provided in this book and you will assuredly make the rest of your life *the best of times.*

William L. Wolcott
Author, *The Metabolic Typing Diet*
Founder, Healthexcel System of Metabolic Typing
Winthrop, WA

CONTENTS

A journey of a thousand miles must begin with a single step.

Lao-tzu, *The Way of Lao-tzu*

Our scientific power has outrun our spiritual power. We have guided missiles and misguided men.

Martin Luther King, Jr., *Strength to Love*

Chapter 1

IF EINSTEIN WAS YOUR DOCTOR

As you patiently sit in the lobby, your gaze drifts to the mirror on the wall adjacent to the magazine rack. You see a vague resemblance of a youthful you and wonder if anyone would recognize you at a high school reunion. Your doctor is always in a hurry, so you mentally cover what you want to tell him before he gives you another drug that has side effects that make you feel as bad as what you've come to see him for. At this point in your life, you realize that your sex drive is hitting a low point, and after following your doctor's dietary advice, you crave more sugar—are gaining weight—and suspect you're the victim of the environmental toxicity that the evening news reported.

Finally, the nurse escorts you into the examining room. She says you'll be seeing an associate of your regular doctor, Dr. Einstein. Couldn't be.

But since he's new, maybe you'll have time to explain how lethargic you feel. Maybe he'll have a better explanation for your inability to control your weight and recommend a diet that really works.

The door opens and you're looking at a small man with an electric hairdo, a rather large nose and a gray mustache.

Cheerfully, he says, "How can I help you today?" The man's eyes have depth and clarity, and you're immediately struck with a sense of wonderment.

Could this be the *real* Albert Einstein, the father of modern science?

"But you look exactly like..."

"That's because I *am* Albert Einstein. And you are about to see how well the principles of quantum physics and the theory of general relativity can be applied to medicine."

You quickly cover your reasons for coming to your doctor while Einstein flips through your chart. After a long silence, he lifts a bushy brow. "I see here that all your lab tests look good."

"Yes, Dr. Einstein, but I just don't feel well. How is it that I feel so lousy, yet my lab tests don't reveal anything wrong with me?"

"Well," Einstein replies, "lab tests are much like mathematics. As far as the laws of mathematics refer to reality, they are not certain; as far as they are certain, they do not refer to reality. Lab tests are often just a very small piece of a bigger reality. Let's start with a look at your home life, relationships and work environment."

"What does that have to do with not feeling well?"

"A human being is a part of a whole, what we call the Universe, apart and limited in time and space. He experiences himself, his thoughts and feelings as a part, living in a sort of delusional state. This delusion can be a prison, restricting us to our personal desires, forcing us to show affection for only the few people nearest to us. Our task is to free ourselves from this prison by widening our circle of compassion, to embrace all living creatures and the whole of nature in its beauty. How much time do you commit to yourself each day? Do you have a hobby, take time to exercise, read and do things that you enjoy?"

"I don't have time for all that. I have bills to pay, a mortgage, car payments and a family to raise. Sure, I enjoy relaxing with a few drinks while watching a late show, but that's about it. My family and friends depend on me. They're the ones who really count."

Dr. Einstein sighs. "Not everything that counts can be counted, and not everything that can be counted counts. You've lost sight of the essence of what creates life, what gives you the vitality and well-being to really live. It's only when you are alive, fully present, self-fulfilled and happy that you are truly doing what counts. What good are you to your family if you burnout? Think of yourself as the sun in the sky, and your family and friends as being dependent upon your light. As the sun, it is your duty to care for yourself so that you never burn out. Like the sun, you can only share the energy that you have. Unfortunately, it has become common for people to burnout while trying to be everywhere and do everything."

Einstein places his hands in the pockets of his lab coat. "If you're not taking care of yourself, your life is out of balance. Subsequently, your family's life is out of balance. And that affects your children in ways that may not be obvious to you. Did you know that nearly 50% of American children are overweight, and the number of Caucasian children who are overweight doubled between 1986 and 1998, with the number of African-American and Hispanic children that have become overweight increasing 120% in the same 12-year period?[1] In addition to the problem of childhood obesity, Type II diabetes among children has increased 10-fold in the past five years. Type II diabetes, rare among children not long ago, presently accounts for 40 - 50% of all cases reported."

"But don't kids get plenty of exercise?"

"Sadly, not always. California law requires school children to take an annual fitness test. Recently, only 23% of students passed what is a reduced version of the test most adults would have taken as a child. In fact, in one Los Angeles school, only 1% passed the test."[2]

Einstein shakes his head. "Adults haven't fared better. The number of obese adults has doubled since 1960; 63% of males and 55% of females now overweight or obese. An interesting statistic, considering the percentage of energy in the diet from fat has decreased during the past 20 years, yet the number of overweight and obese people has skyrocketed."[3]

"Are you saying that cutting fat intake won't necessarily prevent you from being fat?"

"Indeed. Let's take you for example. I see in your chart that your doctor has asked you to reduce red meat, trim the fat off other meats, skin your chicken, and he also suggests you try to eat more good carbohydrates in order to lower cholesterol, blood pressure and body fat percentage. Judging from your weight, reducing your dietary fat is not working for you."

"To make matters worse, I feel tired and lethargic eating this way. And my cravings are stronger. It seems the only enjoyable thing my doctor allows me to consume is my evening cocktail. If I'm already eating right, do you think it's the cholesterol-lowering drugs that are causing the problems?"

"Drugs can be a challenge to the system. And indeed, many American doctors rely too heavily upon them. Europeans eat far more fat—particularly the saturated fat the American diet dictocrats keep harping about—and drink just as much wine. Still, fewer drugs are prescribed in Europe and in general there is less disease than in the U.S. In all fairness, American doctors are commonly pressured by patients with a quick fix mentality. And they suffer more than any other population from a "this for that" attitude. Patients should not go to doctors to get a drug to mask their symptoms, they should go to the doctor to find out what is causing their symptoms and learn what they need to change, whether it be diet or lifestyle, to make them feel better.

"Consider that in the year 2002," Einstein continues, "drug sales worldwide amounted to $430 billion.[4]

Couple those statistics with the fact that in the year 2000, Americans spent more than $110 billion on fast food.[5] And today, Americans drink nearly 600 12-ounce cans of cola per person per year, with a significant number of teenage boys drinking 5 - 6 cans a day. Still, the Coca-Cola® bottling company has the goal of increasing consumption of its products in the U.S. by at least 25% per year."[5]

"But I drink *diet* soda, Dr. Einstein."

"Then it may interest you to know that research has found drinking any soda, even diet, will increase your chance of becoming obese.[6] In light of these figures, it's easy to see why so many people feel just like you.

"Now, I'm sure your doctor's dietary recommendations were based on the assumption that, like most people, you won't consider eating foods you were designed by Mother Nature to eat."

"Foods designed by Mother Nature?"

"My entire career has been spent trying to determine how God built the Universe, how things work in light of a grand view. While there are many opinions on God and on the Universe, I've always considered myself a disciple of philosopher Baruch Spinoza. Spinoza felt that God is Nature and Nature is God, and it is from Nature that we human beings have emerged. The problem is that most patients don't realize that what we eat today has changed more in the past 40 years than in the previous 40,000.[5] The body can't change that fast, and this causes problems. We've got to get back to Mother Nature's basic principles, the same principles that keep animals healthy in the wild, and the same principles that got us this far."

"But we're a modernized society with all kinds of high-tech medicines."

"People aren't machines, and, unfortunately, Western medicine has spent a large amount of its time trying to better Mother Nature's theorems. They try to break things down into their component parts, looking at disease through the lens of a microscope. Unfortunately, they don't listen to what matters most—the patient's explanation of his or her ailment. To show how

a machine works, you take it apart. But to see how a living entity functions, it must be seen as an organism in unity with its natural environment.[7]

"As a doctor, I can wholeheartedly say that education is what remains after one has forgotten everything he learned in school, and one thing I know for sure is that we have more disease and mental disorder than ever before. Unfortunately, most doctors and scientists focus on finding a cure for disease by studying the disease instead of the conditions that favor the presence of the disease. For example, when I look at the stars, it's obvious that there's no life as we know it in our solar system because the conditions are not favorable there. Now, just as plant and animal life doesn't exist on Mercury, Saturn or Jupiter because the conditions are not favorable, health and vitality are not going to develop in your body until you make conditions favorable for them there as well.

"Let's take a brief look at how the approach taken by doctors over the past 4,000 years has changed as they've become more and more isolated in their thinking. To treat an ear infection, doctors used these various approaches:

2000 BC: Here, eat this root.

1000 AD: That root makes you a heathen.
Here, say this prayer.

1850 AD: Prayers are superstitions.
Here, drink this potion.

1940 AD: That potion is snake oil.
Here, swallow this pill.

1985 AD: That pill is ineffective.
Here, take this antibiotic.

2000 AD: That antibiotic is artificial.
Here, eat this root.

2003 AD: Don't eat that root. It is very likely toxic.
Here eat this root. It came from an organic farm."

"So you're saying there's a movement to eat the foods that better match our biological make up."

"We have to come back to Nature. Unfortunately, I can't suggest that you simply cut the junk foods from your diet and expect you to feel better and lose weight. Sadly, we've damaged Mother Nature enough that it may take thousands of years to repair Her. This is why we must stick to organic foods and promote organic farming. To be healthy, you've got to model your eating, exercise and lifestyle after healthy people. While modern medicine has long overlooked the study of healthy people, pioneering health care and agricultural professionals such as Weston A. Price, Sir Robert McCarrison, G.T. Wrench, Innes Pearse, and farmers Sir Albert Howard and Lady Eve Balfour have clearly demonstrated the benefits of organic foods for human health."

"I've never heard of those people."

"Their studies of various cultures and the relationship between nutrition and disease brought out three points of significance with regard to healthy groups of people:

"First of all, these communities lived under harsh conditions, at times with limited resources for food, yet they did not suffer from the physical and nervous disorders now so rife among 'civilized' communities. Secondly, they represented a wide variety of races and environments. Their diets varied greatly in the amounts of protein and carbohydrates consumed. And finally, they consumed mainly whole foods. Processing was minimal, and all edible portions of a food were consumed so as to limit waste.

"Take Lady Eve Balfour, for example. She was a founding member of the British Soil Association, a farmer and lifetime student of nutrition while serving as the director of the longest-run experiment comparing conventional and organic farming methods. She is most likely the person responsible for Great Britain's organic movement. After a survey of Dr. Price's research on the healthiest people in the world she said, 'The only discernible common factor, other than good air, seems to be that the diets of all these groups are 'whole' diets in the full sense of the word.[8]

"There is a complete and continuous transference of health from a fertile soil, through plant and/or animal to man, and back to the soil again. The whole carcass, the whole grain, the whole fruit or vegetable—these things fresh from their source, and that source is fertile soil. Herein appears to lie the secret.

"So," Einstein continues, "I'm going to fine-tune your doctor's recommendations, provided you're willing to follow my advice."

"Of course, Dr. Einstein."

"I won't try to reinvent the wheel, so to speak. Rather, I will build upon what works, moving toward a greater understanding of the whole. I suggest you buy and eat organic produce and meats whenever possible. Organic foods don't contain dangerous chemical residues such as pesticides, herbicides and fungicides. Free-range organic meats are raised on high-quality, pesticide-free feed without toxic hormones."

"Do you think then, Dr. Einstein, that the reason I've not lost weight and felt worse on this diet is because I've been eating commercially farmed produce, commercially raised meats and processed low fat foods?"

"Judging by the way you feel when eating processed foods, you can see that these foods are truly toxic and potentially damaging to the body and mind. While it is important to wean yourself from processed foods and sodas and to drink plenty of good clean water, you must also identify your Metabolic Type. Each of us has different nutritional needs. To feel your best, you must eat what's right for you.

"Later, I'll provide you with a questionnaire that will help me determine your Metabolic Type. You may have been eating the wrong foods and/or in the wrong amounts for your type. Eating wrong for your make-up will shift your body out of a balanced state and can eventually lead to disease.

"Furthermore, by cutting down on the toxins entering your body from poor food and drink choices and by reducing the amount of sugar in your diet, you'll see a dramatic difference. If you eat organic, free-range meats, you don't have to worry about cutting the fat away, and you can eat red meats. In no time, you'll have more energy, your cholesterol levels are likely to normalize, and you'll be far more interested in getting the exercise you need.

"Just as you need to determine which are the right foods and proportions that are best for you, you must also choose the best type of exercise or movement and in the right amount for you. I can refer you to a C.H.E.K Practitioner who can get you started with the stretching and exercise program that will benefit you the most."

"To be honest, Dr. Einstein, I've never really liked to exercise."

"Don't let that stop you. You may be surprised to find that some of the non-traditional approaches to exercise are quite enjoyable."

"It's more complicated than I thought. It's all connected somehow; diet, exercise and state of mind."

"Indeed. Each of the stressors in your body has an accumulative effect. You and your body are a physical, emotional, mental and spiritual component of the Universe. You are very much like a star in a galaxy, comprised of key systems such as the musculoskeletal, visceral (your organs), limbic (emotional) and hormonal, which are linked to each of the more subtle body systems such as the emotional, mental and spiritual.

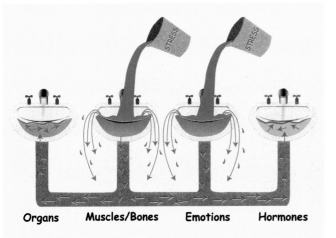

Organs   Muscles/Bones   Emotions   Hormones

"I want you to imagine each of these systems as a separate sink, yet each plumbed together. Now, considering that you are constantly overworking and are rife with financial stress, as an example, you can see how that will result in a lot of stress being poured into the physical and limbic (emotional) sinks. To help your body recover both physically and mentally, you must get to sleep earlier in order to provide your body with adequate repair time."

"The body always wants to find balance and minimize stress on any given body system. As you can see, the natural tendency is for the body to share the stress with the organ systems and hormonal system. This is one reason why so many people go to doctors with seemingly unrelated symptoms, only to be given drugs to treat the symptoms they are asking the doctor to take away. Most drugs, being harmful to the body, put stress on the liver and other organ systems, leading to even more stress to be shared with the rest of the body. Eventually, there's no single major problem in many cases, just a lot of small problems that can grow into bigger ones if left unattended."

"This is amazing, Dr. Einstein! For the first time, I'm really beginning to understand my body. I'm also beginning to understand that maybe I need to take a look at my life from a bigger perspective, like you do! I'm going to follow your advice. But, I'd really appreciate it if you could recommend a book that will reinforce what you've taught me here today. I want to surprise my doctor when I come in for my next check up."

"The book I recommend is titled, *How to Eat, Move and be Healthy!* by Paul Chek, a well known Holistic Health Practitioner."

"Thank you, Dr. Einstein, My time with you has been very enlightening. How long do you think it will take me to get my body shape and my energy back?"

"If you work at it consistently, you can make an amazing transformation in just three to six months, and in a year, you'll look and feel at least ten years younger. But remember, you must make all these things a part of your new lifestyle to continue your quest for optimal health."

Case History
Emma Lane, C.H.E.K Practitioner Level 3, CHEK NLC Level 3, Metabolic Typing Advisor, NMT, a client of Paul Chek

I was a fitness professional, in my 20s and leading what I thought was a very healthy life. I followed the WHO (World Health Organization) protocols for nutrition, was a vegetarian and exercised regularly. Granted, I was quite busy, as I was running multiple businesses, working with clients and presenting at international fitness conferences, but I didn't feel like I was over-stressing my body.

I have since become aware that this so-called healthy lifestyle that I was leading was actually doing me more harm than good. It began in 1998, when I found out that I had cancer. I followed the allopathic route—had surgery—and the cancer was cleared. When the cancer came back in 1999, I decided I wanted to try an alternative route, as clearly the traditional medical approach hadn't worked the first time.

Also in 1999, I was in a serious head-on car collision. The accident left me with numerous injuries: concussion, brain damage, whiplash, very bruised legs and dislocations. Being hyper-mobile, I did not actually break any bones but was completely covered in bruises and was unable to walk for over a week.

I followed a rehabilitation program at the hospital and also worked with a physiotherapist several times a week privately. Eventually I followed my own rehabilitation programs as I felt it would be more effective. After about two and a half months, I was gradually starting to get back to work. I still did not feel well and was on 3-4 strong pain-killers a day, anti-inflammatory drugs and sleeping pills. Even with all of these medications, I was in constant pain.

I consulted with several specialists and was told that, "it would just take time." At this point, I was becoming frustrated. The pain continued, and I was experiencing memory loss and cognition problems which greatly affected my daily activities. I often didn't recognize people who I knew quite well and would zone out during conversations.

Just as I was getting back to work and felt like I was making a bit of progress, I was in another car accident—again someone ran into me. This accident left me in traction for two days. The doctors at first thought that I might have broken my back. Fortunately, I hadn't. Physically, this second accident was not as serious as the first, but my body just crashed. I was in pain in every joint, my whole body ached constantly, and I couldn't make any sense of it because I hadn't actually sustained any major injuries. I felt in a daze most of the time. I would zone out, often losing hours at a time. I couldn't maintain information and had difficulty focusing. I got dizzy frequently and experienced pins and needles in my hands and feet, as well as numbness and total loss of sensation.

I was experiencing severe pain in my knees, back and neck, as well as extreme fatigue. This physical fatigue was not due directly to damage from the second car accident, however; it was my body trying to tell me something!

I had over six months off work. When I eventually returned, it was at a very reduced level. I still felt terrible and was relying on medications to get me through the day and to sleep at night. My pain symptoms were still as intense, but on an intermittent level. The pain would be heightened and worse in different joints most days. Some days my knees would hurt more, while other days it would be my back or my neck that felt worse. It all seemed very strange to me.

I consulted many specialists. Because I had not received serious damage from the accident and my pain and symptoms constantly changed from day-to-day, the doctors couldn't make any sense of my case, since it didn't fit into their known approach. Therefore, I was told that I needed to see a psychologist because it was, "all in my head!" So far the financial cost for my treatments was in the thousands (sterling), and I had not regained any health or quality of life.

When I finally saw Paul in London, I was desperate for help and information on my condition. I had given up on the medical community because I felt it had given up on me. I had to change the focus of my business hugely in order to keep earning a living. I was extremely unhappy and confused. I couldn't function and didn't know why! Paul did!

In the two days I worked with him in London, he did some neuromuscular work on me which gave me immediate relief from the headaches and low back pain. He also educated me on my lifestyle and diet. He made me eat a steak for the first time in 13 years. At the time, looking at the steak made me feel sick, and it took me an hour to eat it, but I did feel substantially better after.

Paul insisted that I needed to go out to the C.H.E.K Institute in California to work with several specialists in the area so that I could start the healing process. I was out in the States within two weeks. After finally being referred to the correct people, I found out what was wrong. Looking back, it is no wonder I felt so bad. Here is a list of things that Paul helped me address:

Toxicity
Atlas (vertebra in the neck) subluxation
Brain damage
Damaged spine
Joint damage:
  • Knees
  • Feet/Toes
  • Elbows
Adrenal fatigue
Postural malalignment
Abdominal wall dysfunction
Hypothyroid
Parasites and candida
Hormonal imbalances
Gluten and dairy intolerance
Chemical sensitivity
Eating according to my Metabolic Type

I was in the States for two months this first visit, working with the **right** people. I made substantial improvements, thanks to a lot of hard work from everyone involved! It wasn't a pleasant experience, at times, as my body was weak and very toxic. It took a long time to detox. I was metabolically

typed when I initially saw Paul and came out as a protein type—hence the steak in London. However, I have changed metabolic types three times since I was so out of balance. I needed to do the advanced level of the testing. I also needed huge supplemental support to help my systems heal.

I totally changed my lifestyle and eating habits for the better—getting to bed by 10:30, drinking enough good water, taking time out for myself, relaxing and eating organic foods. These are just a few of the changes I was advised to make.

Many of the changes I had to make in my lifestyle and diet were difficult to change and stick to in the beginning. However, you soon realize that when you do slip up, the consequences of your actions on how you feel are not worth the few minutes of pleasure you get from eating a muffin, for example. I follow the 90/10 rule now. If I really fancy eating something or doing something that I know my body will not like, I only do it occasionally (the 10%). I accept that I will experience consequences and try to minimize them by supporting my body and doing everything that I know will help it to function optimally (the 90%), and this ultimately makes me feel healthy and vital.

I had to go back to the States regularly to work with the specialists as I was unable to find another brain specialist or NUCCA chiropractor (for my neck) at home. It has been a slow process, but it has proven to be very informative and worthwhile. I have learned so much going through the process of dealing with all the different issues. I am still working on some of the issues, knowing they are going to take time to reach a satisfactory level. However, I am now a fully functioning, happy human being who has been able to learn the techniques and protocols from Paul and the other specialists I have worked with. Although I had to do a lot of work, today I am productive and cancer-free!

I am now able to apply these protocols to other people in pain and have helped many individuals to recover and regain their lives free from pain and symptoms. I would like to thank Paul for giving me my life back as well as for teaching me how to help my clients regain a functional, fulfilled life.

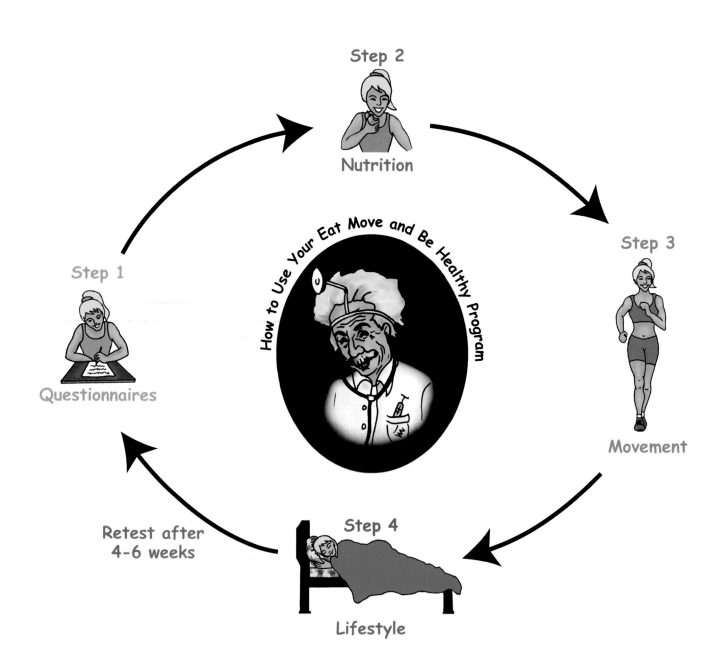

Step 2
Nutrition

Step 1
Questionnaires

How to Use Your Eat Move and Be Healthy Program

Step 3

Movement

Step 4

Retest after
4-6 weeks

Lifestyle

Chapter 2

How to Use Your Eat, Move and Be Healthy! Program

Portions of this book may conflict with previous thoughts on nutrition and fitness. I urge you to consider the material presented here with an open mind. You may wish to conduct your own investigation. It's up to you to decide how to proceed with the information provided.

Perhaps you'll find data here that substantiates what you've heard in the past but that left you with no plan of action. My goal is to lead you towards health and vitality. There are probably as many ways to get there using this book as there are individuals. Whether you already have an active workout routine or hate to exercise, you'll find a plan of action that suits you. We'll explain why no one diet fits all, and, we'll help you develop eating habits that are right for your metabolic type.

This book is organized in modules, so once you've completed the steps below you can either read it straight through, cover to cover, or begin with the sections that will benefit you the most. Your questionnaires will identify which sections to take on first. Follow the steps below to create a customized plan of action:

Step 1:

Complete the Questionnaires
Your scores will identify which of your body systems are stressed.

A. Complete the Nutrition and Lifestyle Questionnaires on pages 28 - 36. Take your time and answer the questions as accurately as possible. These results, together with your current fitness level, will determine the starting point for your exercise program.

B. Chart and total your scores using the Results Graph on page 37.

Step 2:

Complete the Metabolic Typing Test
Develop an eating plan that's right for you.

A. Fill out the Metabolic Typing Test on pages 38 - 41. It's important to take your time and answer the questions as accurately and honestly as possible. To do this, forget about everything you have been told about what you should and shouldn't eat. Answer the questions based on how you would prefer to eat if you could eat what you innately desire.

B. Read Chapter 3, The "No-Diet" Diet (page 43), which shows you how to eat according to your metabolic type, and begin following your diet plan (pages 234 and 235).

Step 3:

Movement

*Build a Personalized Exercise Program
to achieve your goals.*

Stretches

This chapter is a must read for everyone. There are many benefits to stretching. If you don't like to stretch, it probably means that you need to. If you already enjoy stretching, you may learn which muscles no longer need to be stretched and find some that you've been missing.

A. Go through the stretch tests on pages 88 through 95.

B. Place a check mark by each of the stretches listed on your Stretching Test Sheet (pages 96 and 97) when you feel tightness or restriction when performing the test.

C. Begin your workouts, or even your day, with the stretches you checked on your sheet. If time is limited, always choose stretches over exercises to balance your body.

Energy Building Exercises

If you scored high in any of the sections on your questionnaires in Step 1, immediately begin implementing exercises for the zone(s) that corresponds to that section(s). You'll find several exercises to choose from for each zone listed at the end of Chapter 6. **This is also a must-read for anyone who is not interested in traditional exercise, as you'll learn how to "workout" without really "working out."**

A. Implement exercises for each zone that you scored in the High Priority range on your questionnaires. Prioritize your zone exercises by focusing on the zones with high scores to the left side of your score sheet, working to the right as time permits.

B. Experiment with each of the exercises to find ones that you enjoy.

Core Function

A. Perform the Core Function Tests on pages 124 & 125.

B. If you do not pass any of these tests, perform the test as an exercise until you can pass the test.

Exercise Programs

A. Choose the exercise program suited for your body based on the total score from your Nutrition and Lifestyle Questionnaires.

Note: If you scored in the low or medium range but do not currently exercise, start with the TLC or Energizer Programs. If you qualify for the Performance Program, **complete at least one Energizer and one Vitalizer Program from start to finish (4 circuits with 60 - 90 seconds rest between circuits) before beginning the Performance Program**. If you do not feel sore after these workouts, proceed with the Performance Program. If you do feel sore, either immediately after or for up to two days after the workout, stick with that program for a few weeks, or until you no longer experience post-workout soreness, before progressing to the more advanced programs.

B Follow the sample workout schedule for your program (pages 172 - 187).

C. If you have dieted in the past, are a woman who has given birth, or if you have back pain, read the appropriate sections of Chapter 9.

D. If you wish to build your own program, read Chapter 10.

Step 4:

Nutrition and Lifestyle
Fine-tune diet and lifestyle issues to achieve optimal health.

A. Read the chapters recommended for each section in which you scored in the medium or high range on your questionnaires.

B. Begin implementing the recommended strategies immediately! Focus on the highest scores, working from left to right on your score sheet.

Retest:

A. After following your eating and stretching/exercise program for four weeks, it is time to re-test. Complete all of the Nutrition and Lifestyle Questionnaires again.

B. If your total score has dropped into a lower zone and you are not experiencing post-workout soreness, you may safely increase your workout time in circuits, frequency of workouts per week, or progress to the next workout level.

C. If your score has not dropped into a lower zone, review the CHEK Points for each section in which you scored high, and work on fine tuning your eating and lifestyle. Make sure to include Energy Building Exercises in your program as well.

You can achieve anything you want in life if you have the courage to dream it, the intelligence to make a realistic plan, and the will to see that plan through to the end.

Sidney A. Friedman, Speaker and Author

Case History

Jeff, client of Sue Grey, C.H.E.K Practitioner Level 1, CHEK NLC Level 2, Golf Biomechanic, UK

When Jeff called to cancel his game with my husband, I could tell immediately there was something seriously wrong. Jeff's voice, usually so buoyant and always the comedian, sounded flat and despondent. Apparently, a severe attack of breathlessness had taken him to his doctor, who prescribed a course of steroid tablets and armed him with an inhaler. Asthma, he was told. Reduce your stress and change your life!

Jeff was devastated and freely admitted that he had no idea where to start. So I told him about the benefits that I and others had found from following a personally tailored CHEK programme, a holistic approach to health and fitness, where the responsibility for maintaining health is placed with the individual. He was keen to give it a try, so I immediately dispatched him a set of intake forms. Jeff can best fill you in on his background:

"Like most of my peers I have had my share of ups and downs in life; show me a man in his fifties who hasn't. Then, just when my life seemed to be running on an even keel, having found my soul-mate, I was run aground. Completely out of the blue, I started having breathing problems. At first, I put it down to singing in smoky clubs on weekends and stress at work, but then it spread like wildfire through my life. It invaded my golf, my singing, even my ability to play the football I had enjoyed since youth.

Furthermore, answering the questionnaires made me realise that my health must have been silently creeping downhill for years and I had now reached the point where it was even difficult to carry out simple, everyday tasks that had always seemed easy! Let Sue take it from here."

Jeff's immediate concerns, understandably, were about his newly diagnosed asthma and the major impact it was having on his life. The four key priority lifestyle areas he wished to improve in descending order were: his diet and nutrition programme; amount of quiet time and rest; exercise programme; and level of anxiety. His Health & Exercise survey revealed that Jeff was consuming a diet predominantly made up of convenience foods high in carbohydrates, especially grains, coupled with an extremely low fluid intake, comprised of caffeinated beverages and little water. He also confessed to having a serious sweet tooth, and he found himself constantly stopping at garages (convenience stores) for sweets.

Armed with his metabolic type, which we ascertained using the self-test in *The Metabolic Typing Diet* by William Wolcott, Jeff embarked on a four-day food rotation. Gluten and dairy products are often identified as common triggers of asthma, so for the first three months we excluded all gluten products from Jeff's diet, but because his dairy intake was already minimal we left this unchanged except for including dairy in the food rotation. Jeff's ideal water intake worked out at three litres per day; he aimed for 1-2 litres initially. Additionally, Jeff decided to substitute fruit teas for his regular caffeine intake.

At this point, the only other areas we looked at were Jeff's breathing technique and stress coping strategies, more as an aid to better managing any subsequent asthma attacks than anything else. Both he and his wife were 100% committed to Jeff's programme from the start, and it came as no surprise when, three weeks on, I received a somewhat elated call from his wife. I will leave Jeff to share the news with you.

"Right from the start I felt that I had much more energy. Somehow I seemed more awake and alert. The neck tension I had been experiencing, though not of great concern, was considerably reduced. It was my wife who realized that not only had I not had an asthma attack since I started making changes but that I had hardly been using the inhaler.

I ought to admit at this point that my physical shape had been giving me grief, too, especially my abs. I had it as #3 on my priority list, so Sue and I had that next in line to tackle. Sue told me you need to work from the inside out, that I could 'crunch' forever, but if everything is not in good order on the inside, it will make little difference in the long term. I am beginning to see what she means now. Within the first few weeks of starting to rotate my diet and excluding the grains, not only had I lost that bloated feeling after meals but also all the gas! I had dropped just over half a stone in weight, and I felt great!

So I am now four months on, having completed my physical, into which Sue incorporated a 'Whole in One' golf assessment, too! I am fired up and ready to start my exercise programme."

For Jeff and his wife, rotating their food has now become a part of their lives. He has handed in his football boots and decided to concentrate his energies on golf. Jeff feels he has already made great strides toward improving the future quality of his life. He feels more in control of his health and has a better understanding of his body, how it works and how he can take care of it. You can, too!

Nutrition & Lifestyle Questionnaires

IMPORTANT DIRECTIONS (PLEASE READ)

1. Answer each question with the response that best fits you. It is recommended that you either photocopy the questionnaires or record your answers on a separate piece of paper. You will hopefully be using them again to test your progress, and it will be easier if you do not have your previous answers in front of you at that point. It is extremely important to answer the questions as accurately and honestly as possible. There are no right or wrong answers. Supply the response that most accurately describes you, not what you think you should answer.

   When answering these questions, forget everything you've been told about what you should and shouldn't eat. Answer the questions based on your gut instinct to how you would prefer to eat if you could eat what you innately desire.

2. Total your scores for each questionnaire. There are numbers in parentheses after each answer. Add up the numbers corresponding to each of your responses to get your total score for the section.

3. Graph your scores on page 37.

4. Calculate your total score by adding up the scores for each section.

1. Do you shop for food less frequently than every four days?

   ✓ Yes (1)
   ___ No (0)

2. Do you eat more packaged (frozen or canned) fruits and vegetables than fresh?

   ___ Yes (3)
   ✓ No (0)

3. Do you eat more cooked vegetables than raw?

   ___ Yes (3)
   ✓ No (0)

4. Do you eat vegetables with fewer than two meals daily?

   ✓ Yes (5)
   ___ No (0)

5. Do you buy more non-organic vegetables than organic vegetables?

   ✓ Yes (5)
   ___ No (0)

6. How often do you use a microwave oven?

   ___ Never/very rarely (0)
   ___ 1-2 times per week (2)
   ✓ 3-4 times per week (5)
   ___ 4+ times per week (10)

7. Do you eat white bread more often than whole grain breads?

   ✓ Yes (5)
   ___ No (0)

8. Do you eat quick cook grains such as Rice-aroni, Quaker Oats or Minute rice more often than slow cooked organic whole grains?

   ✓ Yes (5)
   ___ No (0)

9. How often do you consume pasteurized/homogenized milk or cheeses?

   ___ Never/very rarely (0)
   ___ 1-2 times per week (1)
   ___ 3 times per week (3)
   ✓ 3+ times per week (5)

10. How often do you eat non-organic yogurts?

    ___ Never/very rarely (0)
    ___ 1-2 times per week (1)
    ✓ 3 times per week (3)
    ___ 3+ times per week (5)

11. Do you eat typical store bought eggs from cage raised chickens (as opposed to free-range eggs)?

    ✓ Yes (5)
    ___ No (0)

12. Do you eat red meat more than once every four days?

    ✓ Yes (3)
    ___ No (0)

13. Do you commonly eat meats (beef, chicken, turkey) from sources other than a free-range and hormone-free source?

    ✓ Yes (3)
    ___ No (0)

14. Do you eat canned fish more frequently than fresh fish?

____✓ Yes (3)
____ No (0)

15. How often do you use commercial salad dressings?

____ Never/very rarely (0)
____ once a week (1)
____ twice per week (2)
____✓ 2+ times per week (3)

16. How often do you use products containing hydrogenated oils?

____ Never/very rarely (0)
____✓ once a week (1)
____ twice per week (2)
____ 2+ times per week (5)

17. Do you eat nuts and/or seeds that are roasted and/or salted?

____✓ Yes (1)
____ No (0)

18. How often do you use white table sugar as a sweetener?

____ Never/very rarely (0)
____ once a week (1)
____ 2-3 times per week (3)
____✓ 3+ times per week (5)

19. How often do you use artificial sweeteners such as Sweet-n-Low, Equal or NurtaSweet?

____ Never/very rarely (0)
____ once a week (1)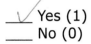
____✓ 2-3 times per week (5)
____ 3+ times per week (10)

20. Do you use standard white table salt?

____✓ Yes (5)
____ No (0)

21. Do you eat TV dinners or highly processed foods more than three times a week?

____ Yes (5)
____✓ No (0)

22. How often do you eat from fast food restaurants like McDonald's, KFC, Wendy's, etc...?

____✓ Never/very rarely (0)
____ 1-2 times per week (2)
____ 3 times per week (5)
____ 3+ times per week (10)

23. How often do you eat snacks from vending machines?

____✓ Never/very rarely (0)
____ 1-2 times per week (2)
____ 3 times per week (5)
____ 3+ times per week (10)

24. Do you drink tap water?

____✓ Yes (10)
____ No (0)

25. How often do you eat some form of store-bought dessert such as ice cream, cookies, donuts, cakes or pies?

____✓ Never/very rarely (0)
____✓ once a week (1)
____ 2-3 times per week (3)
____ 3+ times per week (5)

Total Score: 31

prev page 45
79

1. Do you eat more or less when stressed than when not stressed?

   ✓ More (10)
   ___ Same/less (0)

2. Do you worry over job, income or money problems?

   ✓ Yes (10)
   ___ No (0)

3. Are any of your relationships causing you stress?

   ✓ Yes (10)
   ___ No (0)

4. Do you often feel anxious?

   ✓ Yes (5)
   ___ No (0)

5. Do you often get upset when things go wrong?

   ✓ Yes (5)
   ___ No (0)

6. Do you lash out at others?

   ✓ Yes (5)
   ___ No (0)

7. Do you feel your sex drive is lower than normal for you?

   ✓ Yes (5)
   ___ No (0)

8. Do you feel isolated or lonely?

   ✓ Yes (3)
   ___ No (0)

9. Do you feel stressed due to lack of intimacy in one or more relationships?

   ✓ Yes (5)
   ___ No (0)

10. Have you had reduced contact with friends (feeling antisocial) or an increase in contact because you feel you need to vent your frustrations or stresses to others?

    ✓ Yes (3)
    ___ No (0)

11. Do you take any form of medication prescribed by a physician directly or indirectly related to stress in your life or for a psychological disorder?

    ✓ Yes (15)
    ___ No (0)

12. Do you commonly lose more than two days of work a year due to illness?

    ✓ Yes (5)
    ___ No (0)

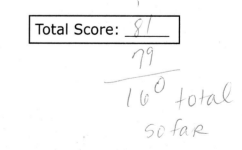

Total Score: _81_

79

160 total
so far

Sleep Wake Cycles

1. Do you live in the same time zone you were born in?

   ____ Yes (0)
   __✓__ No (5)

2. Do you travel across time zones more than once a month?

   ____ Yes (10)
   __✓__ No (0)

3. How often do you wake up feeling un-rested and in need of more sleep?

   ____ Never/very rarely (0)
   __✓__ once a week (1)
   ____ 3 times per week (5)
   ____ 3+ times per week (10)

4. Do you commonly go to bed after 10:30 PM?

   ____ Yes (10)
   __✓__ No (0)

5. Are the times you have bowel movements consistent and predictable on a daily basis?

   ____ Yes (0)
   __✓__ No (5)

6. Do you suffer from reduced memory since moving to a new time zone or since traveling across time zones?

   __✓__ Yes (10)
   __✓__ No (0)

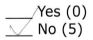

7. Has your sense of hunger changed from being hungry at breakfast (upon rising), lunch (midday) and dinner times (sunset) since moving to a new time zone or traveling across time zones frequently (> once a month)?

   ____ Yes (10)
   __✓__ No (0)

8. How often do you wake up at night between 1 and 4 am and have a hard time falling back to sleep?

   __✓__ Never/very rarely (0)
   ____ once a week (1)
   ____ 3 times per week (5)
   ____ 3+ times per week (10)

9. How often do you tend to have a hard time staying awake in the afternoon after eating lunch?

   ____ Never/very rarely (0)
   __✓__ once a week (1)
   ____ 3 times per week (5)
   ____ 3+ times per week (10)

10. Do you do shift work that requires you to stay up late at night?

   ____ Yes (10)
   __✓__ No (0)

   Total Score: __12__

   (17?)

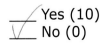

1. Do you frequently skip meals?

   ____ Yes (3)
   __✓_ No (0)

2. How often do you typically go more than four hours without eating?

   _✓_ Never/very rarely (0)
   ____ 1-2 times per week (1)
   ____ 3 times per week (2)
   ____ 3+ times per week (3)

3. How often do you skip breakfast?

   _✓_ Never/very rarely (0)
   ____ 2 times per week (1)
   ____ 3 times per week (5)
   ____ 3+ times per week (10)

4. Do you avoid fats when eating?

   _✓_ Yes (5)
   ____ No (0)

5. Do you frequently eat carbohydrates (i.e. breads, bagels, cookies, pasta, fruit, cereals, muffins, crackers, chocolate, or candy) by themselves?

   ____ Yes (5)
   _✓_ No (0)

6. Do you often get hungry or crave sweets within two hours after eating a meal?

   _✓_ Yes (5)
   ____ No (0)

7. How often do you consume drinks containing caffeine and/or sugar (i.e. coffee, tea, sodas, fruit juices with sucrose, corn syrup or added sugar)?

   ____ Never/very rarely (0)
   ____ 1 cup a day (1)
   _✓_ 2 cups per day (3)
   ____ more than 2 cups per day (5)

8. Have you tried diets to lose weight?

   ____ No (0)
   ____ once (1)
   ____ twice (2)
   ____ three-five times (5)
   _✓_ more than five times (10)

9. Do you have difficulty burning fat around your belly, hips or thighs even with regular exercise?

   _✓_ Yes (3)
   ____ No (0)

10. Do you eat your largest meal in the evening?

    _✓_ Yes (1)
    ____ No (0)

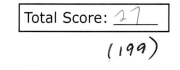

Total Score: 27

(199)

1. How often do you experience lower abdominal bloating?

   ✓ Never/very rarely (0)
   ___ 1-2 times per week (3)
   ___ 3 times per week (5)
   ___ 3+ times per week (10)

2. Do you frequently have loose stools or diarrhea?

   ✓ No (0)
   ___ once a week (1)
   ___ 3 or more times per week (5)

3. How often do you experience constipation or stools that are compact/hard to pass?

   ✓ Never/very rarely (0)
   ___ 1-2 times per week (3)
   ___ 3 or more times per week (5)

4. Do you find that you often burp after meals?

   ___ Yes (3)
   ✓ No (0)

5. Do you frequently have gas?

   ___ Yes (3)
   ✓ No (0)

6. Do you crave certain foods such as bread, chocolate, certain fruit, and red meat if you have not eaten them in a day or two?

   ✓ Yes (5)
   ___ No (0)

7. How often do you have a poor appetite and/or feel worse after eating?

   ___ Never/very rarely (0)
   ✓ 1-2 times per week (3)
   ___ 3 times per week (5)
   ___ more 3 times per week (10)

8. Do you have an excessive appetite and/or sweet cravings?

   ✓ Yes (5)
   ___ No (0)

9. Do you frequently (more than twice a week) experience abdominal pain, cramps or general abdominal discomfort?

   ___ Yes (20)
   ✓ No (0)

10. How often do you have indigestion, heartburn or an upset stomach?

    ✓ Never/very rarely (0)
    ___ 1-2 times per week (3)
    ___ 3 times per week (5)
    ___ more 3 times per week (10)

11. How often do you get a headache after eating?

    ___ Never/very rarely (0)
    ✓ 1-2 times per week (3)
    ___ 3+ times per week (5)

Total Score: ___16___

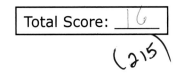

(215)

1. Have you ever been given general anesthesia?

    ✓ Yes (10)
    ___ No (0)

2. Have you ever taken antibiotics?

    ✓ Yes (10)
    ___ No (0)

3. Have you been or are you being treated for any condition requiring that you take medical drugs?

    ✓ Yes (10)
    ___ No (0)

4. In general, are your bowel movements loose, hard or foul smelling?

    ___ Yes (10)
    ✓ No (0)

5. Would you consider your life to be:

    ___ Stress free (0)
    ✓ Mildly stressful (5)
    ___ Very stressful (10)

6. Do you currently suffer from any digestive disorder or frequently have pain in the region above or below the navel?

    ___ Yes (10)
    ✓ No (0)

7. Do you have mercury amalgam fillings in your mouth?

    ___ Yes (10)
    ✓ No (0)

8. Do you have two different kinds of metal in your mouth; i.e., gold and silver or mercury amalgam and gold or silver?

    ___ Yes (5)
    ✓ No (0)

9. Do you experience itching in the ears, nose or rectum area?

    ___ Yes (10)
    ✓ No (0)

10. Do you have or have you had dandruff in the past year?

    ✓ Yes (10)
    ___ No (0)

11. Do you regularly eat or drink products containing sugar, white flour, processed dairy products?

    ___ Yes (5)
    ✓ No (0)

12. Do you crave sugar, fruit or milk if you don't have either of these items for more than three days?

    ✓ Yes (10)
    ___ No (0)

13. Do you find that regardless of how much you eat you get hungry quickly?

    ___ Yes (5)
    ✓ No (0)

55 total
(270)

14. In the past year, have you experienced athlete's foot (itching around the toes, soles or heel of the feet), jock itch or a fungal infection under a toenail (thickening of the toenail)?

____Yes (20)
__✓__No (0)

15. Do you ever get a reddening around the mouth or nose area after eating or drinking?

____Yes (5)
__✓__No (0)

16. Do you experience muscle or joint aches on a regular basis?

____Yes (5)
__✓__No (0)

17. Do you experience mood swings?

__✓__Yes (10)
____No (0)

18. Do you snack on sweets or drink coffee, soda pop or sports drinks most days to keep your energy up?

__✓__Yes (10)
____No (0)

19. Do you suffer from any kind of skin condition?

____Yes (10)
__✓__No (0)

20. Have you ever had sex or close physical contact with anyone who you know had a fungal infection (including athletes foot, jock itch, dandruff) or parasite infection?

____Yes (20)
__✓__No (0)

| Total Score: 20 |

If you score high on this questionnaire, refer to page 239 of the Appendix for more information regarding fungi, parasites and the approach that you should take.

290 total

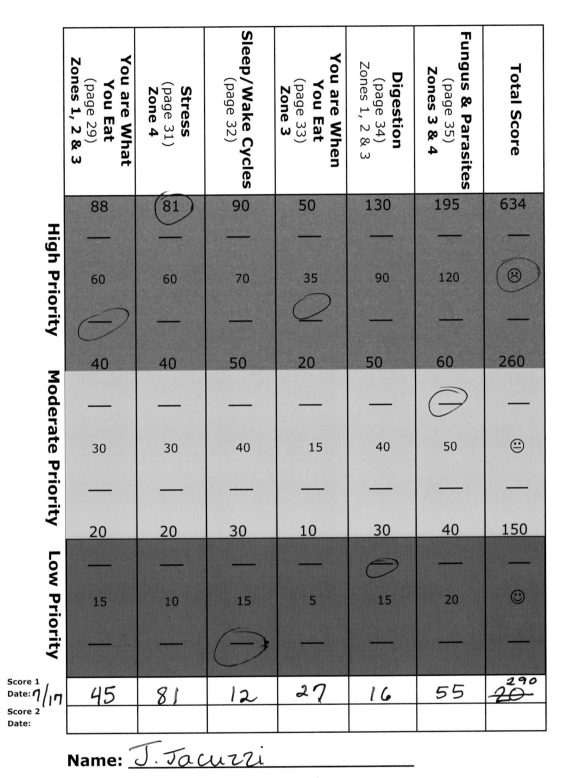

You are What You Eat (page 29) Zones 1, 2 & 3	Stress (page 31) Zone 4	Sleep/Wake Cycles (page 32)	You are When You Eat (page 33) Zone 3	Digestion (page 34) Zones 1, 2 & 3	Fungus & Parasites (page 35) Zones 3 & 4	Total Score	
88	(81)	90	50	130	195	634	**High Priority**
—	—	—	—	—	—	—	
60	60	70	35	90	120	(☹)	
(—)	—	—	(—)	—	—	—	
40	40	50	20	50	60	260	**Moderate Priority**
—	—	—	—	—	(—)	—	
30	30	40	15	40	50	(😐)	
—	—	—	—	—	—	—	
20	20	30	10	30	40	150	**Low Priority**
—	—	—	—	(—)	—	—	
15	10	15	5	15	20	(☺)	
—	—	(—)	—	—	—	—	

| Score 1 Date: 7/17 | 45 | 81 | 12 | 27 | 16 | 55 | ~~20~~ 290 |
| Score 2 Date: | | | | | | | |

Name: J. Jacuzzi

This questionnaire is designed to help you determine the optimal macronutrient ratio (fats:proteins:carbohydrates) to begin the process of fine-tuning your body's feedback mechanisms. For those of you not sure what a fat, protein or carbohydrate is, let me simplify that for you. If the food comes from something that has a set of eyes, it is going to be higher in fats and proteins; fats and proteins most often come together in nature. For example, cows, sheep, birds and fish all have eyes and all provide higher protein/fat foods. Foods like vegetables, fruits and cereals do not come from a source that had a set of eyes and are generally much higher in carbohydrates and lower in fat and protein. There are a few exceptions to this rule such as nuts, seeds and avocados, which have no eyes, yet are high-fat foods.

When answering the questions, circle the answer that best describes the way you feel, not the way you think you should eat! If none of the answers suit you with regard to a particular question, simply don't answer that question. If the answer A suits you some of the time (in the morning, but not the evening for example), and answer B suits you other times, you may circle both provided that the answers refer to how you may feel on any given day, not within a period of over 24 hours.

1. I sleep best:

        A. when I eat a snack high in protein and fat 1-2 hours before going to sleep.

        B. when I eat a snack higher in carbohydrates 3-4 hours before going to sleep.

2. I sleep best if:

        A. my dinner is composed of mainly meat with some vegetables or other carbohydrates.

        B. my dinner is composed mainly of vegetables or other carbohydrates and a comparatively small serving of meat.

3. I sleep best and wake up feeling rested:

        A. if I don't eat sweet deserts like cakes, candy or cookies. If I eat a rich desert that is not overly sweet, such as high-quality full-fat ice cream, I tend to sleep okay.

        B. if I occasionally eat a sweet desert before I go to bed.

4. After vigorous exercise, I feel best when I consume:

    A. foods or drinks with higher protein and/or fat content, such as a high-protein shake.

    B. foods or drinks higher in carbohydrates (sweeter), such as Gatorade.

5. I do best—maintain mental clarity and a sense of well-being for up to four hours after a meal—when I eat:

    A. a meat-based meal containing heavier meats such as chicken legs, roast beef and salmon, with a smaller portion of carbohydrate.

    B. a carbohydrate-based meal containing vegetables, bread or rice and a small portion of a lighter meat such as chicken breast or white fish.

6. If I am tired and consume sugar or sweet foods such as donuts, candy or sweetened drinks without significant amounts of fat or protein:

    A. I get a rush of energy, but then I am likely to crash and feel sluggish.

    B. I feel better and my energy levels are restored until my next meal.

7. Which statement best describes your disposition toward food in general:

    A. I love food and live to eat!

    B. I am not fussed over food and I eat to live.

8. I often:

    A. add salt to my foods.

    B. find that foods are too salty for my liking.

9. Instinctually, I prefer to eat:

    A. dark meat, such as the chicken or turkey legs and thighs over the white breast meat.

    B. light meat such as the chicken or turkey breast over the dark leg and thigh meat.

10. Which list of fish most appeals to you?

> **A.** Anchovy, caviar, herring, mussels, sardines, abalone, clams, crab, crayfish, lobster, mackerel, octopus, oyster, salmon, scallops, shrimp, snail, squid, tuna (dark meat)

> **B.** White fish, catfish, cod, flounder, haddock, perch, scrod, sole, trout, tuna (white), turbot

11. When eating dairy products, I feel best after eating:

> **A.** Richer, full fat yogurts and cheeses or desserts.

> **B.** Lighter, low fat yogurts and cheeses or desserts.

12. With regard to snacking:

> **A.** I tend to do better when I snack between meals or eat more smaller meals throughout the day.

> **B.** I tend to last between meals without snacking.

13. Which describes the way you instinctually prefer to start your day in order to feel your best and to have the most energy?

> **A.** A large breakfast that includes protein and fat, such as eggs with sausage or bacon.

> **B.** A light breakfast such as cereal, fruit, yogurt, breads and possibly some eggs.

14. Which characteristics best describe you:

> **A.** In general, I digest food well, have an appetite for proteins, feel good when eating fats or fatty foods, am more muscular or inclined to gain muscle and/or strength easily.

> **B.** I am more lithe of build, prefer light meats and lower fat foods, am more inclined toward endurance athletics.

Total A answers: _____   **Total B answers:** _____

To score your test, add the questions you circled **A** and the number you circled **B**.

➢ If your number of **A** answers is three or more than **B** answers, you are a Protein Type. (See pages 45 and 46).

➢ If your number of **A** and **B** answers are tied or within two of each other, you are a Mixed Type. (See pages 45 through 47).

➢ If your number of **B** answers is three or more than **A** answers, you are a Carb Type. (See pages 45 through 47).

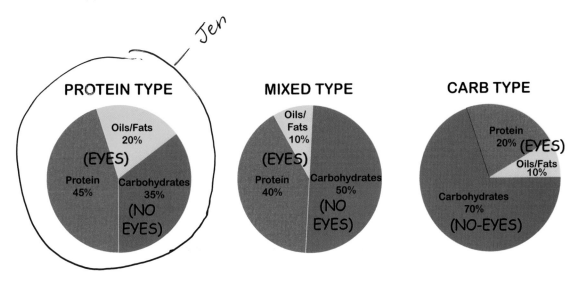

What is Metabolic Typing?

Metabolic Typing is a system that identifies an individual's genetically-based nutrition and diet requirements. There is not one diet that is right for everyone, therefore to achieve optimal health, you must determine what is right for you. You can find out what your Metabolic Type is through the questionnaire on pages 38 through 40. This questionnaire will categorize you as a protein type, a carb type or a mixed type. You may notice that the diet for a protein type is similar to the popular Zone Diet[1] while the diet for a carb type is closer to the Ornish Diet[2]. The great thing about Metabolic Typing is that it will direct you towards the diet plan that is right for your body.

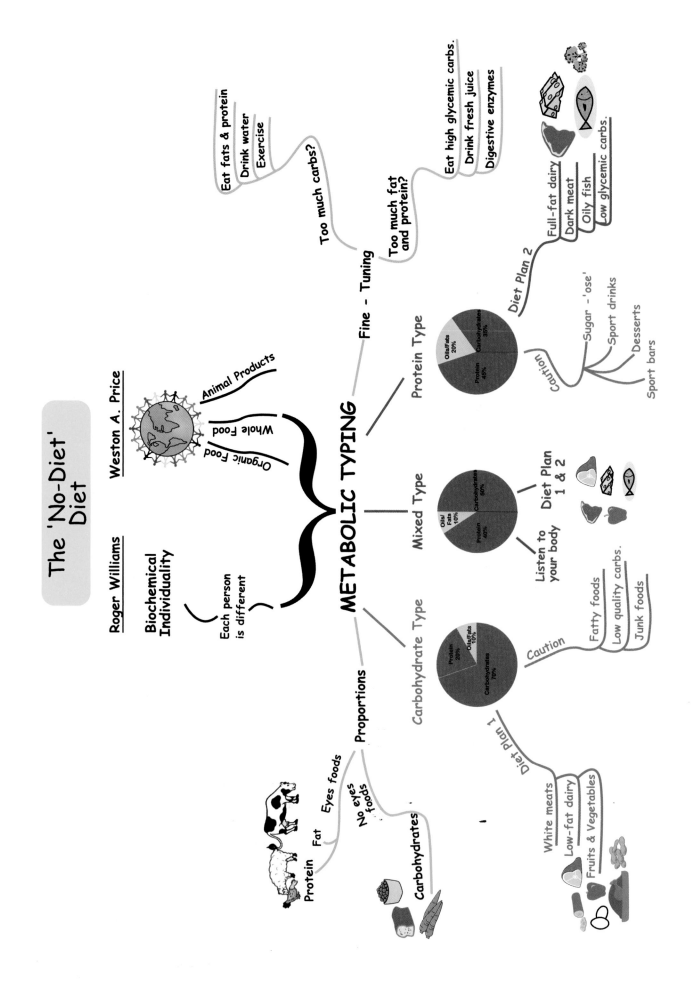

The 'No-Diet' Diet

METABOLIC TYPING

Roger Williams

Biochemical Individuality

Each person is different

Weston A. Price

Organic Food
Whole Food
Animal Products

Proportions

Protein Fat Eyes foods

No eyes foods

Carbohydrates

Carbohydrate Type

Carbohydrates 70%
Protein 20%
Oils/Fats 10%

Diet Plan 1

White meats
Low-fat dairy
Fruits & Vegetables

Caution
Fatty foods
Low quality carbs.
Junk foods

Mixed Type

Carbohydrates 50%
Protein 40%
Oils/Fats 10%

Diet Plan 1 & 2

Listen to your body

Protein Type

Carbohydrates 35%
Protein 45%
Oils/Fats 20%

Diet Plan 2

Full-fat dairy
Dark meat
Oily fish
Low glycemic carbs.

Caution
Sugar -'ose'
Sport drinks
Desserts
Sport bars

Fine - Tuning

Too much carbs?
Eat fats & protein
Drink water
Exercise

Too much fat and protein?
Eat high glycemic carbs.
Drink fresh juice
Digestive enzymes

THE "NO-DIET" DIET

This could be the most important chapter of this book for many readers. There's wide-spread confusion and a lack of understanding regarding how to eat these days—much of it coming from the media. Whether you want to lose weight, reduce body fat or put on muscle, you'll find experts touting all sorts of pills, magic hormone supplements, genie in a bottle shake drinks, even surgical procedures to help you reach your goal. The safest and most effective way to achieve such goals is to eat right for your metabolic type.

You can't fill your car with diesel when it was designed for gasoline and expect it to run at peak performance. If you wish to avoid living through the expression of your potential genetic flaws, you must do your very best to determine which *fuel sources* meet your genetic requirements so that you can accentuate your genetic strengths instead.

The good news is that you can slim down without being hungry while feeding your body what it needs—and when it needs it—so that you have a fighting chance to deal with the social, economic and environmental stressors inherent in modern life. The notion of *individuality* in diet is the key. There can *never* be any one diet or product that works for everyone. We must all discover which formula works for our biochemical and cultural individuality.

A Breakthrough Concept: Biochemical Individuality

In 1956, Roger Williams, a famous biochemist, published a book entitled *Biochemical Individuality*.[1] This unique and highly respected book outlined many of the anatomical variations that exist within each of us. For example, Williams revealed that there are variances in the size, shape, location and capacity of virtually all of our internal organs. He showed that there is a tremendous difference in metabolic rate from one person to the next, even from as early as two years of age. He found wide variations in water content and in oxygen carrying capacity of the blood from one person to the next. In short, just as we all look different on the outside, we also function differently on the inside and have different nutritional needs.

The Pioneering Studies of Dr. Weston Price

Weston A. Price documents the most thorough investigation of dietary variations among primitive peoples in his book *Nutrition and Physical Degeneration*.[2] In the early 1930's, Price traveled the globe investigating the relationships between health and diet among native peoples.

This was a pivotal time, as there were still tribes left to study that were untouched by civilization. His records were extensive in comparing the health of natives who had deviated from their natural diets to those who continued with their traditional ways of eating.

Price identified some 16 diverse cultures whose diets varied greatly depending on where they lived and what foods were available. Some groups, such as the Eskimos, ate diets high in fats and protein, while other groups, such as the Quetchus Indians of South America, ate a small amount of meat and mainly plant-based foods. Food sources varied greatly depending on what was available. In cold regions, some diets were mostly void of plant foods, while others contained a variety of seasonal fruits, vegetables, grains and legumes.

These diets did, however, share several underlying characteristics—all contained **organic foods, whole foods (minimally processed, if at all) and animal products**.

Preservation methods among primitive groups included drying, salting and fermenting, all of which preserve and even increase the nutrient value of the food. Through the selective pressures of nature, native cultures ate what was ideal for their lineage and geographical region—what was right for their metabolic type.

In all of Price's journeys, he did not come across a single healthy tribe or group that existed on a diet completely free of meat. One group that came close to being vegetarian was the Quetchus Indians of South America, who lived largely on a vegetable diet, not because they believed eating meat was bad, unethical or unhealthy, but because meat was scarce.

Price found that *all* primitive diets contained at least four times the quantity of minerals and water-soluble vitamins as the American diet of his day—which was far superior to that of today's diet.

Price, along with other pioneering doctors who studied native cultures during the first half of the twentieth century, found that many of these peoples enjoyed robust health and had excellent physiques—until they adopted what Price referred to as a "white man's diet" (refined and processed foods that included white sugar, flour, pasteurized milk and hydrogenated vegetable oils). A perfect example is the Eskimos and Indians of Alaska. Price wrote on what Dr. Josef Roming (a surgeon who worked among the Eskimos and Indians in Alaska) reported to him.

In his 36 years of contact with these people, he had never seen a case of malignant disease among the truly primitive Eskimos and Indians, although it frequently occured when they became modernized. He found, similarly, that the acute surgical problems requiring operation on internal organs, such as the gall bladder, kidney, stomach and appendix, do not tend to occur among the primitives but are very common problems among the modernized Eskimos and Indians. Growing out of his experience, in which he had seen large numbers of the modernized Eskimos and Indians attacked with tuberculosis, which tended to be progressive and ultimately fatal as long as the patients stayed under modernized living conditions, he now sends them back, when possible, to primitive conditions and to a primitive diet, under which the death rate is very much lower than under modernized conditions. Indeed, he reported that a great majority of the afflicted recover under the primitive type of living and nutrition.[2]

Numerous diet and nutrition 'experts' today seem hell-bent on emphasizing the harm caused by high-protein and/or high-meat diets. If these people were to qualify their concerns based on the status of our meat sources today, I believe their concerns might be relevant. However, this is usually not their reason. How can the American Dietetic Association (among others) tell us to eat multiple servings of grains, cereals and breads when the works of such pioneers like Weston A. Price and others show that our ancestors thrived on a much different diet?

Nutritional experts such as Sally Fallon and Dr. Mary Enig of the Weston A. Price Foundation, along with William Wolcott, author of *The Metabolic Typing Diet*, emphasize the importance of eating balanced meals, both for improved nutrient availability and for purposes of digestive efficiency.[3, 4] The importance of eating balanced meals means something different for each metabolic type.

Though few of us are really sure of our genetic heritage, we need to return to a diet similar to the one that each of our systems is designed to eat. The goal of your metabolic typing test is to determine which foods and in what amounts are best for you. There are a number of factors that influence your optimal macronutrient ratio at any given time. These factors are explained in detail in Wolcott's book, *The Metabolic Typing Diet*. Our goal here is to fine-tune your senses so that you become acutely aware from meal to meal what your body needs to optimize your genetic potential and suppress your genetic weaknesses.

Step 1

Review your Metabolic Typing Questionnaire (page 38) to determine whether you're a protein type, carb type or mixed type. The first step is to determine the optimal fuel ratio for your body. Look at the pie chart (Figure 1) that corresponds to your metabolic type. This will give you a starting point for proportioning your meals.

If you're unsure how to define protein, fat and carbohydrate, here's an easy way to remember:

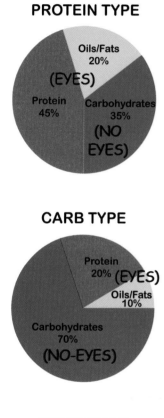

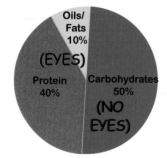

Figure 1: Meal Proportions

Proteins/Fats = Eyes

Proteins and fats usually come from something that has a set of eyes. For example, cows are the source of beef and dairy products—and of course, they have eyes. Pigs have eyes and give us pork. Birds have eyes and most of us love chicken or duck and their eggs. Even shrimp and fish have eyes and they, too, are great sources of protein and fats. Exceptions to the rule are avocados, seeds and nuts, which are all quite high in fat and therefore, placed in the "eyes" group for purposes of balancing your meals.

Carbs = No-eyes

Carbohydrates come predominantly from something that did not have eyes, so I refer to them as the "no-eyes" group. Yes, I realize that potatoes have "eyes," but I am actually refer-ring to eyes that see things. Your carbohydrate-based foods include fruits, vegetables, legumes and grains.

To determine your "eyes" vs. "no-eyes" proportions, simply locate the pie chart for your metabolic type and look at your starting ratio. As you see in the pie chart for a mixed type, meals should be about 50% eyes and 50% no-eyes. You simply arrange each meal or snack (remember to include your drinks) such that about half of what you consume is from the eyes group and half is from the no-eyes group. There's no need to pull out a triple beam scale to weigh things. The goal is not to turn eating into a math class. You'll learn to tune in to your body's messages telling you when you ate the right amounts for you. The Tachometer Form on page 48 will help you interpret some of the symptoms you may experience after an incorrectly proportioned meal.

It's a good idea to write down everything you eat for the first couple of weeks. Make notes on how you feel immediately after you eat and for the period of time up to your next meal. When you eat the right foods in the correct proportions for your metabolic type, you should feel satisfied after eating (not hungry or overly full), and your energy levels should increase. You should not feel hungry again for another four hours or so, and your energy levels should remain stable. (This corresponds to the Power Zone on the Tachometer Form, page 48.)

Your body will tell you when you didn't eat right. You may feel bloated, tired, remain hungry or become hungry soon after you eat. If you experience any of the short term responses listed in the white areas of the Tachometer Form, follow the tips given in the blue arrows and make note of what you last ate. Remember to make adjustments the next time you eat to avoid feeling down. If you're eating the proper proportions for your metabolic type but are consistently feeling unwanted side effects, try keeping a food log to determine if you're feeling this way after eating a specific food. This will help you reveal possible food intolerances (discussed further in Chapter 14).

Step 2

Beyond the quantity of food eaten, equally important is which foods you're eating. Now that you understand the amounts of different foods you should eat, have a look at the Diet Plan for your type (Appendix pages 234 and 235). You'll see that different foods are recommended for different metabolic types.

Carb Type = Diet Plan 1
Protein Type = Diet Plan 2
Mixed Type = Diet Plan 1 & 2

Each of these Diet Plans contains the best foods for your metabolic type. These foods will help support and balance your body chemistry. If a food is not on your list, you shouldn't eat it, or only eat it once in a while. These foods may push your body away from a balanced state. Remember, one man's medicine is another man's poison. An orange, for example, is generally thought of as a healthy food. For a carb type, it is a good food that will help balance the body, but the same orange may push a protein type out of balance.

Tips for Protein Types

Protein types are generally people who *live to eat*. You don't want to get between a protein type and food when they are hungry! When protein types follow the food pyramid or the dietary advice given in most exercise magazines, they can become chunky, fat and downright miserable. Since protein types burn through carbohydrates quickly, they must eat more protein and fat than carbohydrates to slow down the digestion of carbohydrates in their bodies. Protein types also have a higher requirement for *purines*, a type of amino acids prevalent in dark meats such as chicken legs and thighs, red meat, fish roe, sardines and anchovies. They tend to have a greater appetite for salt, which is okay as long as they consume high-quality, unprocessed sea salt, not regular, refined table salt (see page 77).

Protein types, against the advice of many health experts, frequently find that they sleep better and wake rested if they eat a meal that is higher in fat and protein closer to bedtime (within 2 - 3 hours or even less). This is largely due to the fact that protein types tend to rapidly burn carbohydrates in their metabolic pathways, leaving them hypoglycemic (low blood sugar) if they don't consume adequate fat and protein to tie up and slow down the carbohydrates. If your blood sugar drops during the middle of the night, your body is stressed in an attempt to raise blood sugar levels. This often results in a yo-yo fluctuation of your hormonal tides and rhythms throughout the night, which disrupts the release of melatonin (sleep and immune hormone) as well as other growth and repair hormones. As a result, you wake up feeling like you've been wrestling all night and will usually head straight for a pot of coffee to start the process all over again.

This is the very reason why protein types need to be very careful of what they have for dessert and what they drink, particularly within a few hours of bedtime. If they eat or drink too many carbohydrates, they're setting themselves up for visits to doctors and therapists for many seemingly unrelated, nagging conditions for which they often get treated with an arsenal of creams, pills and other medications. I've often seen symptoms such as chronic headaches, depression, chronic fatigue, poor concentration in the morning, back pain, neck pain, constipation and low sex drive clear up by simply balancing blood sugar levels in protein types, particularly at dinner and before bed.

Protein types also need to be wary of performance bars and drinks. Such products generally contain large amounts of sugar (any word ending in "-ose", like sucrose, dextrose or fructose) that will cause problems for a protein type if not balanced by adequate fat and protein. The lack of **quality** fats, protein and sugars in most of these sports nutrition bars is of course a concern for all metabolic types.

Protein types do better on full-fat dairy products. If they eat low-fat yogurts and cheeses, for example, they're usually hungry again in no time. Remember, protein types "live to eat" and if their bodies don't sense satiety, they go back into *hunter mode on the prowl for food!*

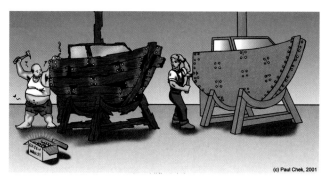

Figure 2: Vitamins as Nails

If protein types are going to drink coffee, they should not add sugar or non/low-fat milk. Remember, protein types go through carbohydrates very fast, easily rendering themselves hypoglycemic. If you need to add something to your coffee, try an organic full-fat cream or even whipping cream (raw if available). Add sugar to caffeine and your poor little adrenal glands start doing back flips. You'll experience the same roller coaster ride as when you eat too many sweets before bed, but this time you get a cognitive experience because you're awake! By adding a little full-fat cream with no sugar you'll at least be able to enjoy your vice without taking a chain saw to your pancreas and adrenal glands. And please, don't use artificial sweeteners because they're poisons, causing a plethora of problems. An alternative sweetener is Stevia (see page 77).

Many protein types, particularly those needing to lose body fat, will find that they do better eating smaller balanced meals more frequently. There is some controversy in literature these days regarding how much protein one can metabolize at any given time, suggesting that it's better for digestion to eat more frequent, smaller meals. Generally, if your post-meal responses are in the Power Zone (see page 48), you're not eating too much protein.

Tips for Carb Types

Carb types have the opposite challenge with regard to their metabolic pathways. Just as protein types don't efficiently metabolize carbohydrates (when eaten alone), carb types don't efficiently metabolize fats and proteins (when eaten alone). A carb type must, therefore, eat a proportionately larger amount of carbohydrates to meter the fats and proteins.

Don't forget, a carb type still needs to eat some fat and protein at each meal.

Just because you're a carb type and can handle more carbs, it doesn't mean you can take a multi-vitamin and have a permanent ticket to the junk food train. Vitamins are like nails, and your macronutrients are like the wood used to build a boat (see Figure 2). It doesn't matter if you use golden nails, building a boat out of junk wood will only result in a useless boat that sinks, taking your golden nails right to the bottom. In your case, they just go right out your bottom! My point is that while carb types feel better on a diet of as much as 70% carbohydrates, the carbohydrates need to be composed of real food, not junk food, no matter what kind of vitamin supplements you take.

Carb types shouldn't feel pressured to eat a huge breakfast. Many won't be attracted to heavy food in the morning and will likely opt for light foods such as a boiled egg, toast and juice (fresh squeezed) or coffee (organic). Their appetite will often kick in by lunch, particularly if they have exercised by then.

Carb types often do well on only two meals a day, which can lead to friends and family members (especially mothers and grandmothers) putting pressure on them to eat against their instincts. To achieve optimal health, the carb type needs to focus on avoiding junk foods, even if they feel good after eating them. They must seek high-quality *organic* foods and remember that they also need to include some fats and proteins in each meal or snack.

The carb type will generally **not** do well eating full-fat dairy products or fatty meats, which often make them feel dull and more likely to resort to stimulants such as coffee and sugar to pick them up. Carb types will fare best eating light meats like chicken breast, leaner cuts of meat and light fish.

Tips for Mixed Types

If your questionnaire identifies you as a mixed type, you enjoy the status of being the easiest to feed, *and the toughest to train.* Mixed types need to read everything here with regard to protein types and carb

Tachometer Form

Responses to too much carbohydrate

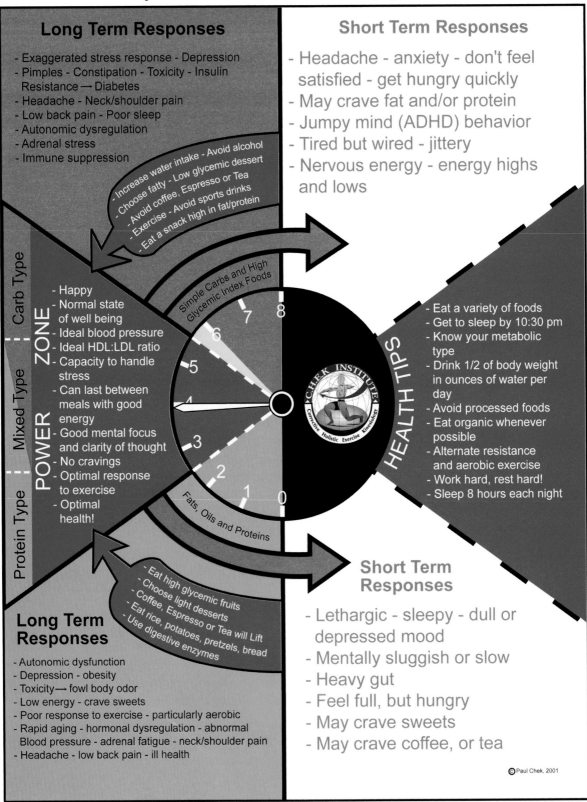

Long Term Responses

- Exaggerated stress response - Depression
- Pimples - Constipation - Toxicity - Insulin
  Resistance → Diabetes
- Headache - Neck/shoulder pain
- Low back pain - Poor sleep
- Autonomic dysregulation
- Adrenal stress
- Immune suppression

- Increase water intake - Avoid alcohol
- Choose fatty - Low glycemic dessert
- Avoid coffee, Espresso or Tea
- Exercise - Avoid sports drinks
- Eat a snack high in fat/protein

Short Term Responses

- Headache - anxiety - don't feel
  satisfied - get hungry quickly
- May crave fat and/or protein
- Jumpy mind (ADHD) behavior
- Tired but wired - jittery
- Nervous energy - energy highs
  and lows

Carb Type

Mixed Type

Protein Type

POWER ZONE

- Happy
- Normal state
  of well being
- Ideal blood pressure
- Ideal HDL:LDL ratio
- Capacity to handle
  stress
- Can last between
  meals with good
  energy
- Good mental focus
  and clarity of thought
- No cravings
- Optimal response
  to exercise
- Optimal
  health!

Simple Carbs and High Glycemic Index Foods

Fats, Oils and Proteins

HEALTH TIPS

- Eat a variety of foods
- Get to sleep by 10:30 pm
- Know your metabolic
  type
- Drink 1/2 of body weight
  in ounces of water per
  day
- Avoid processed foods
- Eat organic whenever
  possible
- Alternate resistance
  and aerobic exercise
- Work hard, rest hard!
- Sleep 8 hours each night

- Eat high glycemic fruits
- Choose light desserts
- Coffee, Espresso or Tea will Lift
- Eat rice, potatoes, pretzels, bread
- Use digestive enzymes

Long Term Responses

- Autonomic dysfunction
- Depression - obesity
- Toxicity → fowl body odor
- Low energy - crave sweets
- Poor response to exercise - particularly aerobic
- Rapid aging - hormonal dysregulation - abnormal
  Blood pressure - adrenal fatigue - neck/shoulder pain
- Headache - low back pain - ill health

Short Term Responses

- Lethargic - sleepy - dull or
  depressed mood
- Mentally sluggish or slow
- Heavy gut
- Feel full, but hungry
- May crave sweets
- May crave coffee, or tea

© Paul Chek, 2001

Responses to too much fat / protein

types because as a mixed type you're both types at the same time and will oscillate back and forth between the two. Depending on sensitivity, your environment and your physical, hormonal and emotional stress levels, this oscillation can occur from meal to meal, week to week or month to month. Simply stated, this means you must master the ability to feel the messages coming from your body. As a mixed type, you'll likely lean toward either a protein or a carb type most of the time, yet you won't feel well if you just stick to one pattern of eating and ignore your internal body language.

The mixed types will start proportioning their meals with 50% from the eyes group (proteins/fats) and 50% from the no-eyes foods (carbohydrates). To maximize the chances of achieving health and vitality, the mixed types need to study and become intimate with the methods of *fine-tuning meals* as presented on the Tachometer Form (page 48).

Fine Tuning Your Meals

I use the analogy of a car's tachometer to represent the speed and efficiency with which your metabolic engines produce energy, because in a very real sense each cell in your body is like a little engine. If your cells run too fast, they become exhausted and if they continue to operate that way, they can become burned out—diseased! If you run your car's engine too slowly and shift gears too soon, the engine becomes sluggish and clogged up with incompletely combusted fuel residues. The cells of your body behave similarly if your fat and protein intake is too great for your metabolic pathways—you feel clogged up and sluggish.

The blue zone on the Tachometer Form is the *Power Zone* and represents the optimal response to any given meal or snack. To the left of the tachometer, you'll see the indicators of having eaten a meal in the correct proportions and composed of the right foods for your body. These Power Zone responses generally appear within minutes of beginning your meal or snack and should last three to four hours or longer. Protein types may need to eat sooner than slow or mixed types. With an ideal meal (the right foods in the correct proportions) comes an improved state of well being. You basically feel good all over.

The red zone is the response to eating too many carbohydrates for your metabolic type. In the top left of the Tachometer Form, you'll see some (there are many more) of the common chronic or long-term responses of eating too many carbohydrates for your metabolic type. The top right of the form gives common acute symptoms, or symptoms that will show up as soon as a few minutes to two hours after eating a meal too high in carbohydrates.

The green zone is the response to eating too much protein and/or fat. In the bottom left corner you'll see some of the many long-term responses to eating too much fat and protein for your metabolic type. The bottom right demonstrates the immediate response to too many fats and proteins.

Health Tips

Within as little as a few minutes and over the two hours following a meal, you'll begin getting signals from your body. Generally, the healthier you are, the faster you get the information and the more information you get.

If you eat too many carbohydrates and experience symptoms written in red on the Tachometer Form, immediately try one of the following remedies:

1. Eat fats and protein
2. Drink water

   or,

3. Exercise

If you eat too much fat or protein, immediately:

1. Eat carbohydrates (high-glycemic if possible, such as below-ground veggies, fruits or grains)
2. Consume fresh-squeezed juice or fresh fruit

   or,

3. Take digestive enzymes containing protease and lypase

The sooner you respond to any of the symptoms listed on the Tachometer Form the better. By taking one or more of the actions directing you back to the Power Zone (the blue arrow) you are more likely to normalize your fuel mix for optimal conversion to energy.

Putting it all Together on Your Plate

You need to be aware of a few facts that can throw you for a loop when it comes to eating right for your metabolic type.

Not All Vegetables Are Created Equal: A general rule of thumb that can be used when proportioning meals is that above-ground vegetables have a lower glycemic index (less sugar) than below-ground vegetables such as beets, potatoes and carrots. Grains and corn also have a high glycemic index. This information is particularly important to protein types because they're the most sugar sensitive and should consume carbohydrates that have a lower glycemic index.

Drinks: Failure to consider the carbohydrate content of drinks is the number one reason why people have less than optimal results when they begin their Metabolic Typing diet plan. For example, a 12-ounce can of Coke has 40 grams of carbohydrates, which is equal to about 12 one-cup servings of romaine lettuce, two servings of homemade potato salad, a cup of long grain rice and 1 ½ baked sweet potatoes! Just six ounces of orange juice from frozen concentrate delivers 21.3 grams of carbohydrates.

Alcoholic beverages, such as vodka and whiskey, don't have the same carbohydrate content that soft drinks or fruit juices do, but many others, such as, wine coolers, liquers and cocktails do have a very high sugar content. Another issue to consider is that drinking alcoholic beverages on an empty stomach—such as when waiting for your meal at a restaurant—can cause hypoglycemia (low blood sugar) due to altered carbohydrate metabolism caused by the alcohol. The typical response to low blood sugar is to eat any foods immediately available, often bread, chips or other displacement foods that are likely to alter optimal meal proportioning for your metabolic type.

A rule of thumb is to consider any sweet or alcoholic drink equal to at least one serving of no-eyes food. If you're a protein type, you have a very important decision to make—coke and a steak or water and a steak and a sweet potato? Remember, you are what you eat, and you can't make or replace anything in your body with soda or processed garbage drinks (more about this in Chapter 4).

Butters, Oil-based Dressings and Gravy: When eating foods such as a potato, adding butter increases your overall fat content and must be considered with regard to the ratio you're trying to maintain. If you're a protein type, adding butter to a potato, particularly in combination with leaner meats, such as chicken breast, can be helpful in maintaining your energy and sense of satiety. Should you be a carb or mixed type, the same butter may make you feel sluggish, dull and even full—but hungry. The carb or mixed type who balances their meal properly, but gets crazy with Thousand Island dressing, slaps a couple pats of butter on their potato and can't resist a little extra gravy, is sure to have an urge for a sweet dessert or a cup of coffee after dinner. These are folks who are looking to rev the engines and keep from going into hibernation on the couch.

In short, to balance your meals effectively and get optimal energy from food, you need to consider the fat content of butter, dressings and gravies. It doesn't have to be complicated. Simply **feel** your response to a given meal and adjust accordingly using your Tachometer Form—either as you feel the changes or at the next meal. Soon, you'll intuitively know just how much gravy, butter or dressings you can use with most any combination of eyes and no-eyes foods to get the ideal response for your body.

Sauces: Just as fatty dressings and toppings can throw your meal ratio off, so can sweet sauces. Many such toppings (teriyaki and sweet and sour sauce) have a lot of sugar in them and can push you over your carbohydrate limit. Remember to take this into account when eating such foods.

Fatty Acid Supplements: While it may seem menial, taking essential fatty acid supplements, particularly those that provide optimal and much needed sources of omega-3's, can throw your meal balance off if you're not careful. This is more often the case for the carb types because they're far more sensitive to fats. If a carb type has prime rib for dinner (or any fatty cut of meat), a salad and a large potato and is feeling great, all that can change as soon as they go the extra mile to be super healthy. Taking as little as two grams of fish oil, for example, could make them feel lethargic, sleepy and may make them crave coffee or sweets. A little experimentation will soon teach you how many fatty acid supplements to take with any given type of protein source or meal combination. Should an EFA supplement be needed for theurapeutic reasons, you many need to adjust and increase the carb content of your meals.

Desserts: Let's face it, most people love dessert. If you're going to have dessert once in a while, make sure to calculate it into your eyes to no-eyes ratio. If you're a protein type, this means that you may need to skip carbohydrates completely with your dinner, or consume only a small amount. By making the switch to organic vegetables, you're more likely to find that the natural sweetness and flavor are so satisfying that your cravings for dessert diminishes or disappears all together.

This may seem like a lot of information, but it's worth it once you get your body chemistry in balance by eating right for your metabolic type. The key points to remember are:

1. Eat the proportions of fats/proteins carbohydrates that **feel** right to you.

2. Eat the right foods for your type (see diet plans).

3. Retest your Metabolic Type every couple of months, it is common to change types as you become healthier.

Rowing harder doesn't help if the boat is headed in the wrong direction.

Kenichi Ohmae

Case History
Katie, a client of James Williams,
CHEK NLC Level 2, London, UK

When I was first introduced to Katie in July 2002 she was a bubbly 23-year-old with several ongoing health conditions and the desire to lose some body fat. Her doctor had told her that she had Myalgic Encephalitis (M.E., also known as Chronic Fatigue Syndrome) and Endometriosis. Katie experienced several different 'symptoms' that made life uncomfortable and tiring.

"With M.E., every day is like having the flu. My body aches all over and I am tired and depressed all the time. There is no medication available except anti-depressants—a route that I took and gained 1½ stone! The weight gain didn't help my depression and I entered into a downward spiral."

Katie's mum, Marian, was so impressed with the results she'd had with basic Metabolic Typing that she suggested I consult with Katie, who wanted help before returning to university.

During our consultation, it became obvious that the university was going to provide Katie with all her meals and that there was no practical way of helping her eat according to her Metabolic Type. I felt uneasy about it, but I gave her general advice about the types of food to eat and how to raise her energy levels by eating a low glycemic diet. We agreed to meet the following May, after her course, when Katie would be in a position to make her own meals.

I had since completed the C.H.E.K Institute's Nutrition and Lifestyle course, and Katie's health

had gotten worse. Marian brought her along to one of my holistic weight loss groups.

"By April of this year my weight was really causing me problems. I lost all my self-confidence, was unhappy and felt like I was at a 'dead-end'. I didn't want to go out with my friends, and the thought of a summer holiday having to wear swimsuits horrified me."

Katie was determined to improve her health and to lose a stone or two, so Marian gave her the Metabolic Typing questionnaire from Wolcott's book to complete. Katie turned out to be a protein type. I agreed it was a great start towards rebuilding Katie's health, and so she carried on eating a high fat, high protein diet. When I had Katie's health assessment questionnaire back and produced the graph, 21 out of 27 of her body systems were in the high priority. Katie's body was so stressed it was approaching meltdown, yet to her credit she remained focused and strong-willed and took the result in her stride.

A week before she went back to university for the exams, potentially the most stressful part of her course, Katie visited her doctor. She'd made the appointment long before we'd met up again and went along to ask his advice for fat loss. He asked her what she'd had for breakfast that morning and when she told him about her fat and protein feast he said, "Your diet is all wrong, you're eating too much fat and should take a good look at your diet." Katie adds, "He implied my weight gain was a result of my eating habits and nothing to do with my illness or any other changes in my body."

In addition, he gave her information about pharmaceutical pills that had the potential for some rather unpleasant side effects. His response did not exactly encourage Katie. "He offered me slimming pills, which disgusted me. I couldn't believe he wasn't willing to investigate my weight gain. I went to him for help, but I just left feeling disheartened and upset."

Katie assured me that her doctor is usually a bit more supportive than he was on that occasion, and she put it down to him having a bad day and continued eating her Protein Type meals.

Katie had also been the patient of an experienced Upledger-trained CranioSacral therapist who had been working on her for a year. Just days before Katie and I met, the therapist (Zakia Collins), had worked on Katie. Through a technique known as SomatoEmotional Release, the cause of Katie's health problems was located. It was suspected that Katie's hypothalamus and pituitary gland had not been communicating properly and that this was linked to trapped emotions after her Grandfather's death 13 years earlier. The emotional trauma of the death had remained in her body and, like a time bomb, had been ticking away for years, slowly eroding her health. Zakia had helped Katie's body release the trapped emotions, which played a part in restoring proper function to these two vital parts of her brain. When Katie told me what she'd experienced, it perfectly explained many of her health problems and the stress her body was under.

Days before she went back to university, Katie and I agreed on some easy-to-introduce lifestyle changes that would lessen the stress on her body. Even though she only had five weeks of hard study and exams left, we had to act and got her to ask the canteen staff for more protein. They took Katie under their wing and were soon offering her extra rations of meat. Although it was far from organic, it was the best option.

To rest and rebuild her tired body, we ordered several supplements specifically for her metabolic type. The only adjustment I had to make to her MT diet was to recommend lean meats to rest her liver and gallbladder because they, too, were highly stressed. The final part of our plan was to ensure she drank enough water, and, amazingly, Katie just started drinking what she needed, three litres daily without any resistance.

Five weeks later we met again and the improvement was just jaw-dropping. In fact, I'll let Katie tell you how she felt: "I was amazed with my weight loss, especially as I couldn't follow the diet 100% at university. Now that I am at home, I find it easy to follow and enjoy the foods that I am allowed. My self-confidence is gradually coming back, although I am aware that I have a great deal more weight still to lose. I have previously lost weight with Weight Watchers and Slimming World, but I only managed to keep it off for a few months. I am hoping that the MT diet will be different; it's not just a diet, but a lifestyle change – one which will hopefully change my life forever."

While at university Katie lost 12 pounds in five weeks. This was at the time of writing and she also reports that she has more energy, is less depressed and feels more emotionally secure – so much so that chocolate hasn't passed her lips for five weeks!

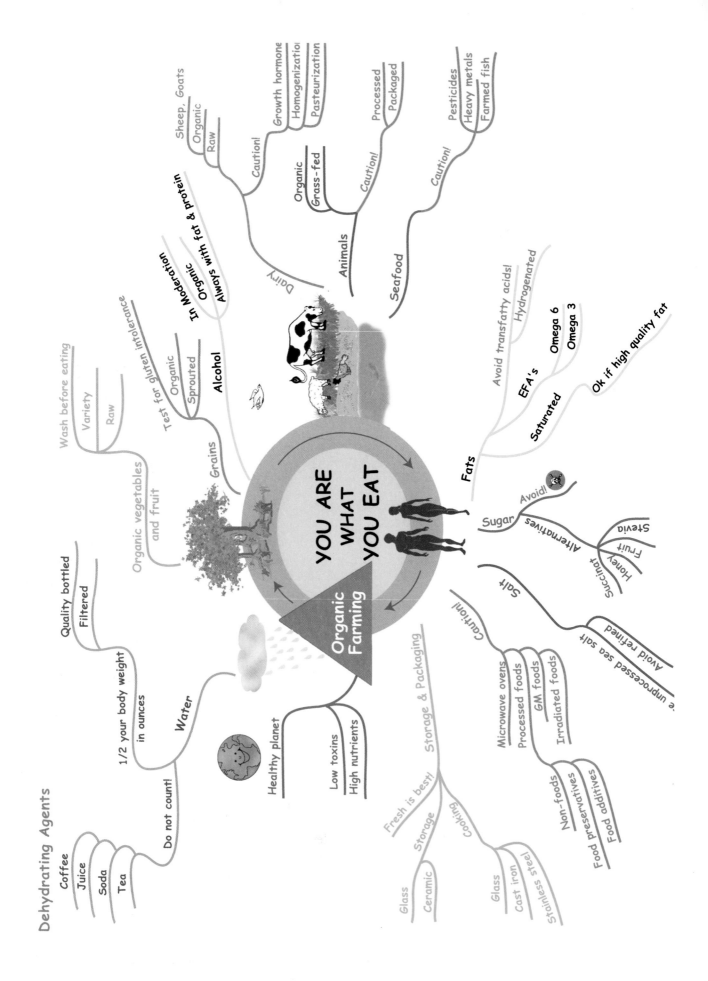

Dehydrating Agents

Coffee
Juice
Soda
Tea
Do not count!

Water
1/2 your body weight in ounces
Quality bottled
Filtered

Organic vegetables and fruit
Wash before eating
Variety
Raw

Grains
Test for gluten intolerance
Organic
Sprouted

Alcohol
In Moderation
Organic with fat & protein
Always

Dairy
Sheep, Goats
Organic
Raw
Caution!
Growth hormone
Homogenization
Pasteurization

Animals
Organic
Grass-fed
Caution!
Processed
Packaged

Seafood
Caution!
Pesticides
Heavy metals
Farmed fish

YOU ARE WHAT YOU EAT

Organic Farming

Healthy planet
Low toxins
High nutrients

Fats
EFA's
Avoid transfatty acids!
Hydrogenated
Omega 6
Omega 3
Saturated
Ok if high quality fat

Sugar
Avoid!
Alternatives
Succinate
Honey
Fruit
Stevia

Salt
Avoid refined
Use unprocessed sea salt

Storage & Packaging
Caution!
Microwave ovens
Processed foods
GM foods
Irradiated foods
Non-foods
Food preservatives
Food additives

Cooking
Fresh is best!
Storage
Glass
Ceramic
Cast iron
Stainless steel
Glass

YOU ARE WHAT YOU EAT

Let's face it—we live in a crazy world. Our air and water is polluted, the United States alone sprays two billion pounds of pesticides a year on crops to compensate for poor farming practices, and most people place a higher priority on driving a nice car than eating high quality food. Many organic farmers are barely able to keep their businesses going. So few people are conscious of the benefits of organic foods and most shop for groceries as if they were gasoline or motor oil—searching for the *cheapest eggs, meats, produce* and so on. Do you think people would be in such a rush to buy the cheapest food available if they realized that within hours whatever they put in their mouth is replacing cells somewhere in their body? That's right—*you literally are what you eat!*

In this chapter, we'll cover the dangers of modern food packaging and processing and provide a number of tips that will help you develop health and well-being from the inside out.

Organic vs. Commercially Farmed

I am passionate about organic farming. Organic food is grown without the use of toxic pesticides, herbicides, fungicides or chemical fertilizers. Organic foods are better for your health, and they're produced in ways that support a healthy environment; organic farming works with Mother Nature, not against Her!

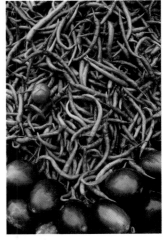

Before achieving organic certification in the U.S., fields must be farmed for a minimum of three years under guidelines handed down by the organic committee of the farmer's state. This three-year period assures that microorganisms have time to digest and eliminate chemical residues that may be left in the soil from previous exposure. Farmers operating in this three-year grace period can label their food as "organically grown," yet there may still be pesticides in their soils, so it is best to purchase "certified organic" products.

Nutrient Values

The media generally report that there is no significant difference in the nutritional value of organic foods when compared to conventionally grown produce. This is virtually impossible if you consider what organic farming entails.

Dr. Virginia Worthington reviewed 1,230 published comparisons between organically grown and conventionally grown crops. The results of her survey indicated that organic crops had higher nutrient levels or lower levels of toxicity in 56% of the comparisons.[1]

While many of these studies proved that organic foods had more nutrients, it's interesting to note that there was still a high percentage of researchers who claimed that conventionally grown crops were better. Those studies must be closely scrutinized. The British Soil Association analyzed 109 studies on organic and conventionally raised foods. They determined that only 27 of the studies were valid comparisons—almost all of which found organic foods to be significantly better. In many of the other studies, the organic produce was flown in and was much older than the locally grown conventional crops, therefore decreasing its nutritional value.[2]

Secondary Nutrients

The nutrients gener-ally mentioned when comparing convention-ally grown and organic foods are *primary nu-trients* such as water, fiber, proteins, fats, carbohydrates, vitamins and minerals. Among the differences cited between conventional and organic foods are notable increases in the amount of *secondary nu-trients* in organic foods.

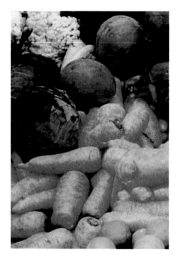

There are some 5,000 – 10,000 secondary com-pounds in plants. While secondary nutrients have not been classified as, or known to be, *essential* for health, there is a wealth of information suggesting numerous health benefits. The British Soil Associa-tion's "Organic Farming, Food Quality and Human Health" report alone cites 57 references supporting both increased levels of secondary nutrients in or-ganic produce and their beneficial effects.[2]

Research from Copenhagen University suggests that organic food may help prevent cancer. Organic foods were found to contain high levels of a potent group of antioxidants called *phenolic compounds*—a group of secondary nutrients. According to the researchers, phenolic compounds are ten times more efficient at mopping up cancer-causing free radicals in the body than other antioxidants like vitamins C and E.[3]

The beneficial effects of secondary nutrients are also well known among Naturopaths and holistic medical practitioners. Many doctors and healing clinics include an organic diet in their approach to treatment. The healing effects of these organic foods are associated with the superior secondary nutrient content and quality as well as with increased vita-min, mineral, trace mineral, protein and enzyme content.

Protein Quality

One of the largest studies on organic food, the Haughley Experiment, found that cows fed organic produce ate less but consistently produced more milk. Some feel this is due to the quality of protein in the grass. Protein is dependent on the range of amino acids in its composition. Plant proteins may or may not contain certain amino acids that are es-sential for human and animal nutrition. Whether they do or not depends largely upon the soil con-ditions in which the plant is grown. The plant is dependent upon minerals, trace minerals and trace elements—and their availability is dependent upon microorganisms in the soil. These essential mi-croorganisms are depleted by as much as 85% in conventionally farmed soils, usually as a result of chemical fertilizers, pesticides, herbicides and fun-gicides. The protein composition of plants growing in the depleted soil are, therefore, inferior.[4]

Fewer Toxins

Despite the controversy over the nutritional differ-ences between organic and conventionally farmed produce, meats and poultry, one thing is indisputable, even under scientific scrutiny—organically raised foods should be free of the harmful chemical residues present on commercial farms. This alone makes them worth the extra time and money they may take to acquire. Still, we are now at the point when even or-ganic foods are sometimes in contact with chemicals from irrigated water and the air, so it's hard to say that they're 100% free of chemicals.

Critics of organic foods say that they are not worth the extra money. I find this shocking, especially when these statements come from individuals with industry credentials, whom the public tends to trust.

Manfred Kroger, Ph.D., a Quackwatch consultant and Professor of Food Science at Pennsylvania State University, stated:

> Scientific agriculture has provided Americans with the safest and most abundant food supply in the world. Agricultural chemicals are needed to maintain this supply. The risk from pesticide residue, if any, is minuscule, is not worth worrying about, and does not warrant paying higher prices.[5]

First off, if this is true, why are there volumes of documented information, some dating back 60 years or more, proving otherwise? Surely it can't *all* be wrong. Secondly, consider our society's current state of health. The more chemicals and toxins we are exposed to, it seems that the worse our health becomes.

If you are eating conventionally farmed/raised foods, you had better hope that Professor Kroger is right and pesticides are not "worth worrying about." Here are just a few examples of how prevalent pesticide residues are in our food supply.

This first study I would like to share, tested a typical school lunch of a New Zealand student.[7] When you read these findings, keep in mind that New Zealand has much stricter food and farming standards than most countries, including the U.S. and the U.K.

Ingredients found in lunch items:

Sausage: DDE (a metabolic derivative of DDT), Chlorpyrifos-methyl, fenitrothion, Pirimiphos-methyl

Tomato: Alpha-endosulfan, beta-endosulfan, endosulfan-sulphate, chlorothalonil, dithiocarbamates, iprodione, procymidone, vinclozolin

Butter: DDE

White bread roll: chlorpyrifos-methyl, dichlorvos, fenitrothion, malathion, pirimiphos-methyl.

Apple: chlorpyrifos, captan, iprodione, vinclozolin.

For the sake of economy, let's focus on the apple. Most people think of an apple as a healthy food item, but what about when it is laden with chemicals? Research has revealed these potential effects from the chemicals found above:

Chlorpyrifos: endocrine disruptor, impairs immune response, reproductive abnormalities, damage in developing nervous system and brain

Captan: carcinogenic, genetic and immune system damage

Iprodione: carcinogenic

Vinclozolin: carcinogenic, genetic, endocrine and reproductive disruptor, dermatitis [6, 7, 8]

A study of 110 urban and suburban children in Washington state found that children who ate primarily organic foods had significantly lower organophosphorus pesticide (nervous immune system disruptor) exposure than children on conventional diets. Out of the children tested, only one did not have measurable levels of the **pesticide** in their urine. **This child was on an all-organic diet**. Other children eating mainly organic foods had exposure levels below the EPA's (Environmental Protection Agency) "safe" level, while the children eating conventional foods were above this level.[9]

Better for the Environment

From the soil up, organic farming is better for the environment. We survived for thousands of years on organically grown foods. Modern "advances" in farming such as chemical fertilizers, pesticides, herbicides and fungicides, are destroying our soils, which results in destruction of the plants, animals and ultimately the humans dependent upon them. There are numerous sources of information covering the benefits of organic products. Remember, when you spend a bit more to buy organic, you're not only doing yourself a favor, you're helping to improve the environment.

An ounce of prevention is worth a pound of cure!

Processed Foods

Most shopping carts today are filled with what I call **non-foods**. A non-food is any food that costs more in nutritional value to digest, absorb and eliminate than it delivers. Most processed foods fall into this category.

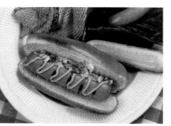

Before you read the next paragraph, go to your cupboard or refrigerator and have a look at how many packaged food items are there. Then pull out:

1. A dessert item

2. A boxed item, such as cereal or cookies, and

3. Any other item that is flavored, such as salad dressing or sauces

Look at the labels to see how many ingredients you either can't pronounce or don't know what they are. The vast majority of these multi-syllable words look more like the ingredients of super glue or fingernail polish than food.

The gigantic and often strange words listed on packages are the various concoctions used to color, stabilize, emulsify, bleach, texture, soften, preserve, sweeten, add or cover smells and, in the manufacturer's words, flavor! In case you were wondering just how many of these little chemicals were sneaking into your mouth, the U.S. Food and Drug Administration (FDA) currently lists about 2,800 international food additives and about 3,000 chemicals that are deliberately added to our food supply each year. Including chemicals used in food production from ground to stomach, the number rises to between 10,000 and 15,000! [10]

Perhaps you already read labels to avoid chemicals. While you may not think you're eating too many food additives, you may very well be getting duped. Since the FDA doesn't require any food additive *Generally Regarded as Safe (GRAS)* to be listed on the label, all you'll see is "artificial flavor," "artificial coloring," or even the word *natural*. The average American eats approximately his or her body weight in food additives each year, or about 150 pounds (about the same for most English speaking countries).[10] Of that amount, as much as 15 pounds or more will be flavoring agents, preservatives and dyes—hundreds of which are on the FDA's GRAS list. Before you get comfortable with the GRAS signifier, you should realize that to save time and money, the FDA *allows the food and additive manufacturers to notify them of the GRAS status of their additives and they're allowed to provide their own evidence to support their claim!* That's a bit like asking a cigarette or drug manufacturer to make sure they provide evidence that their products are safe.

The food and additive manufacturers, like drug manufacturers, are running the largest study in history— *and the general public are the guinea pigs.* An additive is removed from the GRAS list only after reports accumulate citing its damaging effects. With that in mind, what are the chances of a doctor notifying the FDA that a patient suffered adverse reactions to *acetaldehyde, acetic acid or agar* when neither is listed as anything other than a "food additive" because they're on the GRAS list? Acetaldehyde is known to be an irritant to mucous membranes (which line your entire digestive tract), is a central nervous system depressant and in large doses may cause death. Acetic acid may cause gastrointestinal distress, skin rashes and eye irritation. Agar may cause flatulence, bloating (goodbye abs) and may have the same effect as a laxative. Please realize, these are just a few of the food additives that I randomly selected from the book *Food Additives, A Shopper's Guide to What's Safe & What's Not,* by Christine Hoza Farlow, D.C.[11] There are hundreds of GRAS additives that read like something you could buy on the black market—yet we buy and eat these additives every day.

Don't be fooled by the use of the term *natural.* Insects, insect larvae, monkey guts and even mercury are all "natural" and are just a few of the natural items that end up in your food. In his book *Fast Food Nation,* Eric Schlosser nicely sums it up by quoting Terry Acree, a professor of food science technology at Cornell University, who says, "A natural flavor is a flavor that's been derived with an out-of-date technology." [12]

Food manufacturers like to play with your perception of what given words mean, and they know that if they can label an additive as natural, the health conscious consumer is much more likely to purchase it, yet just because something is natural doesn't mean it's better for you. After all, alcohol, tobacco, marijuana and cocaine are all natural, but none of them are necessarily *good for you.*

To better demonstrate my point, consider the ingredients commonly used in a typical fast-food restaurant strawberry milk shake. They are not listed because they are GRAS:

> Amyl acetate, amyl butyrate, amyl valerate, anethol, anisyl formate, benzyl acetate, benzyl isobutyrate, butyric acid, cinnamyl isobutyrate, cinnamyl valerate, cognac essential oil, diacetyl, dipropyl ketone, ethyl butyrate, ethyl cinnamate, ethyl heptanoate, ethyl lactate, ethyl methylphenylglycidate, ethyl nitrate, ethyl propionate, ethyl valerbate, heliotropin, hydroxyphrenyl-2butanone (10% solution in alcohol), α-ionone, isobutyl anthranilate, isobutyl butrate, lemon essential oil, maltol, 4-methylacetophenone, methyl anthranilate, methyl benzoate, methyl cinnamate, methyl heptine carbonate, methyl naphthyl ketone, methyl salicylate, mint essential oil, neroli essential oil, nerolin, neryl isobutyrate, orris butter, phenethyl alcohol, rose, rum ether, γ-undecalactone, vanillin, and solvent! [12]

Now that you've seen the chemical tricks behind strawberry flavoring, can you imagine what Neapolitan ice cream would look like on paper? You'd need a small booklet and a short course in chemistry even to begin to understand what you're eating. The liver must process all these chemicals. If your liver becomes overworked, these chemicals and additives can end up in your blood stream, with almost unlimited access to the cells of your body, as well as placing strain on your systems of detoxification. This can, and often does, lead to many unpleasant

symptoms such as weight gain, skin disorders and eventually auto-immune diseases. Many young people today, don't realize that things didn't use to be this way.

Dr. Weston A. Price, dentist, researcher and author of *Nutrition and Physical Degeneration*, traveled the globe studying indigenous populations and correlating their dietary habits with their incidence of disease and dental caries. He noted that cancerous diseases and the like were relatively unheard of in many cultures. In his study of native peoples, he consistently noted that the processing of foods was minimal.[13] Primitive people mostly used fire to cook meats, but not all. The Eskimos, for example, commonly ate many portions of animals and fish raw. Salts, lacto-fermentation and pickling were among the very few methods of processing foods for storage and, not surprisingly, these methods have been found to *increase* the nutritional value of many foods.[14]

Dr. Price's research was consistent with the research of Francis Marrion Pottenger, author of *Pottenger's Cats*.[15] In his extensive studies of cats, Pottenger demonstrated that consumption of pasteurized milk and/or cooked meats resulted in rapid onset of disease and bodily malformation. His clinical observations suggested that similar results occur in humans. Because of his findings, Dr. Pottenger stated, "Nutrition becomes one of the most important elements in preventive medicine." Regardless of which disease process is studied, the link between poor nutrition and disease, including cancer, clearly exists in studies and clinical observations of animals and man.

Avoid Genetically Modified Foods

If ever there was a great idea that could go very *bad*, genetic engineering of foods is likely to be the one. Genetic engineering (GE), also called genetic modification (GM) is the manipulation of plant and animal development by altering the gene expression. The products of genetic modification are often called *genetically modified organisms* (GMOs). I am sure you're familiar with the concept of farmers breeding prize bulls with prize cows to get *superior cows.* Or, as my father spent many years doing, breeding black rams with black ewes, both of which are known to produce off-spring with black wool to get a higher percentage of black sheep. These are examples of genetic manipulation, but within the confines provided by Mother Nature. But you're not likely to have heard of a farmer mating a bull with a sheep to get *giant* lamb chops. Or, a fish mating with a dog so the fish will come when you whistle. While this may sound ridiculous, *it's a direct analogy for what the biotech industry is doing with your food.*

Biotech scientists attempt to splice genes from bacteria and insects among other things, as well as other plants, into a given plant or species. Most genetically engineered crops planted worldwide are designed to either survive exposure to a certain herbicide or to kill certain insects. One of the big problems with this very powerful technology is that the mechanisms by which it works *or doesn't work* are not even understood by the scientists themselves. Genetic engineers certainly know much more about genetics than you or I, but they actually *don't know* with great certainty what will result from their manipulation of genes — Mother Nature's Laws. Genetic engineers are falling prey to the same arrogance that led to conventional farming methods—*they think they can "improve" on Mother Nature, or out-smart Her!*

While the mechanisms by which genetic engineering takes place are very complicated, particularly with regard to the scope of this book, it's safe to say that there are some real concerns. Genetic engineering can introduce an allergen into a food that previously did not contain it. For example, a soybean engineered with genes from a Brazil nut, designed to make it *tastier*, was found to produce allergic reactions in individuals with nut allergies. Some people apparently reacted violently to the GM soy. Nut allergies can be life threatening. This brings up another *big* problem. The biotech industry, supported by the U.S. government, doesn't want mandatory labeling of foods containing genetically modified organisms (GMOs). While they worry it may hurt sales, some of you could *die* from an allergic reaction, or some other reaction we simply can't predict, since scientists producing GM foods are not required to prove the safety of the foods before selling them to you.

After all, when genetic engineering causes a familiar food to start producing a substance previously not present in the human food supply, it's impossible to know who may have an allergic reaction to it.

The lack of quality research supporting GM crops is a real concern. However, one of the most comprehensive animal studies on the consumption of GM was done by Arpad Pusztai.[16]

Pusztai's research found that genetically engineered foods may also produce unexplained health effects in laboratory animals. Pusztai conducted studies with a GM potato. Galanthus Nivalis Agglutinin (GNA), which is ordinarily found in snowdrops (a type of flower), was added to potatoes to increase the plant's resistance to certain insects and other pests. The results showed that the GM potatoes had significantly less protein than the non-altered potatoes. The levels of starch, glucose and anti-nutrients were also significantly different. The GM potatoes were also associated with abnormal organ development and immune responsiveness in the rats that served as the subjects in the study. Pusztai concluded that his research, and that done by others, did not conclusively show that GM foods were safe for human consumption at that time. He recommended that further research be done.

Pusztai reported his findings in a television interview. He stated that, "It is very unfair to use fellow citizens as guinea pigs. Guinea pigs should be in the laboratory, and GE foods should be properly tested before they are approved for the market." Pusztai began his studies to prove that GM foods were safe, but when he exposed his results which proved otherwise, he lost his funding and assistants.[16]

Avoid Irradiated Foods

Let's say I invited you over for turkey dinner and told you that before cooking the meal, I'd be using my new food sanitizer. My new sanitizer happens to deliver 450,000 RADS of radiation, which is about 150 million times more radiation than the standard chest X-ray. The radiation source will be cobalt (Co-60), or possibly caesium (Cs-137), the remains of spent military nuclear fuel, and if you get too close to my new

Dr. Joseph Mercola, a highly regarded osteopathic physician specializing in natural health, cites the following 10 reasons for opposing food irradiation on his popular web site **www.mercola.com**:

1. In legalizing food irradiation, the U.S. Food and Drug Administration (FDA) did not determine a level of radiation to which food can be exposed and still be safe for human consumption, which federal law requires.

2. In legalizing food irradiation, the FDA relied on laboratory research that did not meet modern scientific protocols, which federal law requires.

3. Research dating to the 1950s has revealed a wide range of problems in animals that ate irradiated food, including premature death, a rare form of cancer, reproductive dysfunction, chromosomal abnormalities, liver damage, low weight gain and vitamin deficiencies.

4. Irradiation masks and encourages filthy conditions in slaughterhouses and food processing plants. Irradiation can kill most bacteria in food, but it does nothing to remove the feces, urine, pus and vomit that often contaminate beef, pork, chicken and other meat. Irradiation will not kill the pathogen that causes mad cow disease.

5. Irradiation destroys vitamins, essential fatty acids and other nutrients in food—sometimes significantly. The process destroys 80 percent of vitamin A in eggs, but the FDA nonetheless legalized irradiation of these products.

6. Irradiation can change the flavor, odor and texture of food—sometimes disgustingly so. Pork can turn red; beef can smell like a wet dog; fruit and vegetables can become mushy; and eggs can lose their color, become runny and ruin recipes.

7. Irradiation disrupts the chemical composition of everything in its path—not just harmful bacteria, which the food industry often asserts. Scores of new chemicals called "radiolytic products" are formed by irradiation—chemicals that do not naturally occur in food and that the FDA has never studied for safety.

8. The World Health Organization did not follow its own recommendation to study the toxicity of "radiolytic products" formed in high-dose irradiated food before proposing in November 2000 that the international irradiation dose limit—equal to 330 million chest x-rays—be removed.

9. Soon, some irradiation plants may use caesium-137, a highly radioactive waste material left over from the production of nuclear weapons. This material is dangerous and unstable. In 1988, a caesium-137 leak near Atlanta led to a $30 million, taxpayer-funded cleanup.

10. Because it increases the shelf life of food and is used in large, centralized facilities, irradiation encourages globalization and consolidation of the food production, distribution and retailing industries. These trends have already forced multitudes of family farmers and ranchers out of business, reduced the diversity of products in the marketplace, disrupted local economies in developing nations, and put American farmers and ranchers at a great economic disadvantage.

machine you could get one hell of a tan. Now, how excited would you be about tasting my turkey?

If this sounds ridiculous, you may want to take a seat for this—I've just described the radiation dose for meats as approved by the U.S. FDA. While there are other sources of radiation that can be used on your food, such as the use of a costly linear accelerator 'E-beam' technology left over from President Reagan's Star Wars Program, the U.S. Department of Energy (DOE) has aggressively promoted food irradiation for decades. The DOE sees food irradiation as a way of reducing disposal costs of spent military and civilian nuclear fuel by providing a *commercial* market for caesium nuclear wastes.[17]

Food irradiation is touted as a "needed" means of food sanitation by government agencies such as the International Atomic Energy Agency (IAEA), FDA, U.S. Department of Agriculture (USDA), DOE (Department of Energy), World Health Organization (WHO), Food and Agriculture Organization (FAO) and the World Trade Organization (WTO). These organizations are the main players streamlining the legislation for yet another technology that threatens your health and vitality.

Both the FAO and WHO insist that food irradiation makes more "safe" food available to the world's hungry. According to the WHO, ineffective regulation has in many countries overwhelmingly contaminated the food chain with pathogens such as salmonella, listeria or E. coli 0157. The cost of remedying this problem at its very root would be enormous. These organizations say that food irradiation reduces the incidence of food-borne diseases. All the while, experts have raised serious questions about the validity and necessity of food irradiation, such as the *absence of toxicological and carcinogenicity testing* by the FDA. As it turns out, the FDA approved irradiation based on five studies selected from 441 studies published prior to the early 1980's. To this day, these early studies remain the basis for their claims that irradiation is safe.[18]

A wide range of independent studies prior to 1986 clearly identified mutagenic and carcinogenic radiolytic products in irradiated food, and confirmed evidence of genetic toxicity in tests on irradiated food. Studies in the 1970's run by India's Institute of Nutrition reported that feeding freshly radiated wheat to monkeys, rats, mice and to a small group of malnourished children induced gross chromosomal abnormalities in blood or bone marrow cells and mutational damage in the rodents.[19]

Food irradiation results in major micronutrient losses, particularly vitamins A, C, E and the B complex group.

Foods approved for irradiation in the U.S.
The following list of foods is currently approved for irradiation by the FDA: [20]
- Seeds (used for sprouting—like alfalfa and clover. The sprouts will NOT be labeled as irradiated unless they are also irradiated.)
- Beef
- Pork
- Lamb
- Poultry
- Fruits
- Vegetables
- Wheat/Wheat Flour
- Eggs (in the shell)
- Herbs and Spices
- Dried Vegetable Seasonings

Foods not yet requested for irradiation are:
- Dairy (which is already pasteurized),
- Dried Legumes/Beans
- A few single-category foods like Honey and Coffee

Bacon was approved for irradiation in 1963, but the approval was rescinded in 1968 because animals fed irradiated bacon showed adverse health effects. These effects were probably due to fat oxidation (the fat becomes rancid quickly), which explains why nuts are not approved for irradiation in the U.S.

Organic foods cannot be irradiated, but the term "natural" for foods does not exclude irradiation. Some nutritional supplements like garlic are irradiated. To avoid irradiated foods, always ask store and/or restaurant managers if they sell or use irradiated foods.

Vegetables and Fruit

Eat as much raw produce as possible within the confines of the macronutrient proportions for your metabolic type.

Weston A. Price noted that many native cultures did only a minimal amount of cooking. Much of their diet consisted of raw foods. Many cultures even ate much of their meat raw. Cooking was used to soften fiber in some vegetables, making them more digestible or to make meat more digestible.[13]

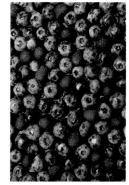

The process of cooking kills vital enzymes that are needed to aid in digestion. Generally, these enzymes cannot survive in temperatures beyond 118° F (48° C). Many vitamins and secondary nutrients in foods are also heat sensitive. Consuming predominately cooked foods increases your risk of becoming both vitamin and enzyme deficient, which often results in compromised digestion.

Raw foods and juices have been used for thousands of years to recover from illness and detoxify the body. Quite simply, *it takes life to give life*. If everything you eat is dead, you'll soon be one of those people who *die* at age 35 but whose corpse continues to walk around for another 35 years, bouncing from doctor to doctor.

Juicing is an excellent way to get nutrients from your raw veggies and fruits. Many of the essential nutrients in fruits and vegetables oxidize very rapidly upon juicing, it's therefore important to drink your juices immediately after juicing. Drinking them later in the day basically leaves you with sugar water. I recommend avoiding store-bought juices, as most have been pasteurized—a process that kills vital enzymes.

Consume a variety of fruits and vegetables.

We developed eating a vast variety of foods. Today, many people eat the same foods day in and day out. Different plants provide us with different essential nutrients. By consuming an array of different fruits and veggies, you will get a better variety of nutrients

as well as limit your chances of acquiring food intolerances. The deeper its color, the more antioxidants a fruit or veggie will likely provide. Remember to keep within your Metabolic Typing diet plan. The longer you stick to this way of eating the more balanced your body will become. At that point, you may begin eating more vegetables and fruits that may not be on your diet plan.

Wash your produce with a non-toxic soap before eating or juicing.

Even if your fruits and vegetables are organic, it is still a good idea to wash them before consuming. A non-toxic soap will help get rid of possible parasites that may be hiding on your food and also any residues from transporting. You will find fruit/veggie washes at most natural food stores, or you can make your own with vinegar and water.

Remember to choose organic produce whenever possible.

Grains

The story of grains goes part and parcel with the story of bread, neither of which the human machinery is designed to function optimally on. While I'm sure this is a surprise to some of you, significant amounts of scientific evidence suggests that for most of human evolution, until about 10,000 years ago, the

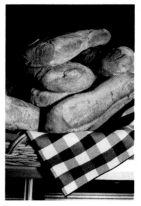

primary staple in the diets of most civilizations was animal meat. Generally, consumption of fruits, vegetables, nuts and seeds was seasonal and supplementary.[13, 21, 22] Most of the animals we preferred to eat, such as deer, were herbivores. These animals served to *condense* nutrition in their meats, one pound of meat containing the nutritional equivalent of several pounds of vegetables.[23] Such a dense nutrient source provided a sustaining food source during the winter months, when there were minimal food storage methods other than the cold itself. Although many argue (mostly from an emotional bias) that we must have carbohydrate sources to function, biochemistry reveals that we have the capacity to convert some fat molecules (glycerol) into carbohydrates.[24]

While there are many controversial theories as to why we began farming, most agree that farming practices, or nurturing the growth of specific plant species and domesticating animals, began no more than 20,000 years ago and more likely as recently as 10,000 years ago.[22] Since then, there's been a progressive increase in the amount of grains consumed—especially highly refined grains. Yet this time period is but a flash in the scope of human evolution, during which our digestive machinery was formed.

The process of sprouting grains changes the composition of the grain in numerous ways to make it more beneficial as a food. Sprouting increases the content of vitamins, such as vitamins C, B2, B5 and B6 and Carotene increases dramatically—sometimes eight-fold. Even more important, especially considering how many suffer from indigestion, is that phytic acid, a mineral blocker, is broken down in the sprouting process. Present in the bran of all grains and the coating of nuts and seeds, phytic acid inhibits the absorption of calcium, magnesium, iron, copper and zinc. These inhibitors can neutralize our own digestive enzymes, resulting in digestive disorders.[25] Complex sugars responsible for intestinal gas are also broken down during sprouting and a portion of the starch in grain is transformed into sugar. In addition, sprouting inactivates aflatoxins, which are toxins produced by fungus and are potent carcinogens found in grains.

For individuals who are not gluten intolerant, whole-grain cereals and breads are nutritious and provide fiber, which aids in detoxification. But processed wheat and white flour (which is just bleached wheat flour) is nutritionally deficient. Levels of zinc, chromium, manganese, iron and vitamin E are all reduced in processed flour compared to whole grains. Since the 1950s, conventionally-farmed American grains have been low in protein quality and quantity. The U.S. tried *giving* its surplus grains to countries with starving populations, but they would not accept grains from the U.S. if grains from any other countries were offered. This was because the deficient U.S. grains did little to maintain or improve the health of the starving.[26]

After 130 years of consuming highly processed grains in the form of breads, pastries and cereals, chronic disease is rampant among most industrialized nations. The greatest prevalence of rheumatic disease is in England, which has the greatest consumption of white flour, white sugar and tea per capita, while the U.S. runs a strong second.[27]

CHEK Points on Grains

1. Test yourself for gluten intolerance. Exclude all grains except corn, rice, buckwheat and millet for two weeks. If you feel a noticeable improvement in how you feel, you're probably gluten intolerant and should avoid all gluten-containing grains.

2. Minimize consumption of commercially processed grains and grain-based products.

3. Choose organic whole or sprouted grain products.

Alcohol

We were not designed to drink alcohol. Very few people actually like the taste of alcohol the first time they try it. Anyone who says alcoholic beverages of any kind are good for you is seriously misinformed. If there were to be any benefit from an alcoholic beverage, it would not be the alcohol, but the 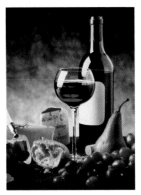 grapes or source material it was made from, nothing else. There was some nutrition in beer fifty years ago, but today, even the best beer hops are grown on the poorest soils, assuring minimal nutritional value. Further, to make beer light and clear, a number of chemical agents are added.

Americans consume more than 37 gallons of alcoholic beverages per person each year in the United States. In other words, the average American drinks about 11.4 cups of an alcoholic beverage each week or 1.6 cups a day. For every person who doesn't drink alcohol there is someone else around the corner who drinks 74 gallons a year![28]

Alcohol, being a simple chemical structure, is rapidly absorbed through the stomach and small intestine. That is why it is used as a carrier agent for many medical drugs and tinctures. Research shows that the metabolism of alcohol in the liver may not only disrupt the liver's ability to produce energy. It may also drastically affect blood sugar balance leading to hypoglycemia, particularly if consumed on an empty stomach.[29]

Take, for instance, most any restaurant in the world. The first thing offered, while you are in a state of hunger, is alcohol. Why? Drinking alcohol, particularly beverages that have sugar added, results in a rapid rise in blood sugar. This causes your pancreas to release insulin in an attempt to balance your blood sugar. Insulin circulates and does its job, leaving you hypoglycemic (lacking blood sugar) just about the time you are ready to order. Hypoglycemia often produces significant hunger pangs and even behavioral changes, making one aggressively pursue food. By this time, you're likely to have *eyes that are bigger than your stomach!*

Alcoholic beverages also serve as displacing agents. Each time you drink one you're displacing the intake of health-giving fluids and foods such as water and live vegetables, fruits or quality fat and protein sources. You're taking on *empty* calories, which are non-food calories, as I've described previously. If that's not enough, alcohol, particularly when consumed near or at mealtimes, serves as a blocking agent, prohibiting the absorption of several vitamins and minerals.

Moreover, regular exposure to alcoholic beverages, particularly when consumed without fat and protein to slow down absorption and balance the ratio of carbohydrates to proteins and fats, can cause damage to the stomach and linings of the small intestine. Alcohol, along with many medical drugs and high stress levels, are the primary sources of *leaky gut syndrome* (explained in Chapter 14).

CHEK Points on Alcohol

1. If you choose to drink alcoholic beverages, drink in moderation.

2. Consume alcoholic drinks made from organic sources when available.

3. Always eat fat and protein with alcohol (for example, cheese, nuts and meat).

Dairy

Pasteurization

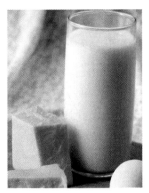

Milk was first pasteurized in Chicago, the first American city to pass a law that stated milk must be pasteurized. The year was 1908, and reasons for the law revolved around fears of tuberculosis, botulism and myriad other diseases spreading through the milk supply. While this may have been a legitimate concern during that time, there were, and still are, many health professionals against pasteurization. Louis Pasteur, himself, the man who developed pasteurization, later admitted the germ theory was not sound.[30] While the dairy industry maintains that the prevention of disease is the motive for pasteurizing milk, it's highly unlikely. We now know that the naturally occurring lactic acid-producing bacteria in raw milk protects it from pathogens—until it's killed by pasteurization, that is! In fact, all outbreaks of salmonella from contaminated milk in recent decades (there have been many) occurred in pasteurized milk. One outbreak in Illinois affected 14,000 people, resulting in at least one death.[14]

The pasteurization process involves heating milk for 30 seconds at 63° C (~145° F), for 15 seconds at 72° C (~162° F), or 1 second at 89° C (~192° F). The idea is to kill potentially harmful bacteria. The problem is that the heat kills important enzymes as well as damaging or destroying vitamins and amino acids. In fact, milk is declared pasteurized when the chemist finds no enzymes present in the milk![31]

Many people are wary of consuming raw dairy products. Yet raw milk actually contains lactic acid-producing bacteria that protect us against pathogens. Unlike pasteurized milk, which will putrefy when bad, raw milk turns to buttermilk and sour cream. There are many beneficial qualities to the fats in raw dairy. People with sensitivity to dairy can often tolerate raw milk and milk products because the enzymes that aid in the digestion of the milk are left intact, as are the vitamins and other trace elements that serve as enzyme cofactors.

Homogenization

Homogenization is a process whereby milk is passed through a fine filter at pressures equal to 4,000 pounds per square inch, making the fat globules smaller by a factor of 10 times or more. These fat molecules become evenly dispersed within the liquid milk so that after 48 hours of storage at 45° F (about 9° C), there is no visible cream separation in the milk.[32] According to some experts, this ensures that the protein hormones in milk survive the normal process of protein digestion/breakdown in the stomach. But homogenization causes fat molecules to become smaller and allow substances to bypass digestion, so proteins that normally would be digested and broken down in the stomach are not broken down, increasing the chances of incomplete protein digestion in the small intestine. This allows some milk proteins to be absorbed into the bloodstream intact. This could very well sensitize the immune system and lead to milk allergy and intolerance.

Growth Hormones

Another problem with commercially produced milk is that dairy farmers commonly inject cows with a growth hormone to make them produce more milk than is normal. After giving birth, a cow normally produces milk for about 12 weeks, at the expense of her own tissues. During this time she loses weight, is infertile and is more susceptible to diseases such as mastitis (inflammation of the udder). By giving a cow rBGH (recombinant bovine growth hormone, a genetically modified growth hormone), a farmer can extend milk production for another 8 – 12 weeks, meaning the cow is stressed to produce milk for this time period. The labeling on the Prosilac (rBGH)

package insert says, "Cows injected with Prosilac are at an increased risk for clinical mastitis." By the way, when cows get mastitis, the pus from the udders may end up in your milk. Many farmers refuse to inject their cows with this new hormone because it increases risk of infection by almost 80%. Farmers then have to give their cows antibiotics to treat infections.[33]

While there have been a number of attempts by farmers and retailers to let the consumer know their milk was "free of rBGH hormone," the FDA warned grocery stores not to do so. Monsanto, the producer of rBGH, sued two milk processors who labeled milk as free of the hormone. Of course, all organic dairy products will be free of this growth hormone. Some companies, including Trader Joe's, still label their milk as rBGH free. If you can't get organic dairy, make sure to find a brand that provides products that are rBGH free.

The use of rBGH is approved in the U.S. by the FDA, which states that, *"no significant difference has been shown between milk from treated and untreated cows."* This statement, which is found on milk labels, is based on minimal, short-term research done on rats, mostly by Monsanto scientists—*this is akin to asking the Devil to run studies on evil!* Studies on rBGH also have inconsistencies.[33] For example:

- The only human study involving rBGH was done over 50 years ago, in which dwarves were given the hormone to see if they would grow—they did not.

- In one of the studies, cows treated with the hormone were getting sick and gave birth to cows with genetic deformities, though the FDA withheld much of this data. Monsanto said that out of 10,000 dairy farmers and 800,000 cows, they only received 95 complaints (those were from the farmers, but there were likely many more from the cows). The FDA actually received complaints concerning nearly 9,500 cows contracting mastitis—*the infection that creates pus which can in turn pass into milk.*

- Enormous spleen growths (in rats) were considered to be "statistically insignificant." The spleen is part of the lymphatic and immune systems, which manufactures red and white blood cells.

- In one study conducted by Monsanto, all of the animals treated with rBGH got cancer, even the animals orally ingesting this new hormone. This study was reviewed by ex-Monsanto employees who were working for the FDA at the time the study was conducted.

Another issue with the use of rBGH is that it increases levels of IGF-1 in the cow's milk. IGF-1 is a powerful growth hormone in the human body and is identical in both cows and humans. One of the major concerns with milk containing increased concentrations of IGF-1 secondary to rBGH use is that the growth hormone makes existing cancers grow. Pasteurization has little effect on IGF-1 levels. Humans receive the IGF molecule from a cow through consuming its milk and the human body will treat it as its own. Drinking one glass of untreated milk will nearly double levels of IGF in the body. One glass of treated milk will increase IGF levels even more, as much as nine-fold, according to Robert Cohen, author of *Milk the Deadly Poison*.[33]

Increased IGF concentrations have been associated with breast cancer, human colorectal tumors and colon cancer growth.[34] IGF-1 is an autocrine and endocrine growth regulator that *accelerates* various types of cancer.[35] IGF-1 activity is significantly higher in cancer extracts, suggesting that higher IGF-1 activity in cancer tissue is involved in regulating growth of thyroid cancer cells.[36]

So you can see that there are some real concerns to be had with conventional dairy farming practices and with both national and international governmental policies regarding our food. *We must support a return to local, small, organic or biodynamic farms!*

Yogurt

Yogurt has been consumed for thousands of years. When cultured with beneficial microorganisms such as lactic acid-secreting *acidophilus* and *bifidus*, it's very helpful to the colon. Friendly bacteria, available in high quality yogurt, assists in the maintenance of an optimal friendly bacteria count, which is necessary for the production of several vitamins. Friendly flora manufacture vitamins such as biotin, thiamine (B1), riboflavin (B2), niacin (B3), pantothenic acid (B5), pyridoxine (B6), folic acid and vitamins A and K. The lactic acid-secreting bacteria available in quality yogurts also increase the bioavailability of calcium, copper, iron, magnesium and manganese. Since the friendly microbes change the environment of the colon by making it more acidic, they actually reduce chances of infestation or food poisoning by unfriendly bacteria, which prefer an alkaline environment.[37]

Those who cannot digest dairy products can often consume yogurt with no side effects. Yogurt is easier to digest because the yeast culture actually eats the lactose in the source milk. But, before you get excited and hijack a yogurt truck, there are several things you need to know about your run-of-the-mill, store-bought yogurt:

- Yogurt is only as good as the source material it's made from. Many yogurts are made from commercial cow's milk, which commonly contains antibiotics and rBGH. Choose yogurts made from organic, raw milk when possible.

- Yogurts with fruit added should be avoided for two reasons. First, when fruit is added to yogurts, sugar is usually added as well. Second, the fruit added to most yogurts is over-ripened and/or too damaged to sell in the stores.[38]

- A great majority of the yogurts in supermarkets today should really be reclassified as another form of *liquid candy*. When you have *chocolate yogurt*, you basically have the same sort of nutritional oxymoron you have with a *candy-apple*. If you are consuming such foods, you are merely using an *impersonation of a health food*!

- If you have problems with yogurts from cow's milk, try sheep or goat's milk yogurt.

CHEK Points on Dairy

1. Wherever possible buy *raw, certified organic* dairy products. There are companies that sell milk from organic grass fed cows, which is important because the type of feed the cows eat influences the quality and quantity of protein and fats in the milk. There are states that don't allow the sale of raw milk, such as Vermont, yet some of these states have co-op opportunities where you

can actually buy a percentage of a cow. Because you actually *own* the cow, so to speak, you can legally buy and drink the raw milk it produces.

2. If you can't get raw dairy products, the next best thing is Certified Organic. This way, although the milk may be pasteurized or homogenized, it won't contain antibiotics, hormones or pesticide residues.

3. If you are intolerant to dairy, try goat's and/or sheep's milk products. Many people who are sensitive to cow's milk can handle these other varieties. (If you have taken antibiotics, raw goat's milk is excellent for restoring friendly bacteria in your gut.)

4. If you can't get high quality organic dairy—*stay away from the stuff*! Dairy products are not necessary for a healthy diet. You can get plenty of calcium from other sources, such as leafy green vegetables.

5. If you are gluten intolerant, avoid dairy (along with gluten) for 3 - 6 months to allow the gut to repair itself to digest dairy again.

Animal Products

I believe meat is essential for optimal health. The amount of animal products that you should consume will vary greatly depending on your metabolic type and other lifestyle factors. One thing is consistent: always choose high-quality sources when consuming animal products.

Grass-fed

Cows, sheep, buffalo, etc., are designed to eat grass. However, most commercially raised cows are fed grains (wheat and corn) that quickly make them fat. These animals are not designed to eat grains. When their entire diet is made up of

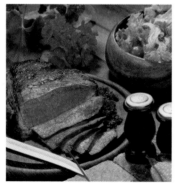

grains, the animals often become sick and the quality of the fats and protein in their meat declines. Michael Pollan's *New York Times* article, "Power Steer" describes how when calves are weaned from their mothers and forced onto a diet of corn and grain, they require antibiotics, and many become so sick they nearly die.[39]

Some commercial meat producers have begun research trials adding cardboard, newspaper and sawdust to cattle feeding programs to reduce costs. Food and Drug Administration (FDA) officials say that it's not uncommon for some feedlot operators to mix industrial sewage and oils into feed to reduce costs and fatten animals more quickly. There are numerous reports of animal cruelty emanating from investigations of factory farming. Most of the chickens and pigs that end up on your dinner table today are raised in extremely tight cages, restricting exercise. Many factory-farmed animals are raised in giant barns and commonly never see the natural light of day. They're fed a constant supply of antibiotics to aid in both rapid growth and to keep them alive, as they literally live their entire lives in their own feces.[40]

You may be wondering about the consequences of raising animals this way. In 1998, the USDA inspections and safety system reclassified an array of animal diseases as being "...defects that rarely or never present a direct public health risk," and said "unaffected carcass portions" could be passed on to consumers by cutting out lesions. The agency said the following animal diseases do **not** present a health danger to humans:

• Cancer

• A pneumonia of poultry called airsacculitis

• Glandular swellings or lymphomas

• Sores

• Infectious arthritis

• Diseases caused by intestinal worms

• Tumors (In the case of tumors, the guidelines state: "remove localized lesion(s) and pass unaffected carcass portions.") [41]

Organic

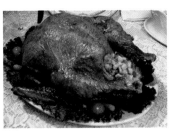

Meat and poultry companies can now apply to the U.S. Department of Agriculture (USDA) to have their products labeled as "Certified Organic." Under the rule, meat and poultry must be certified as "organic" by one of 33 private or 11 state-run groups approved by the Agriculture Department's Food Safety and Inspection Service. Certified meat should have "no antibiotics, no growth hormones, and the animals have to be fed 100% organic feed." [42]

There is one problem that you should be aware of with organic meats. Just because it's organic, doesn't mean that it's grass fed. Even if an animal is fed organic grains, it's still getting a diet that is less than ideal for its makeup. Some people who are gluten intolerant find that they do not feel well when consuming meats and poultry from grain fed sources. Your best option is to get organic, grass fed meats. If you can't find that, grass fed would be your second best option.

Not Just Any Egg

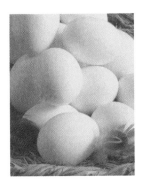

Eggs were considered to be one of the most complete and pure sources of protein by many pioneering nutritionists. Unadulterated eggs are, in fact, not only an excellent source of protein, they're also a great source of dietary fats. In his book *Foods That Heal*, Dr. Bernard Jensen describes eggs as *having the right nutrients for the brain, nerves and glands.* [43] My grandfather, whose hobby was the study of nutrition, told me when I was a boy to always eat eggs. He correctly predicted that more and more doctors would tell their patients not to eat eggs secondary to the cholesterol scare. He emphasized that despite claims that eggs have too much fat or cholesterol, a healthy egg contains

adequate lecithin to emulsify the fats in an egg, making the whole egg a well balanced, natural food source that is *healthy*.

The problem today is that the egg is *only as good as the bird*, which is *only as good as it's environment* and the food it ate, which is *only as good as the soil it was raised on*. Chickens that live a natural life, by the design of Mother Nature, produce eggs *composed of quality proteins and an optimal omega-3:omega-6 fat ratio* (see page 73). A free-range egg will have a ratio between 1:1 and 1:4 while a typical commercially raised chicken egg will be as high as 1:16-30. This presents a problem for those who eat too many conventionally raised eggs, as too much omega-6 fatty acid in your diet facilitates the process of inflammation in our bodies.

There was a big scare regarding cholesterol content in eggs during the 1980s. However, many don't understand that cholesterol is a key building block for all cells and is produced by our bodies as a response to stress. When there's an inflammatory process, there's an elevated need for cholesterol. Stress, alcohol, medical drugs and many food additives are all capable of causing inflammation in the gut, significantly elevating the body's need for cholesterol. But when a trip to the doctor reveals high cholesterol, you're often prescribed medication and told to stay away from the foods that you actually need to produce adequate cholesterol to heal the damaged cells. Doctors seldom look into the potential causes of elevated cholesterol.

To test the difference between a cage-raised chicken and an organic free-range bird, try this demonstration: Compare the effort it takes to break the leg away from the thigh on a typical commercially raised chicken versus a free-range chicken, or even better, an organic free-range chicken. You'll probably be amazed to find that it is three or four times harder to break the ligaments of the free-range bird's knee joint. I've seen the exact same problem with many athletes on garbage food diets that get muscle, ligament or connective tissue injuries and can't heal, sometimes after *years* of therapy.

Seafood

As recently as 100 years ago, our oceans produced an excellent source of edible organic plant and sea life. Today, most of our oceans are toxic. Billions of pounds of sewage and industrial wastes are dumped into the oceans by industrialized nations every day. This irresponsible behavior not only poisons fish, it's coming back to get us. According to Stephanie Hawks-Johnson, an orca researcher at the University of Washington, the lack of salmon today and the presence of PCBs (polychlorinated biphenyls—pesticides) appear to be the primary reasons for the decline in the killer whale population. An orca needs 40-120 kg of salmon a day, and if it doesn't get it, it draws from its blubber, which causes PCBs (stored in fat to protect the whale's liver) to enter its system. PCB-contaminated blubber in turn affects the whale's immune, neurological and reproductive systems.

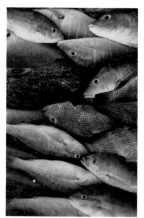

The Inuit people on Baffin Island live about as far north as one can go. They consume mostly marine mammal meat as an essential staple of their diet. The Inuits were found to be consuming up to 20 times the recommended safe limit of the pesticide chlordane. A sugar cube-sized piece of maktaaq, the skin and surface fat from the beluga whale, contains the accepted maximum weekly limit of PCB's. In one week, it is normal for some Inuit people to eat *one hundred times* that amount.[44]

Destroying our ecosystem makes fish unsafe to eat. In fact, the National Academy of Sciences estimated in 1991 that the risk of cancer to the average consumer who eats seafood can be some 75 times greater than normally acceptable guidelines.[45]

Our drugs, industrial chemicals and pesticides are affecting the lives of every living creature on earth, be they in the soil, on the soil, in the water or in the air. We are making them all sick and progressively killing them! More living species are dying and becoming extinct than ever before in the history of man.[46]

Concerns about Farmed Fish

As our oceans become *fished out* (to use a fisherman's term) and toxic, the environmental situation and demand for fish, forever considered a healthy food, has resulted in a boom of fish farms. Unfortunately, eating farm-raised fish isn't as safe as it may sound. Fish farming methods are quite similar to those of the commercial cattle industry. As with cattle, fish are fed grains and soy and are given a wide range of antibiotics and other drugs. As a result, farm-raised fish are likely to contain residues of a wide variety of animal drugs, some of which are carcinogenic.[45] Furthermore, when you buy farm-raised fish, you have no idea where the farm is located, in most cases. If the fish farm is anywhere near—and I mean within 100 miles of—a major industrial complex or commercial farming operation, on the same coast line, or anywhere near a river that feeds into the coast line, you run significant risk of eating farm-raised fish that is high in pesticide and industrial chemical residues. Chemicals commonly found in seafood, *be it from fish farms or otherwise*, are benzene hexachloride, chlordane, DDT, dieldrin, dioxin, heptachlor, hexachlorobenzene, lindane and polychlorinated biphenyls.

How to Safely Eat Fish

Rotating sources of protein will minimize chances of over-exposing yourself to any given pesticide, antibiotic or drug residues that may have tainted your food, not to mention heavy metal contamination. (See rotation diet plan on page 236.)

Be aware that swordfish, shark, tuna and other deepwater fish (particularly the bigger ones) accumulate more mercury than smaller fish with shorter life spans. Today, many of these fish, fresh off the boat, have been found to have mercury levels so high that eating them more than once a week is considered dangerous by many health experts. The greatest concern appears to be fish from the inland waters of the U.S. midwest and the state of Florida.[45, 47]

When cooking fish, particularly the bigger fish that accumulate heavy metals, it's a good idea to grill or broil them to allow the juices to drip out. This allows pesticide residues and other chemicals to escape as you cook the fish. This is due in part to the fact that many industrial chemicals and pesticide residues that accumulate in fish are stored in the fat of the fish (the same is true of animals and man), which begins to drip away when heated to cooking temperatures. Any time you can trim the fat off of fish, it's a good idea.

Avoid fresh water fish unless it comes from high mountain lakes and streams, far from commercial enterprises. Avoid farm-raised fish. In addition to the concerns I've presented above, there is a difference in the omega 3:6 fatty acid ratios in farm raised fish vs. natural freshwater or ocean fish. With few exceptions, the fat ratios in farm-raised fish are about the same as a cage-raised chicken egg. Typically, this is between 16 and 30 omega-6 for every 1 omega-3 fat molecule. Remember, research on developmental man suggests we should eat a ratio of one to four omega-6:one omega-3. We can't outsmart Mother Nature—*it just doesn't work.*

Processed and Cured Meats and Fish

Have you ever read the ingredients listed on the labels of cured fish and meats such as bacon, ham, beef jerky, salami or packaged luncheon meats? You'll find verbiage there that looks like a foreign language—not like a normal part of any food. Two such ingredients in many cured and/or packaged meats are *nitrites* and *nitrates*. Both of these additives are commonly used in the meats mentioned above, as well as fermented sausages, bologna, frankfurters, deviled ham, meat spreads, potted meats, spiced ham and smoked fish products. Nitrates and nitrites are used primarily as a color fixative, to give meats a blood red color, to convey a tangy effect to the palate and to prohibit the development of clostridium botulinum spores. Both additives have been found to cause cancer and tumors in test animals. According to *The Safe Shopper's Bible*, researchers reported that children who ate hot dogs cured with nitrite a dozen or more times monthly have a risk of leukemia ten times higher than normal. Furthermore, children born to mothers who consume hot dogs once or

Important Types of Fats

Saturated fats
- Found in animal fats and tropical oils
- Do not normally go rancid, even when heated for cooking
- Made in our bodies from carbohydrates
- Constitute at least 50% of the cell membranes; they give cells stiffness and integrity
- Needed for calcium to be effectively incorporated into skeletal system
- Protect liver from alcohol and other toxins
- Enhance immune system
- Needed for proper use of EFAs

Sources: animal products, coconut and palm oil

Monounsaturated fats
- Tend to be liquid at room temp
- Do not go rancid easily and can be used in cooking at moderate temperatures

Sources: olive oil, almonds, pecans, cashews, peanuts and avocado

Polyunsaturated fats
- Contain linoleic acid (omega-6) and linolenic acid (omega-3)—essential because our bodies cannot produce them
- Liquid, even when refrigerated
- Should never be heated

Sources: vegetable oils, fish oil, eggs and walnuts

Cholesterol
- Gives cells stiffness and stability
- Precursor to steroid hormones and vitamin D
- Acts as an antioxidant
- Needed for proper function of serotonin receptors in brain
- Low cholesterol levels have been linked to aggressive and violent behavior, depression and suicidal tendencies
- Role in maintaining health of intestinal wall
- High-serum cholesterol levels often indicates that the body needs cholesterol to protect itself from high levels of altered free-radical-containing fats

Sources: animal products

more weekly during their pregnancy are twice as likely to have childhood brain tumors.[45]

Germany banned nitrites and nitrates in 1997 except for use with certain fish species, while in the U.S. the FDA revoked its proposed phase-out because manufacturers said there was no adequate substitute. I suspect that what the manufacturers were really saying is that there is no *cheap* substitute for nitrites, so even though they're known to produce disease in test animals, we'll keep feeding them to you anyway.

Processed meats also trigger *false food allergy* for many people. Some of the preservatives in meats, and the meats themselves, produce histamine. You're probably familiar with histamine. It's what makes your nose run when you have a cold—hence the use of *anti-histamine* in medications. The addition of wheat to numerous processed meat products is another problem. If you're gluten intolerant, make sure to read labels on any deli meats and sausages, etc.

CHEK Points for Safe Meat, Fowl, Fish and Egg Consumption

1. ALWAYS go out of your way to purchase organic, free-range products. They're far more nutritious as well as free of pesticides, hormones and antibiotics.

2. If organic meats are not available, the next best choice is grass fed, free-range meats. At least they were free to roam, got exercise and ate what they were designed to eat.

3. Avoid farmed fish.

4. Read all labels, eliminating, or at least minimizing the consumption of processed meats.

5. Minimize consumption of smoked meats and fish.

6. Rotate meat sources.

7. Do *not* fear the fat in the meat, or on the body of any protein source that is from an organic, free-range source. That is the fat that got us here!

Fats and Oils

Fats and oils are essential to optimal health. They are important building blocks for the cells of your body, as well as for key hormones. Just as with all foods, you must consume high-quality fats and oils for your body to effectively use them. If you're not familiar with the different types of fats, please see the side bar on page 73.

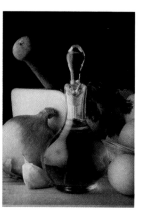

Fats to Avoid

Many processed foods, even those touted as *healthy,* are laden with trans-fatty acids (TFAs). Structurally, trans-fatty acids are closer to plastic than fat. TFA consumption has been linked to heart disease and elevated cholesterol levels. TFAs are also thought to impair lipoprotein receptors in cells, impairing the body's ability to process low-density cholesterol (LDL), increasing their rate of synthesis and eventually elevating LDL levels in the blood. This is generally considered to be unhealthy. Upon discovering elevated total cholesterol and elevated LDL levels, doctors often tell people to restrict animal fats, butter, cheese, eggs, to eat a low-fat diet high in grains and vegetables, and to replace butter with margarine. Unfortunately, this often makes the problem worse.

Margarine is a vegetable oil-based product designed to compete with butter in the marketplace—it's notorious for high levels of TFAs. In an eight-year Harvard Medical School study of 85,000 women, margarine was linked to heart disease.[48] Dr. Mary Enig, a world-renowned expert on dietary fats, analyzed the TFA content of some 600 foods. She noted that Americans eat between 11 and 28 grams of TFAs a day—or one-fifth their total intake of fat.[49] This is a lot of plastic to put in the body!

Essential Fats

Essential fatty acids (EFAs) are fats that our bodies are unable to manufacture. We must, therefore, acquire them from dietary sources. These fats fall into two groups; omega-3 and omega-6 EFAs. Omega-6

EFAs are readily available in grain products, meats and many commonly used cooking oils such as corn, safflower and sunflower. Omega-3 EFAs are found in leafy green vegetables and oily fish, and comparatively small quantities are available in walnuts, eggs and animal meats. Again, the ideal ratio of omega-3:omega-6 fatty acids is 1:4.

Omega-3 fatty acids are vital to the development of a child's brain and nervous system and for the maintenance and repair of the adult brain and nervous system. Studies in which mice were timed through a maze showed that eating a diet low in omega-3 fatty acids (basically the American diet) led to a *dumbing down* effect when compared to those fed adequate omega-3s. While there are a number of behavioral and learning disorders associated with a lack of omega-3 fatty acids in the diet, or an imbalance between omega-3 and omega 6 EFAs, other currently recognized disorders include: [50]

- Heart attack
- Stroke
- Cancer
- Obesity
- Insulin resistance
- Diabetes
- Asthma
- Arthritis
- Lupus
- Depression (even among children!)
- Schizophrenia
- Attention deficit hyperactivity disorder
- Postpartum depression
- Alzheimer's disease
- Chronic inflammatory disorders
- Reduced cellular detoxification

The Saturated Fat Myth

Politically Correct Nutrition, meaning what the "government would have you eat" or what the typical college-educated dietitian would have you eat, is based on the assumption that we should reduce our intake of fats, particularly saturated fats from animal sourc-

Cooking with Oils[68]
Always use unrefined organic oils!

No Heat (up to 120° F/49° C)
- Flax Seed Oil
- Borage Oil
- Hemp Seed Oil
- Cod Liver Oil

Low Heat (up to 212°F/100°C) - Baking*
- Safflower Oil
- Sunflower Oil
- Pumpkin Oil

Medium Heat (325°F/163°C) - Light sauteing
- Sesame Oil
- Pistachio Oil
- Hazelnut Oil
- Olive Oil

High Heat (375°F/190°C) - Frying**, browning
- Coconut Oil
- Ghee (clarified butter)
- Palm Oil
- Lard

* When baking breads and muffins at temperatures around 325° F/163° C, the moisture keeps the inside temperature under 212° F/100° C.

** When frying, always put oil into a cold pan and turn the heat up gradually.

es. Fats from animal sources also contain cholesterol, presented as the twin villain of the civilized diet.

Although hydrogenation of fats began in 1912, coronary heart disease was rare in America before 1920—so rare that when a young internist named Paul Dudley White introduced the German electro-cardiograph to his colleagues at Harvard University, they advised him to concentrate on a more profitable branch of medicine. The new machine revealed the presence of arterial blockages, thus permitting early diagnosis of coronary heart disease. But in those days, clogged arteries were a medical rarity, and White had to search for patients who could benefit from his new technology. During the next forty years, however, the incidence of coronary heart disease rose dramatically, so much so that by the mid-fifties heart disease was the leading cause of death among Americans. Today, heart disease causes at least 40% of all deaths in the U.S. If, as we have been told, heart disease results from the consumption of saturated fats, one would expect to find a corresponding increase in animal fat in the American diet. Actually, the converse is true. During the sixty-year period from 1910 to 1970, the proportion of traditional animal fat in the American diet declined from 83% to 62%, and butter consumption plummeted from eighteen pounds per person per year to four. During the past eighty years, dietary cholesterol intake has increased only 1%. During the same period, the percentage of dietary vegetable oils in the form of margarine, shortening and refined oils *increased about 400%,* while the consumption of sugar and processed foods *increased about 60%.*[51]

The much-maligned saturated fats—which Americans are trying to avoid—are not the cause of modern diseases. If they were, and if the saturated fat/cholesterol myth were true, none of us would be alive today because saturated fat was the primary energy source for most of our ancestors. Studies of North American Indians, Eskimos and other tribes suggest that as much as 80% of their daily caloric intake was from fat, most of which was saturated animal fat.[51]

CHEK Points for Healthy Fat Consumption

1. Good sources of quality fat include: olive oil, coconut oil/butter, palm oil, butter (raw is best), ghee (clarified butter, good if you are allergic to casein, the protein in dairy), organic, grass-fed animal fats (lard, tallow), fish oil (be careful of source), seeds (especially flax seeds), avocados and nuts (raw, organic).

2. Always choose organic foods for safe fats. Remember, many industrial chemicals and commercial farming chemicals are fat soluble and are stored in the fats of animals, fowl, fish and plants.

3. Fats to avoid: trans-fatty acids, hydrogenated or partially hydrogenated oils, vegetable oils (the high temperatures used to produce such oils will destroy the nutrients in the oil), fats from conventionally raised animals/fish.

4. When purchasing EFA supplements, contact the manufacturer to determine the carrier oil if it isn't listed on the label. Soy oil is commonly used because it's cheap. The carrier oils are often rancid and draw the antioxidant qualities from the good oil in the capsules. When you open a new bottle of EFA supplements, bite one capsule open to taste and smell the oil. You would be amazed at how often brand new bottles contain a batch of rancid oils.[52]

5. Avoid eating roasted nuts because the roasting process causes the fats and oils to go rancid, increasing free-radical damage in your body. In other words, *they make you age faster.*

6. Avoid non-organic dairy sources. In many cases milk is loaded with the same sort of fat-soluble chemicals you find in meats. Use the resources in this book to see if you can have raw butter, raw cream and milk shipped to you. If you can't get raw, and you can't find organic, *avoid dairy.*

7. Avoid any and all deep-fried foods unless you prepare them yourself and you use lard, coconut or palm oil—even then frying and deep frying should be kept to a minimum!

8. Always use heat stable fats and oils for cooking (see table on page 73). Avoid using the polyunsaturated oils commonly recommended by diet dictocrats.

9. It's simply best to *never* eat from fast food restaurants. They use low quality foods and fats, many of which are highly processed.

10. Mothers must go out of their way to assure their children get adequate omega-3 EFAs. Whatever it takes, feed your children organic food.

Sugar

How Much Sugar Are We Consuming?

As recently as 400 years ago, refined or simple sugars, with the exception of small amounts of honey, were not available to man. We ate only 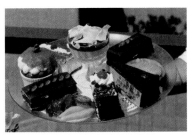 naturally occurring, whole foods that provide complex carbohydrates, which convert to energy relatively slowly when consumed as natural food sources (this is because they get tied up with simultaneously occurring fats, proteins and fiber). Producing *simple* or *refined* sugars such as packaged *white* or *brown sugar* from sugar cane or sugar beets required so much work to manufacture that only the rich could afford to buy them. About 100 years ago, the average yearly intake of simple sugars was only about 4 pounds per person.[53] Today, the average American or Englishman consumes 150 to 170 pounds of sugar per year, and those in most industrialized nations are not far behind.[14, 54] It's said that for every American who only eats five pounds of sugar each year, there's one who eats 295 pounds per year. This statistic is hard to deny since about 60% of the U.S. population is now overweight or obese.

Effects of Sugar

If sugar were nutritious, being addicted to it would be analogous to being addicted to carrots or some other food source that delivers adequate nutrition to be considered "healthy." In reality processed *sugar is not only a drug, it's a poison.* In 1957, Dr. William Coda Martin pondered: "When is a food a food and when is it a poison?" His working medical definition of "poison" was, "Any substance applied to the body, ingested or developed within the body, which causes or may cause disease. Physically: Any substance which inhibits the activity of a catalyst (which is a minor substance, chemical or enzyme that activates a reaction)." The dictionary provides an even broader definition for poison: "To exert a harmful influence on, or to pervert." [54, 55]

Dr. Martin classified refined sugar as a poison because it has been depleted of its life forces, vitamins and minerals. What is left is pure, refined carbohydrates. The body cannot effectively utilize this refined starch and carbohydrate unless the depleted proteins, vitamins and minerals are present. When we eat sugar in absence of the nutritional factors necessary to compensate for digestion, metabolism and elimination, incomplete carbohydrate metabolism results. Pyruvic acid accumulates in the brain and nervous system, and the abnormal sugars accumulate in the red blood cells. These metabolites interfere with the respiration of the cells. They simply can't get sufficient oxygen to survive and function normally. In time, some of the cells die. This interferes with the functioning of that part of the body and is the beginning of degenerative disease.[55]

Daily intake of sugar produces a continuously overacid condition. Consequently, minerals are required from body tissues (such as bones and teeth) in order to buffer the acidic environment and rectify the imbalance. In order to protect the blood, so much calcium is taken from the bones and teeth that decay and general weakening begin. Excess sugar eventually affects every organ in the body.

In the liver, excess sugar is stored in the form of glucose (glycogen). Since the liver's capacity is limited, a daily intake of refined sugar soon makes the liver expand. When the liver is filled to its maximum capacity, the excess glycogen is returned to the blood in the form of fatty acids. These fatty acids are then taken to every part of the body and stored—as fat—in the most inactive areas: the belly, the buttocks, the breasts and the thighs.

When these areas are completely filled with fat, fatty acids are then distributed among active organs, such as the heart, liver and kidneys. These organs begin to slow down—finally their tissues degenerate and turn to fat. The whole body is affected by their reduced ability, and abnormally high blood pressure results. The autonomic nervous system (ANS) is affected because processed sugar is a powerful stimulator of the *sympathetic* branch of the nervous system (Chapter 11). The circulatory and lymphatic systems are invaded, and the quality of the red blood cells begins to change. An overabundance of white cells occurs and tissue creation slows down.

When you ingest processed sugars without adequate amounts of quality fats, proteins, vitamins and enzymes, your blood sugar levels will become elevated. The body responds by releasing insulin, a hormone that rapidly reduces blood sugar levels. Unfortunately, the feedback mechanism that tells the brain that blood sugar has returned to normal is slow, commonly resulting in a blood sugar crash, or *hypoglycemic* state. The body must respond to this immediately. If not, your brain will run out of blood sugar to operate on and you'll go into a coma. This emergency situation results in the release of powerful stress hormones, one of which is *cortisol*. In the midst of all this, most people respond to the hypoglycemic, or low-blood sugar state by drinking coffee or soda, or eating something sweet.

Meanwhile, cortisol has triggered the release of stored glycogen from the liver to quickly raise the blood sugar levels again. This results in an inflow of sugar from the liver as well as from *the sweet thing you just ate or drank, starting the whole process over again.* Many live their lives on this roller coaster ride all day, every day. This creates a big problem because after a while, your body can become insensitive to insulin—the first sign being an accumulation of fat around the middle, giving your midsection an apple like appearance. This results in what is commonly called *Syndrome X*, and is the first major step toward becoming diabetic.

The constant hormonal roller coaster ride caused by the typical sugar-laden junk food diet overworks the adrenal glands. They finally become exhausted from producing excessive cortisol. When the hormonal system becomes disturbed and unbalanced due to the stress of eating processed sugars, numerous other pathological conditions soon manifest—degenerative disease, allergies, obesity, alcoholism, drug addiction, depression and behavioral problems. Our ability to resist disease progressively decreases as processed sugars displace the nutrient dense foods we were designed to thrive on. The chances of acquiring one of the following diseases or side effects skyrockets:

- Kidney disease
- Liver disease
- Atherosclerosis
- Coronary heart disease
- Attention Deficit Disorder (ADD) and Attention Deficit Hyperactivity Disorder (ADHD)
- Behavior problems
- Violent tendencies
- Overgrowth of Candida, yeast and fungi
- Cancer (tumors are enormous sugar absorbers)
- Bone loss - osteoporosis
- Tooth decay
- Chronic fatigue syndrome
- Food intolerance
- Numerous psychological disorders, such as schizophrenia
- Neurological disorders and associated pain syndromes
- Colon cancer
- Diseases of malnutrition

Artificial Sweeteners Aren't the Answer

Aspartame has resulted in more complaints to the FDA due to side effects than any food additive ever approved in FDA history. Artificial sweeteners tell your taste buds that, "sweet stuff has arrived," which to the brain means, "nutrition has arrived." When the artificially sweetened drink or food reaches the small intestine, the receptors find no nutrition. A message is then sent back to the brain saying, "We've been tricked—there's no nutrition here." The appestat (the part of your brain that triggers satiety) sends the message to "keep eating because we need nutrition to help process all this fake food and run your body." And that, ladies and gentlemen, is one of the ways we ended up with fat, starving people across the world today. Some artificial sweeteners have also been found by researchers to be *neurotoxins* that can damage the brain and nervous system.[56]

Sugar alternatives

Honey: Use only *unprocessed, unfiltered* honey. You can't miss it because it has chunks of bees wax in it, and you can't see through it. Used in moderation, this type of honey is supportive of good health and immune function. If honey has been pasteurized and/or filtered, you're not eating a food—it's a by-product. Avoid cooking with honey as it's not heat stable.

Stevia: Stevia is an herb and is about 1000 times sweeter than sugar. Additionally, Stevia is known to assist in balancing blood sugar levels, making it ideal for anyone coming off of caffeinated beverages or weaning themselves from sweets.

Fruit: Use in-season fruit or dried fruits to sweeten foods. It's a good idea to rehydrate dried fruits and berries by soaking them for 8 to 12 hours before using. Then bring them to a flash-boil to kill any unfriendly bacteria, parasites and/or insect eggs that may have been laid on them during the drying process. Only use *un-sulfured* dried fruits and berries.

Below-ground vegetables: By adding properly cooked or, when possible, raw under-ground vegetables, you often get a beautiful natural sweetness to salads and other foods. For example, a cooked organic sweet potato, shredded raw carrots or beets are quite sweet and make great additions to salads and sandwiches.

Turbinado Sugar and Succinat: These are two acceptable forms of sugar, as they're minimally processed and raw. Raw date sugar is also acceptable, but again, *sugar is sugar*, so consume in moderation.

CHEK Points for Becoming a Sugar Detective

1. READ LABELS! Food manufacturers know there's an increased awareness with regard to the negative health effects of sugar. To throw you off, they use big words to hide total sugar content. For example, instead of just listing sugar as the first or second ingredient on the list (the order in the listing indicates relative quantity), they'll include words like *sucrose, maltose, dextrose, fructose, galactose, glucose, arabinose, ribose, xylose, deoxyribose, lactose, trehalose* and the like. In reality, all are sugars. Seeing "-ose" on the end of ingredients listed on the label of any food is an indicator of how much sugar the product contains. Quite often, you'll see as many as five or six different types of sugar in one product. When you add all the sugars up, *sugar is frequently by far the greatest source of calories.*

2. Beware of the term "natural." A *natural sugar* is still sugar. You must be aware of how much sugar you're consuming, particularly with regard to your metabolic type.

3. Avoid **all** sweet drinks, *including juices that are not freshly juiced*! The biggest mistake people make, *particularly parents,* is falling for the marketing hype from juice manufacturers. They want you to think their "fresh orange juice" is actually good for you. If you read the package you'll see *from concentrate*, which could easily be translated to mean *from syrup*.

Salt

Salt comes in the form of sodium chloride, two elements that combine to create something unique and useful to our bodies. While many have downplayed the need for salt, it serves the body in a number of key roles:

- Salt is vital to the extraction of excess acidity from the cells of the body, particularly the brain cells.

- Salt aids in balancing blood sugar levels.

- Salt is needed for the absorption of food particles through the intestinal tract.

- Salt clears the lungs of mucus plugs and sticky phlegm, particularly in those suffering from asthma and cystic fibrosis.

- Salt is a strong, natural antihistamine.

- Salt can aid in the prevention of muscle cramps.

- Salt is needed in order to make the structure of the bones firm.

Refined vs. Natural Salt

There's a big difference between typical refined white table salt sold at the grocery store and unrefined sea salt. Traditional medical doctors, the media and the food manufacturing industry seldom bring this up. First off, refined table salts often contain anti-caking agents, some of which are aluminum-based—aluminum is linked with heavy metal toxicity and possibly Alzheimer's disease. Other additives, such as *dextrose* (a sugar) are used in *iodized* salt (salt with iodine added) to keep the salt from turning purple. Sodium silico-aluminate, added to processed table salt, is thought to be associated with kidney problems and mineral malabsorption. Sodium acetate, also added to processed table salt, may cause elevated blood pressure, kidney disturbances and water retention.[11]

There are two common sources of salt: Land mined and sea salt. Land mined salt from Utah, for example, contains about 98% sodium chloride (NaCl) and the remaining 2% is composed of iron, calcium and smaller amounts of aluminum and strontium. The sodium from land-locked sources or refined salts hardens and has altered molecular structure. This sodium often remains in the body long after it's done its job, causing joints to swell and kidney problems to develop. Unprocessed sea salt is about 78% NaCl plus 11% magnesium chloride and smaller amounts of magnesium and calcium carbonate. There are many trace minerals in quality unprocessed sea salt, such as *Celtic Sea Salt*, that are beneficial to your body, serving many important regulatory and nutritional functions.

Salt and Your Health

Salt consumption, like carbohydrate, protein and fat consumption, is surrounded with controversy and differing opinions from all sectors of the medical and health care community. The medical community generally believes that over-consumption leads to high blood pressure and increased chances of heart disease. Indeed, there are a plethora of studies to suggest this is true. However, most of the research on salt is done on refined salt, not on natural, unprocessed sea salts.

Renowned cardiac surgeon Richard Pooley, M.D., doesn't restrict salt or saturated fat intake with his cardiac patients because he has not seen indicators that either cause problems.[57] Dr. F. Batmanghelidj, a medical doctor famous for his ground breaking work on water, recommends that we add a pinch of high quality salt to each liter of drinking water.[58]

Roger Williams, a renowned researcher in the field of biochemical individuality, found a difference of more than 30% in the sodium content of blood cells among individuals, as well as a four-fold variation in salivary sodium. Because it's often our taste for salt that dictates how much we apply to a given food stuff, it's important to note that Roger Williams' research found that taste threshold values varied between individuals *over a 20-fold range*![59] Consider these figures, in addition to William Wolcott's research on *metabolic typing* and individual differences of foods and nutrients needed by those with differing metabolic types, and it's easy to see why you can walk out of a medical library with your head spinning.

CHEK Points for Healthy Salt Intake

1. Use unprocessed sea salt. Celtic, French or New Zealand are good sources. Due to pollution around much of the world, sea salts can contain mercury and other toxic heavy metals, yet New Zealand's seas are considered some of the safest.

2. Always salt your food **after tasting** it to avoid adding too much salt.

3. If you have a good diet of primarily raw organic produce and quality free-range animal meats, using a quality sea salt to taste will add nutrition for your bodily needs.

4. If you drink adequate amounts of water, adding a pinch of quality sea salt to each liter bottle of water you drink will assist in maintenance of electrolyte and energy levels. If you salt your foods liberally or eat processed foods, salting your water may actually cause more harm than good.

5. Athletes who experience electrolyte loss through sweating may find that using a quality sea salt on their foods and in their water improves energy levels. Becoming light-headed upon standing (due to low blood pressure) is a symptom related to low electrolyte levels. This can often be prevented by following the guidelines above.

Water

Though water covers 2/3 of the Earth, only 3% of the Earth's water is fresh and of that percentage, *only 1% is accessible to humans*. An interesting correlation between humans and the Earth can be made with regard to water content: Almost 70% of the Earth is covered by water, most of which is ocean, and humans are composed of about 75% water—our blood containing roughly the same salinity as ocean

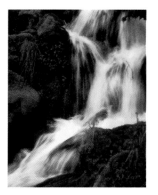

water. While water plays many key roles in our bodies, water's chief functions are to maintain a stable environment inside and around our cells, allowing us to acquire sufficient nutrition and aiding elimination of waste in cells. To provide an optimal environment for life, the water we consume through food and drink must be clean and should supply the body with needed electrolytes, but is this the case today?

Sources

Today, we have a very unique situation as living beings totally dependent upon Mother Earth for our survival—*we have polluted almost every single water supply in the world!* It's hard to find a municipal water supply not contaminated by agricultural chemicals. The U.S. Environmental Protection Agency (EPA) has identified over 700 pollutants that regularly occur in drinking water, both from municipal sources and from water taken directly from the earth through wells or springs. The EPA monitors eight inorganic and ten organic chemicals, leaving approximately 30,000 possible hazardous pollutants without regulation![60] Due to the cost and time required to test for the vast amount of chemicals in our water supplies, we're left on our own to determine where to get safe water. The EPA also reported that agriculture (commercial, not organic) is the biggest polluter of America's rivers and streams, fouling more than 173,000 miles of waterways.[61]

Human and industrial waste discharge and agricultural runoff places a major restriction on the uses of available fresh water. Ninety per cent of the "developing" world's wastewater is discharged untreated into local rivers. In China, 80% of the country's major rivers are so degraded they no longer support fish. Many Eastern European rivers run yellow with industrial poisons. Three hundred million gallons of raw or partially treated sewage is discharged around England's coastline each day and 2 million tons of toxic wastes are dumped into the sea annually.[62] The pollution in our waterways from industrial agriculture has become so bad that when people see a stream, river or lake that's clear blue they stop and stare—because it's so rare!

I recommend using a whole-house filtration system to minimize exposure to heavy metals, chlorine and other waterborne toxins. If it's on your skin, you're basically drinking it, so you want to make sure the water you bathe in is as clean as the water you're drinking.

Dr. Martin Fox, author of *Healthy Water*, suggests the most health-giving waters have a hardness factor of 170 mg/L or greater and a Total Dissolved Solids (TDS) of 300 or greater.[63] Many bottled waters will provide these statistics on the labels. Frequently, because of unfounded beliefs and fears of hard water or solids in water, you'll find that a number of the top brands are *soft* in comparison to these recommendations from Fox as well as lacking in Total Dissolved Solids. Don't worry—simply add a pinch or two of sea salt or a bit of clay (see Resources on page 248) and both the total dissolved solids and hardness are likely to be well within the ideal range.

Store water in a dark, cool area and in glass, if possible. Never purchase water from smoky plastic containers, because they leak all sorts of chemicals into your water. If you're consuming water from a plastic container, make sure it is clear, and take extra effort to keep it out of direct sunlight. Consume water at room temperature. Cold water will sit in your stomach until it reaches body temperature.

How Much Water Should You Drink?

The C.H.E.K Institute has adopted F. Batmanghelidj, M.D.'s hydration guidelines.[58] Dr. Batmanghelidj suggests that for normal hydration, determine your body weight in pounds, divide it by two and drink that many ounces of water each day. (Body weight (in kg) x 0.033 = how much water to drink in liters). For example, a 200 pound man would need to drink 100 ounces of quality *water* each day, possibly more if in hot climates and/or exercising. Again, he recommends a pinch of salt in each liter of water if you don't salt your food. I've also found that many people have a hard time drinking adequate amounts of water until after adding some unprocessed sea salt. The sea salt, when just a pinch or two is added, can't be tasted but gives the water a nice *mouth feel*. Most people also find that adding a pinch of seasalt to their water reduces the frequency of urination.

Milk, Juice, Sodas and Coffee

We're designed to drink water, nothing else. In the past 10,000 years, raw milk became recognized as a nutritious food staple, as did raw, unprocessed fruit juices. Although I am not a proponent of processed milk and fruit juice, most mothers see milk and fruit juices as a staple food source. Americans today drink *twice as much soda as milk and nearly six times more soda than fruit juice*.[28] This clearly demonstrates the power of advertising and certainly serves as a banner for the addictive powers of both sugar and caffeine, particularly when combined.

Adverse health effects from displacing water with soda pop, processed juice and/or coffee include:

• Tooth decay
• Sugar addiction
• Caffeine addiction
• Insulin resistance, Syndrome X and diabetes
• Increased chances of osteoporosis
• Increased severity of kidney stones
• Nervousness
• Insomnia
• Attention deficit disorder.

Where to Get Good Water

Supermarkets are loaded with water choices, but don't be fooled into thinking that because it's in a bottle it's good for you. Many companies have been caught bottling tap water. Regulations on bottled water vary from state to state and country to country. Some of the top quality brands are: Evian, Volvic, Vittel, Fiji and Trinity. Water from an artesian (water naturally flows to the surface) well is ideal.

Storage and Packaging

How often do you shop? If your answer is the most common reply, "once a week," here are a few important tips.

Shop every 4 to 5 days. Once picked, produce quickly loses its nutritional value, especially conventionally raised products. An estimated *80% of the food in supermarkets is already stale*.[64] More frequent shopping will at least yield relatively fresher foods. Shopping at a farmer's market or a shop that sells locally grown/raised products is ideal.

Purchase fresh certified organic foods whenever possible. Certified organic produce not only has a better shelf life, but according to research done by Ehrenfried Pfieffer, it'll improve its nutritional profile for 7 to 10 days after being picked. In contrast, Dr. Pfieffer stated that conventionally farmed produce begins losing nutritional value from the moment it's picked. Meats purchased fresh will last several days when properly refrigerated and will maintain good nutritional value when frozen. Remove only enough from your freezer to last 24 hours. If you live in a region with distinct climate changes and produce is seasonal, purchasing certified organic flash-frozen foods will provide the best nutritional value and eliminate chances of pesticide exposure at the same time.[26]

Schedule your purchases of produce, dairy and meats on the day that they arrive at the market. Check with the store manager for the days that they receive orders.

Store food in glass or ceramic containers. Packaging foods in plastic wrappers and containers, as well as in cans, is risky business. A study performed in the UK found that two thirds of canned foods contained low levels of the potent carcinogen and estrogen-mimicking compound, *bisphenol A* (BPA). A number of toxic solvents used to clean cans and various food containers prior to being filled may also be present. Similar estrogen-mimicking compounds are found in plastics and can leach into your foods, especially when the plastic becomes heated—even just from the sun. These substances, particularly when we're repeatedly exposed to them, can damage our bodies.[65]

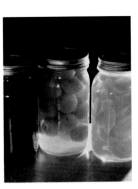

Use stainless steel, glass or cast iron for cooking. Never heat or cook foods in plastic containers, aluminum pots and pans or cheap cookware. Most non-stick cookware (as well as tin cans) is lined with Teflon. Manufacturers would like you to believe that Teflon lining in cans, pots and pans is safe and won't leach toxins. But here's a little test that will prove them wrong: Put a cup or two of water in a non-stick pot (the water should be about half an inch deep). Bring it to a boil and simmer for about one minute, then add a teaspoon of baking soda. Remove a spoonful of the water and smell it. You'll likely smell Teflon—not a pleasant scent. When the water is cool, taste the water, but don't swallow it! You may be shocked to taste how nasty that water is after having only reached boiling temperature. Imagine what is happening when frying an egg, vegetables or meat at double the temperature.

Microwave Ovens

When I ask my clients why they use microwave ovens, they invariably reply, "Because it's fast and it's easy." If your child was to say, "I've devised a fast and easy way to do my homework," or, "I've come up with a fast and easy way to make money," what's your gut reaction? You'd probably think their plan isn't as good as it may sound and that they'll likely end up in some sort of trouble. That's the innate wisdom of a parent. Most doctors and therapists also begin to develop an innate wisdom with regard to what is and is not health giving. Some ignore it because their innate wisdom competes with their materialistic desires, yet others will investigate concerns. This is exactly how

my investigation of the microwave oven and the food that comes out of it began.

I recall being at my grandparents home many years ago when my grandmother offered eggs for breakfast. She cracked a couple eggs open, scrambled them and poured them into a microwavable dish. A minute or so later, a bell rang and she served my eggs. I was rather shocked having grown up on a farm, where I was never exposed to such technology. The first thing I noticed was the color was very light in comparison to the eggs I had eaten before. I took a bite and was perplexed with the almost Styrofoam consistency. I remember picking the eggs up, which was easy because they held a shape almost exactly like a hockey puck. While I was several years from beginning my career in the health and fitness fields, *my gut response was that something was amiss with microwaving food.*

As the years passed, I came to have a family of my own. My concern over the microwave lingered in the background, yet I, too, fell prey to the notion of using the microwave oven in order to save time. I was, however, continually reminded by the little voice inside my head each time an egg came out of a microwave. Then I read Robert O. Becker M.D.'s book *The Body Electric*, which enlightened me to the potential dangers of even standing near a microwave oven.[66] Once activated, they emit electromagnetic pollution of a greater magnitude than most electrical appliances. Listening to my inner voice, and knowing that eggs should not have the characteristics of a hockey puck, I resolved to using the microwave to heat water *while I stood at a distance.*

My concerns about the microwave made a quantum leap toward justification a few years ago when I began studying a nutrition course by a well-respected nutritionist and naturopathic physician in San Diego, David Getoff. In his course, he described some of the harmful effects of the microwave and raised a number of concerns, including: [52]

- The microwaves produced by microwave ovens damage the cell wall of foods to such a degree that the gut receptors are not likely to recognize microwaved food particles as food, resulting in an immune response.

- Microwave ovens heat foods from the inside out by the use of alternating current to produce electro-magnetic radiation. This alternating current, driven by microwave radiation, reverses the polarity of the atoms, molecules and cells of the foods or waters being heated 1 - 100 *billion* times a second. *Atoms, molecules or cells of organic systems are not able to withstand such a violent destructive power for any extended period of time, not even in the low energy range of milliwatts.*

- Microwave technology is used in the field of gene altering technology to weaken cell membranes.

Heating breast milk, even at a low setting, can destroy some of its important disease-fighting capabilities. John A. Kerner, M.D., found that using the microwave to heat breast milk causes the milk to lose lysozyme activity and antibodies as well as fostering the growth of more potentially pathogenic bacteria. Milk heated at a high setting (72 - 98° C) lost 96% of its immunoglobulin-A antibodies (agents that fend off invading microbes). As for heating breast milk using the "low" setting, Dr. Kerner surmised, *"...adverse changes at such low temperatures suggests microwaving itself may in fact cause some injury to the milk above and beyond the heating."* [67]

Some hospitals have banned the use of microwave ovens for the purpose of heating baby foods or formulas of any kind. Since they don't allow the use of microwave ovens for a baby's food, I cannot understand why they continue to use them to feed everyone else in the hospital. For anyone with an ounce of logic, this should raise some serious questions, the first one being: *if microwaved foods and breast milk suppresses immune activity and may be damaging to a baby, why should other foods be any different?*

Microwavable Packaging

Though the FDA has not developed and implemented specific regulations, they've recognized that chemical components of adhesives, polymers, paper and paper-board products used in microwave packaging migrate into food. According to *The Safe Shopper's Bible*, micro-waving some packaging may cause it to disintegrate, allowing carcinogens and other uncharacterized chemicals contained in the packaging to enter food. [45] While the migration of chemicals from such packaging into foods is as yet poorly studied, one such chemical, dimethyl terephthalate, has shown evidence of being a carcinogen. Heat susceptor packaging (packaging that helps retain heat for browning), in particular, is used for microwaving such products as popcorn, pizza, French fries, fish sticks and waffles.

Slow and Steady Wins the Race

I know this is a lot to take in. Don't feel like you have to make all of the changes I suggest overnight. Choose a few issues to address at a time. Remember, living healthy is a lifestyle. I'd rather you take things slowly and stick to your plan for the long term than to dive in and quit because it was too hard. The good news is that the more positive changes you make in regards to your eating habits, the better you will feel and the more energy you will have to happily continue your quest for optimal health!

The Stack family of Fitter International, clients of Paul Chek and Janet Alexander, C.H.E.K Practitioner Level 4, Golf Biomechanic, C.H.E.K Faculty

Background: Tynan Stack, age 6, had experienced significant hip pain and dysfunction for several years prior to seeing Paul. A physiotherapist recommended stretching, a chiropractor suggested regular visits, and the orthopedic surgeon mentioned that surgery might be required. Paul's evaluation revealed that the pain was likely the result of pelvic instability coming from abdominal wall dysfunction due to intestinal inflammation.

Hi Paul,

After we left your office, our lives went through a major transformation. We had promised the kids that we would take them out to pizza that night, which we did. After eating, all four of us felt horrible—over-full and grouchy. Knowing what we had just eaten and the effect that it was having on all of us was a big eye opener.

The first thing that I did when we got home was to go through our cupboards to see how far gluten had invaded our lives. I pulled out everything that included the grains and flours that I knew contained gluten. The next thing I did was go to our local organic food store. The shop was able to provide me with a list of forbidden foods and a list of additives and fillers that are gluten in disguise. I was astounded at what needed to be removed from our diet. Back I went to my kitchen for a second purge. Now we have lots of room in our cupboards!

I purchased a cookbook, *The Gluten-Free Gourmet* by Bette Hagman, which has proven to be a godsend. I can duplicate most of the foods that my family usually ate using various gluten-free flours and substitutes. This has been very important to the kids, as rather than say that they can't have a particular food, it has become that they can have it if we make it.

So, we really became gluten-free within a couple of days of leaving Encinitas. The difference in Tynan was almost immediate. He has always been a very content little soul, but after he was off gluten for only a few days, if you asked him how school was he would literally gush, "Oh Mom, it was great!" It is so obvious that he feels good. He is extremely cautious about what he eats now. At six years old, he realized that he is not able to eat gluten products and loses all interest in a food once you tell him that it contains gluten. We have successfully negotiated both Halloween and Christmas buffets with very little strife.

Ty just turns to me and says, "Mom, can you make it at home?"

The first month to six weeks, we could literally not feed Tynan enough. Louis and I finally figured out that he was so accustomed to feeling bloated when he had eaten that he thought that he was not getting enough. His tummy is now soft, even after he eats, and he was not familiar with this feeling. He knew what he thought he should feel like after eating, and was trying to eat enough to get that feeling again. He has now become familiar with the fact that he shouldn't feel packed full when he leaves the table, and his eating has stabilized.

As far as the pain in his hips goes, Ty has not complained at all since he began eating a gluten-free diet. As a family, we get a lot of questions about why we are eating this way and what differences we have noticed. I had a friend ask, "Why?" and Tynan piped in to say, "You shouldn't eat gluten because then your hips won't hurt." Big testament to how it makes him feel.

We eat out far less now than we used to. It is much easier for me to know what goes into foods if we have prepared them. In addition, most foods targeted at children are all gluten! Everything is either breaded, pasta, or comes in a bun. The thing that we have found that Tynan has developed a real taste for is sushi. We now store our own bottle of gluten-free soy sauce at the sushi restaurant we frequent.

As far as myself, I feel great. I have since discovered that my Dad's brother was diagnosed as celiac, and his daughter is celiac to the point that she gets physically ill if she ingests gluten. I have read somewhere that if celiac disease is in your genetic make-up there is a 70% chance that you will be sensitive as well. This certainly seems to be the case with our family.

Louis has also noticed that he feels much better with gluten out of his diet, although he has not been able to give up beer completely, so he is getting some gluten there. Both Louis and I have noticed that our body shapes have changed, although weight has not. The program that Janet gave me is really helping me to feel much stronger and more sure of my body. The pain in my hip has also gone away. Whether that is a gluten-free thing again, or more of a mechanical issue, I am not sure.

Love,
Margaret

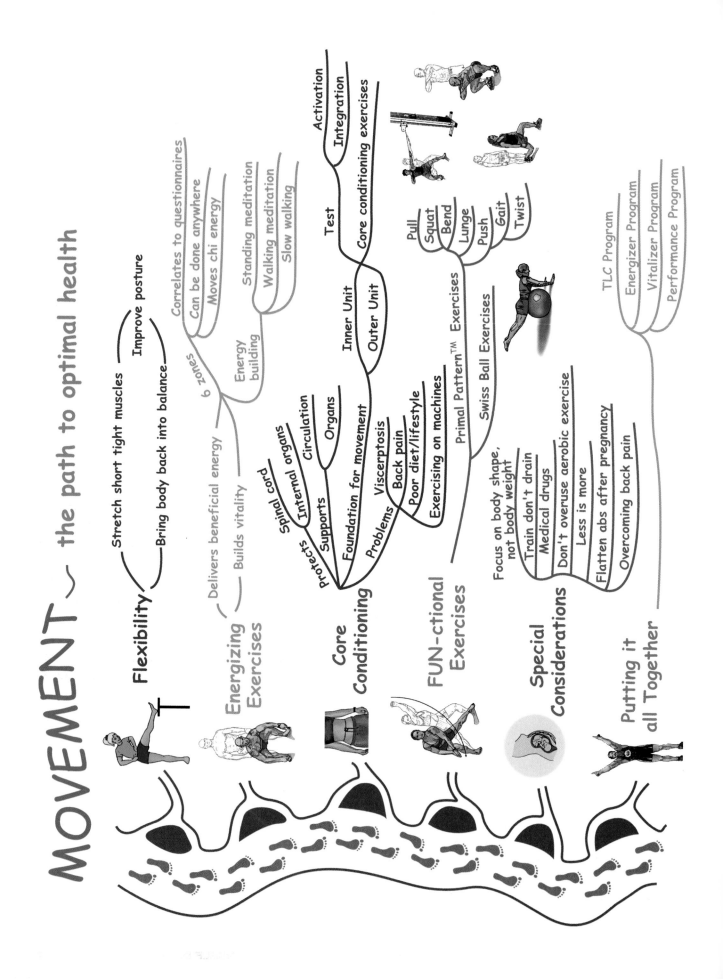

MOVEMENT ~ the path to optimal health

Flexibility
- Stretch short tight muscles
  - Improve posture
- Bring body back into balance

Energizing Exercises
- Delivers beneficial energy
- Builds vitality
- 6 zones
  - Correlates to questionnaires
  - Can be done anywhere
  - Moves chi energy
- Energy building
  - Standing meditation
  - Walking meditation
  - Slow walking

Core Conditioning
- Protects
  - Spinal cord
- Supports
  - Internal organs
  - Circulation
  - Organs
- Foundation for movement
- Problems
  - Viscerptosis
  - Back pain
  - Poor diet/lifestyle
  - Exercising on machines
- Inner Unit
- Outer Unit
  - Test
  - Activation
  - Integration
  - Core conditioning exercises

FUN-ctional Exercises
- Primal Pattern™ Exercises
  - Pull
  - Squat
  - Bend
  - Lunge
  - Push
  - Gait
  - Twist
- Swiss Ball Exercises

Special Considerations
- Focus on body shape, not body weight
- Train don't drain
- Medical drugs
- Don't overuse aerobic exercise
- Less is more
- Flatten abs after pregnancy
- Overcoming back pain

Putting it all Together
- TLC Program
- Energizer Program
- Vitalizer Program
- Performance Program

Chapter 5

You Don't Have to Tie Yourself in Knots

Almost everybody, from office workers to athletes, can benefit from stretching. But don't worry, you don't have to be able to tie yourself in knots! People typically migrate toward activities they're good at. If you're flexible, you probably don't mind stretching, but if you aren't flexible, the thought alone is enough to make you avoid any form of flexibility training.

People commonly make the mistake of stretching muscles that don't need stretching and not stretching the ones that do need it. If you're stretching correctly and you don't feel tightness, that muscle doesn't need that particular stretch.

What Is Optimal Flexibility for You?

Watching a well-limbered instructor can be discouraging if you're as stiff as a board. But remember, we're all different. What's right for some may not be right for you. Most people don't need to have the flexibility required for advanced yoga moves. You do, however, need a certain level of flexibility, which many people lack. The stretches at the end of this chapter will help you determine which of your muscles need stretching in order to balance out your body.

If you're naturally tight and want to participate in a sport or leisure activity that requires more flexibility than you currently have, becoming more flexible will help you avoid injury. Many people spend most of their day sitting—on the job, in the car, at the dinner table—only to spend their evening watching TV. Sitting for extended periods day in and day out, without adequate stretching and movement, will lead to decreased flexibility and muscle imbalances. It won't take long before you lose so much flexibility that bending over to pick up your socks becomes a challenge. Here are two examples in which inadequate flexibility can lead to pain and/or injury.

Tennis: Tennis is what I call a multi-pattern sport, meaning to play it effectively you must squat, lunge, bend, push, pull, twist and run. If you're too tight to perform any of these movements at speeds natural to tennis, you're likely to avoid certain shots to protect yourself, or you may get hurt forcing your body to do things it's not currently equipped to do. Tennis players often find themselves moving very quickly into a lunge while bending, reaching, and twisting to make a forehand (push pattern) or backhand (pull pattern) shot. Figure 1A shows a tennis player who has adequate flexibility while the player in figure B does not. In figure 1B, the red arrows indicate areas in which the player is at greater risk of injury due to inflexibility.

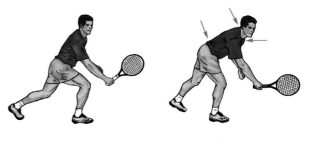

Figure 1A   Figure 1B

Daily activities: A lack of flexibility can also cause injuries while performing simple household chores, day-to-day activities or even gardening. In figure 2A, a woman bends over to pick up a water bottle with good body mechanics. Figure 2B shows the same woman lifting incorrectly because of a lack of flexibility. Back injury is a likely result particularly when the hip and hamstring muscles are tight, relative to the back muscles.

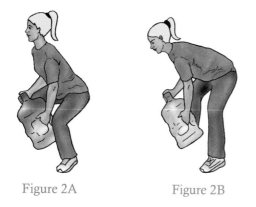

Figure 2A   Figure 2B

Posture and Stretching

Most of you were probably told to "stand up straight" by your parents or teachers. You may wonder what posture has to do with flexibility. Good posture keeps muscles in balance and your body well aligned, allowing optimal efficiency of body systems. Poor posture places abnormal weight on joints and stresses muscles and tendons, often leading to pain. Additionally, poor posture does not adequately support internal organs, circulation is hampered and an environment more favorable for disease and dysfunction is created.

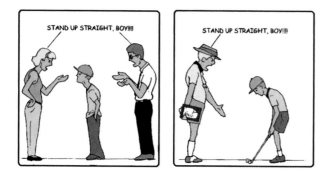

Muscles act as pumps to move fluids through the body. When good posture deteriorates, many of your muscles can't effectively pump fluids. To better appreciate the importance of good posture, muscle function and fluid flow, think of a pond. If a pond doesn't have a steady source of fresh water coming in and a stream taking water away, it becomes stagnant. With that in mind, look at yourself in the mirror. If your posture is such that you can project a line up from just in front of your anklebone and have it run midway between your hip, shoulder and ear, your posture is quite good. If your posture is poor, you'll see increased or decreased curves in the spine, the belly may protrude and the head will often be forward. Poor posture **always** indicates the need for a stretching program to lengthen short muscles and an exercise program to tighten weak/loose muscles.

Poor posture and muscle imbalances are a result of misuse. Some of our muscles react to faulty loading by shortening, tightening and becoming hyperactive; they are called *tonic* or *postural* muscles. Other muscles do the opposite; they become longer and weaker when exposed to the same stressors. These are called *phasic* or *mover* muscles.

The tonic muscles, by design, have a tendency to be workaholics, while the phasic muscles are naturally lazy. When exposed to stressors that either directly hurt the muscles or cause holding patterns, such as a chronic emotional stressor, the tonic muscles will shorten and tighten while the phasic muscles in the same area will often lengthen and may weaken. This is why those who experience traumatic events like a car accident, a fall from a bicycle or a hard

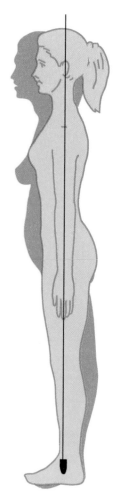

Figure 5:
Good Posture vs.
Poor Posture

tackle in football often end up with chronic muscle and joint problems and may develop poor posture over time.

Address Imbalances Before Exercising

To better understand how muscle imbalances affect your body, think of a bicycle wheel. If a bicycle wheel is out of balance (Figure 6) and you take the bike out for a ride, chances are the bicycle won't handle well. The stress of riding on a crooked wheel could cause the wheel to fall apart. To get a crooked bicycle wheel to roll *straight* or *true*, you must *shorten/tighten the loose spokes and lengthen/loosen the tight ones.*

If you have poor posture or have been injured, the tonic muscles tend to get short and tight while the phasic muscles tend to lengthen and weaken, pulling you out of balance just like the bicycle wheel in Figure 6. If you expose yourself to the stressors of exercise you must attempt to lengthen the short tonic muscles and strengthen or tighten any long or weak phasic muscles to bring your body back into balance, like the wheel in Figure 7. The last thing you want is to turn your attempts to achieve a healthy body through exercise into long-term aliments.

Body Balancing Stretches

To determine which stretches you should complete before beginning your workouts, simply perform each of the stretches exactly as directed on pages 88 through 95. If you perform any of the stretches as outlined and the muscle(s) do not feel tight, that means you *do not* need to include that stretch in your program. Only include those stretches that give you the feeling that there are tight muscles to be released when doing that particular stretch. Record your results on the Stretching Check List on pages 96 and 97.

I suggest re-testing yourself every two to four weeks. By identifying muscles that have become loose and no longer need stretching, as well as identifying muscles that may have become tight from participating in your exercise program, you'll know exactly which stretches keep your body in balance. Stretching muscles that are already loose is like loosening the spokes on a crooked wheel—it will leave the body loose and crooked. Not stretching at all before you exercise leads to your body becoming tight and crooked. You want to stretch the muscles that are tight to avoid either of these situations.

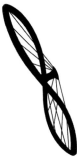

Figure 6:
Bent Wheel

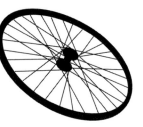

Figure 7:
Balanced Wheel

STRETCHES

Note: Many of the stretches below will use a **contract-relax** method. The three basic phases of a contract-relax stretch are:

1. Move into initial stretch. You should feel the muscles being stretched, but it should not be uncomfortable.

2. Contract the muscle being stretched. Use either your hand or the floor to provide resistance. Use only a light force when you contract.

3. Relax, moving immediately into the stretch position after you release the contraction. You should find that you can move farther into the stretch.

Performing this process 3 - 5 times per muscle each session is optimal.

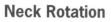

Neck Side Flexion

• Sit with good posture.

• Grasp the end of the bench or the edge of a chair and lean away until your shoulder is depressed. Make sure to maintain an erect posture.

• Use the opposite hand to gently draw your head away from the anchored shoulder.

• Inhale and gently push your head into your hand for 5 seconds.

• Exhale and immediately lean further away, while depressing your shoulder. Then gently move your head and neck further away from your shoulder.

• Hold the stretch position for 5 seconds.

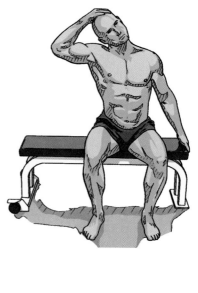

Neck Rotation

• Sit with good posture.

• Rotate your head to one side.

• Place the opposite hand on your cheek. Inhale and gently rotate your head into your hand while keeping the hand firm.

• Look in the direction that you are turning.

• Hold for 5 seconds and exhale as you look behind you and rotate your head into the stretch.

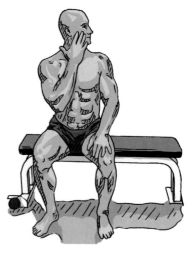

Levator Scapulae

- Reach one arm as far down between your shoulder blades as possible.
- Look as far as you comfortably can to the opposite side.
- Take a deep breath in and hold for 5 seconds. As you exhale, look downward as far as you comfortably can toward your shoulder.

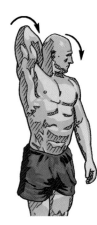

Neck Extensors

- Maintain an upright posture, either sitting or standing, and let your head drop toward your chest.
- Place one hand on the back of your head and one on your chin.
- Tuck your chin and gently stretch the back of your neck by drawing your head toward your chest.
- Take a deep breath and lightly press your head into your hand, without letting your head move.
- After 5 seconds, relax as you exhale and gently move your head toward your chest.

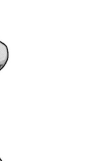

Chest

Pec major: (larger chest muscle)
- Place your forearm on a Swiss ball.
- Keep your shoulders parallel to the ground and drop your body toward the floor. When you reach a comfortable stretch, inhale and press the forearm into the ball for 5 seconds.
- Exhale and move immediately into the stretch.
- There should be no pain felt in the shoulder joint.

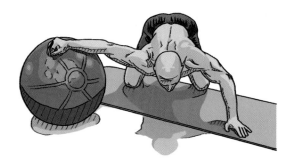

Pec minor (smaller muscle beneath the pec major, that has a tendency to get tight)
- Place your shoulder on the ball instead of your forearm.
- As you drop your upper body downward, allow your shoulder blade to move toward your spine.
- Inhale and press your shoulder into the ball for 5 seconds. Exhale and lower into a new stretch position. Keep your torso parallel to the floor.

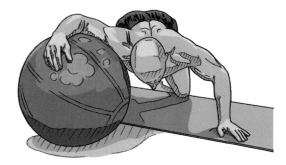

Rhomboids (muscle between shoulder blades)

- Kneel in front of a Swiss ball and place your elbow on the ball.

- Bring your arm across your body as it rests on the ball.

- Inhale and press into the ball with your elbow as you attempt to draw your shoulder blade toward your spine. Use your opposite hand to hold the ball still.

- Hold for 5 seconds and release as you exhale and move farther into the stretch, allowing the shoulder blade to move away from your spine. Use your opposite arm to roll the ball across your body.

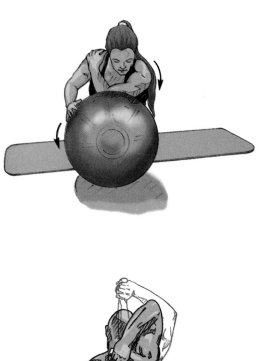

Scratch Stretch

- Stand with good posture, holding a towel behind your back as shown in the picture.

- Use the bottom hand to pull downward until you feel a comfortable stretch.

- Hold that position with your lower arm.

- Inhale as you try to pull upward with your top arm against the fixed resistance of the lower arm.

- Hold that contraction for 5 seconds. Exhale and pull down with the lower arm to further stretch the upper arm.

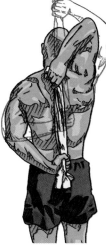

Trunk Rotation

- Lie on your back with your knees bent and pointing up at the ceiling.

- Your lower legs should be relaxed. Place your hand on your thigh while keeping the other arm stretched out to help you stabilize.

- Slowly let your legs roll to that side until you feel a comfortable stretch in your lower back. Inhale and reduce the support from your arm slightly to activate your trunk muscles.

- Hold for 5 seconds and repeat to the other side. Continue to practice this stretch until you can comfortably place your thighs on the ground, or until you are no longer improving your range of motion.

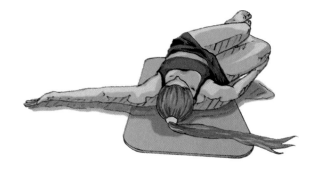

Middle Back and Abdominals

Caution: If you experience dizziness when looking up toward the sky (for example, watching an airplane fly by or when putting something away in a high cupboard), you may also experience dizziness when performing this stretch. It is very important that you stop the stretch immediately if you feel any unusual symptoms. If you do not have sufficient spinal extension (backward bending), you may compensate by over-extending your neck. This may result in nausea, dizziness or changes in vision. Any unusual symptoms indicate the need to see your doctor for a complete evaluation of your neck to rule out occlusion of the vertebral artery. Should your neck be cleared as normal, you should have an ear, nose, throat specialist assess your inner ear function.

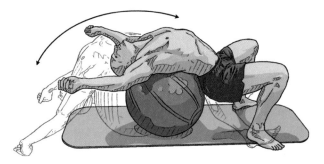

- Perform this stretch on a non-slip surface.

- Sit on a Swiss ball, then walk your legs out and roll backwards until you are lying over the ball.

- Extend your arms over your head. To increase the stretch, slowly straighten your legs. Hold for one minute.

Obliques

- Sit on a Swiss ball and carefully roll down the ball and onto your side.

- You may use a wall to anchor your feet.

- Grasp the wrist of your top hand as your arms are extended over your head.

- Gently begin rolling the upper body forward and then backward while slightly tugging the upper arm downward. When your feel a tight area, inhale and gently attempt to side bend back up, pulling against your lower arm. You don't need to actually move, just activate the muscles.

- Relax into a new stretch position as you exhale.

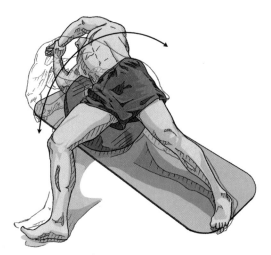

Squat

- Stand with a comfortable stance next to a stable object that you can hang onto.

- Squat down until you are completely relaxed, letting all the tension out of your back and letting your torso rest between, but not supported by, your thighs.

- If you can do this without hanging onto anything, that's great. If you are too tight in the ankles, knees, butt or low back, you can hold onto a stable object so that you can completely relax.

- Gently rock back and fourth between the balls of the feet and the heels for one minute.

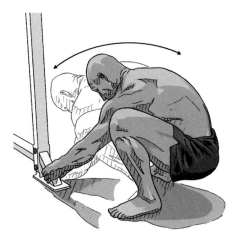

Lunge

- Assume a lunge position, making sure your front foot stays in front of the knee.

- Draw your belly button in toward your spine and tuck your tail under (this will flatten your low back). (1)

- Begin to move your whole pelvis forward, keeping it square to the front. (2)

- To increase the stretch, reach the arm on the trailing leg side over your head and bend your trunk to the side. (3) Rotating your pelvis toward the front leg will also increase the stretch.

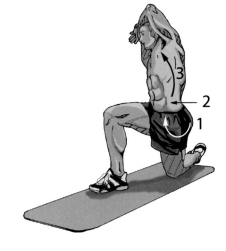

Waiter's Bow

- Stand with your feet parallel and close together.

- Keep your legs straight and stick your bottom out until you have an arch in your low back.

- Bend forward from your hips while holding your low back arched until you feel a comfortable stretch on your hamstrings. To help you maintain the correct position, you may tape your back as described on following page.

- Hold for 20 seconds.

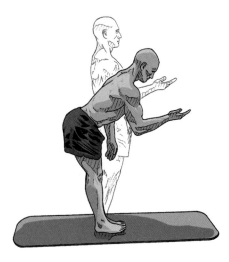

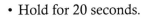

Hamstrings

- Lie on your back with a small, rolled-up towel under your back at the belt line level.

- The towel, when compressed, should be the width and thickness of the fattest part of your hand.

- Grab one leg with both hands, just below the knee, and bring the bent leg up until the thigh is perpendicular to the floor. Extend your toes back toward your shin and slowly straighten your leg without letting the thigh move in your hands or letting your back come off the floor.

- Hold a comfortable stretch for 20 seconds.

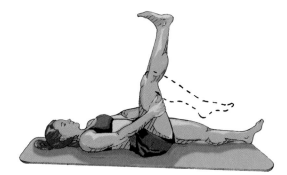

90/90 Hip Stretch

Special Note: If you are tight in the hips, you will find it hard to keep the lumbar curve during this stretch. To help maintain this position, have someone run a strip of athletic tape along your back muscles, on either side of your spine, from the level of your bottom rib to the top of your pelvis while you are standing with good upright posture, as seen in the picture. This modification is very important for anyone with a history of back pain, especially lumbar disc bulges, because it prevents you from over-stretching the lower back.

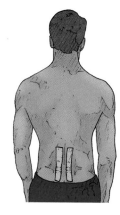

- Sit on the floor with both your front and back legs bent to 90°.

- The angle at your groin should also be 90°.

- Place your hand on the ground next to your hip.

- Tip your pelvis as though it was a bowl and you were trying to pour the contents out over your belt line. Imagine sticking your butt backwards, like Donald Duck.

- You should have an increased curvature of your lower back. Keep the curve in your low back and your chest and head up as you move forward over the front leg.

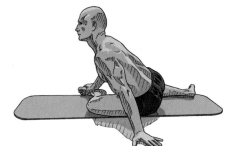

- When you feel a comfortable stretch in your outer thigh and hip, inhale and press the front knee and ankle firmly into the ground for 5 seconds. Exhale and move farther forward into the stretch.

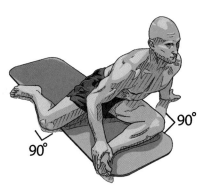

Groin

- Assume a kneeling position and spread your knees as far out as you comfortably can.
- Rock forward, breathe in and gently squeeze your knees into the ground for 5 seconds.
- Exhale and relax as you sink forward.
- Rock backward and use the same contract/relax procedure for any other tight areas you find.

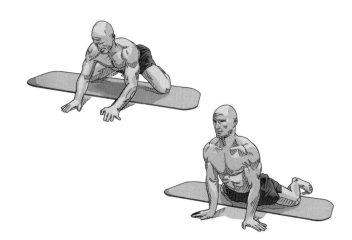

Swiss Ball Quad Stretch

- Begin in a sprinter's start position, with the foot and ankle of the leg to be stretched on the ball.
- Slowly rise upward.
- You may place one hand on the ball or use a chair for support.
- Draw your belly button in toward your spine and roll your pelvis under so that your back flattens to increase the stretch.

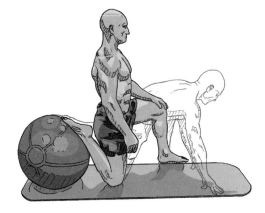

Calves

- Stand on the edge of a step.
- Drop your heel toward the floor and off the step, keeping the leg straight and toes angled upward. (1)
- Hold for 20 seconds and switch sides. Then, repeat with a bent leg on each side. (2)

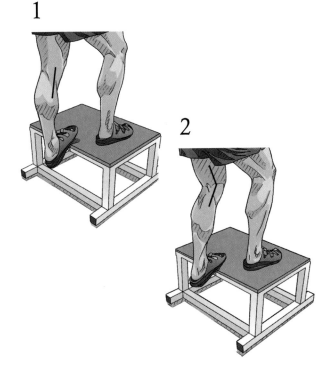

McKenzie Press-up

- Lie on your stomach with your hands just outside the tops of your shoulders as in a push-up position.

- Inhale deeply and begin pressing your upper body upward off the floor, but make sure your hips stay on the ground.

- As you push your body upward, exhale, pretending you are blowing yourself up off the floor.

- It is important to relax your buttocks, legs and spinal muscles.

- Hold the top position until you need to take a breath.

- Inhale as you slowly lower your body to the floor and repeat 10 times.

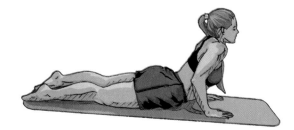

IT Band

- Stand next to a wall and step forward of your inside leg (this is the leg that you will be stretching) as shown.

- Keep both feet flat on the floor.

- Use your inside arm for support against the wall and place the other hand on your hip.

- Press your hip straight towards the wall and slightly downward as it moves toward the wall.

- You should feel a stretch on the outside of the leg closest to the wall and in the hip.

- If you do not feel a full stretch, bring your hips forward slightly and rotate your pelvis toward the front.

- If you are performing the stretch correctly, taking your outside hand off the hip at any point will eliminate the stretch in the hip. You should not feel a stretch in your low back.

- Hold for 20 seconds. Stretch each side up to 3 times.

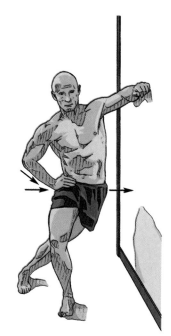

STRETCHING TEST SHEET

☐ Neck Side Flexion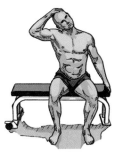

☐ Rhomboids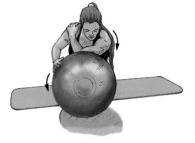

☐ Neck Rotation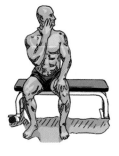

☐ Scratch Stretch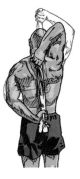

☐ Levator Scapulae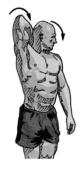

☐ Trunk Rotation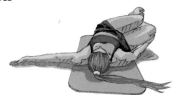

☐ Neck Extension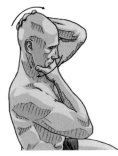

☐ Middle Back & Abdominals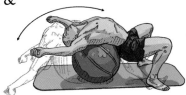

☐ Chest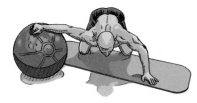

☐ Obliques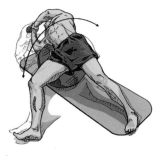

☐ Squat

☐ Groin

☐ Lunge

☐ Swiss Ball Quad Stretch

☐ Waiter's Bow

☐ Calves

☐ Hamstrings

☐ McKenzie Press-up

☐ 90/90 Hip Stretch

☐ IT Band

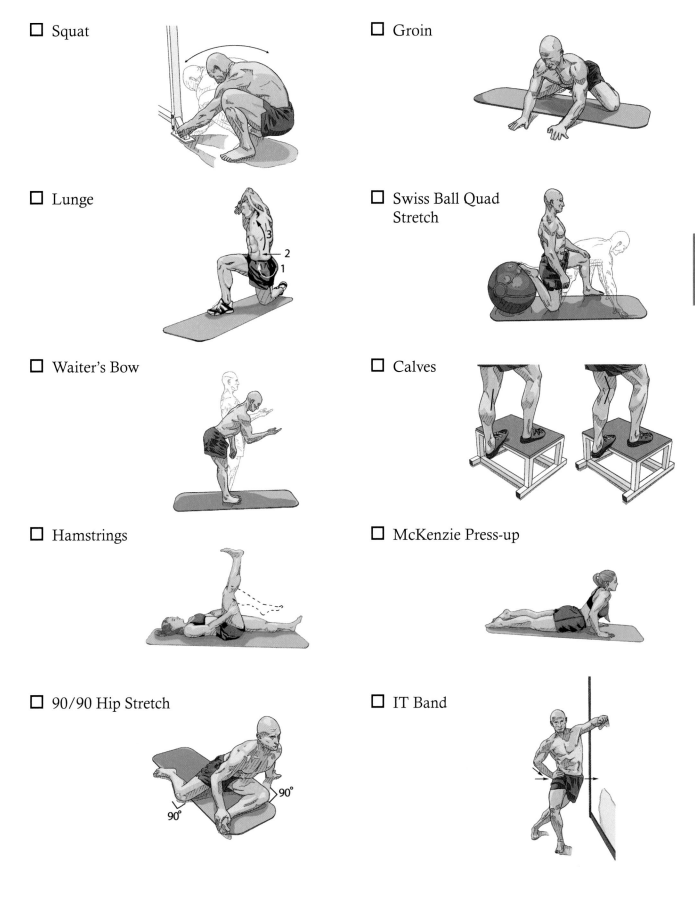

To do nothing is sometimes a good remedy.

Hippocrates

Chapter 6

ENERGIZING EXERCISES

We live in stressful times as many of us deal with information overload, long commutes, deadlines and bills. It's no wonder most people cringe at the thought of trying to squeeze exercise into their busy schedules. Moreover, many despise the idea of going to a gym either for fear of not knowing what to do there, or because they don't feel comfortable working out in front of others. These are legitimate concerns.

Then there are those who feel exercise is like folk medicine: *The good stuff always tastes bad, so just take your daily dose, like it or not.* Fear not! This is the 21st century, and I am about to share a *smarter*, not *harder*, method of increasing your energy and vitality. Changes can be made in just *minutes* a day! Energy Balancing Exercises are about to make all of these anxieties a thing of the past.

Building energy and vitality in your body is a lot like investing. Just as it takes money to make money, *it takes energy to make energy.* As demonstrated throughout this book, your body is a co-dependent, linked system of systems. Just like the heating and air conditioning system in your house or the electrical system in your car, all body systems are energy dependent, even the ones that produce energy. Your circulatory, digestive, hormonal and musculoskeletal systems are all body systems that not only use energy, *they produce it.*

Expending energy to inhale brings air into your body. Your lungs take oxygen from the air you breathe and attach it to iron particles in your red blood cells to be delivered to all parts of your body by the heart via arteries. The oxygen in the air you breathe carries a very strong positive charge, acting like the positive pole of a magnet, while your body tissues and the water in your body (about 75% of your body is water) act like the negative pole of a magnet. As you may remember from science class, wherever you find a positive and negative pole, there's *energy* and *work potential.* Breathing oxygen into the body creates energy or work potential. This energy is called *Prana* by East Indian Yogis and mystics, or *Chi or Qi* by masters of Tai Chi, Qigong and the many martial arts.

Freshly oxygenated blood goes from your lungs to the heart, where two important things happen. First, the heart acts like a powerful generator—producing an electromagnetic field approximately 5,000 times stronger than that of your brain.[1] The heart's electromagnetic field is so powerful that it not only permeates every cell in your body, it can be measured eight to ten feet away by sensitive detectors called magnetometers. Research scientists at the Institute of HeartMath have demonstrated that the powerful electromagnetic field of the heart is used to send information to the brain. Acting like a pump, the heart performs a second very important function, delivering the added charge to your body cells and systems. This form of energy informs your brain and each of your cells about your *heart state* (happy, sad, excited, depressed, etc.) and serves as a form of energy that cells use to perform vital functions.

When you eat quality food (Chapter 4), you *spend* energy to chew and digest it. Metabolized food molecules provide both chemical and electrical charges that help the body perform work, such as building hormones.

The hormonal system is composed of special glands. Each hormonal gland uses energy from breathing and the building blocks from digestion to produce specific hormones, which carry out important work functions in the body. The thyroid gland, for example, produces thyroid hormone, which regulates cellular metabolism. The adrenal glands produce adrenaline and cortisol (stress/activating hormone), which assist your body in getting work done.

Much of the energy produced by breathing and eating is used to run your muscles so you can move, have fun and produce more energy. The method by which your muscles produce energy is seldom considered because most people only associate muscle work with *fatigue or loss of energy*. Fatigue and loss of energy result from excessive use of the muscles and body systems that support activity—particularly when there is an imbalance between the amount of work or exercise relative to the amount of rest time.

Muscles help energize the body by producing electromagnetic energy and by acting as pumps to assist the action of the heart. When your muscles contract, tension is placed on the connective tissues that house your muscles, as well as on the actin and myosin proteins that cause your muscles to contract. When tension is placed on the connective tissues of the muscles, tendons and even the skin over the muscles, an electrical current called a *piezoelectric current* is created.[2] Piezoelectric current is yet another form of energy the body can use to run its systems. To experience this in your own body, try this exercise. Stand up and relax for a second, taking notice of how your body feels. Once you have a sense of your body, tighten your right thigh muscle as tight as you can for five seconds and then quickly relax. Pay immediate attention to the sensation of energy (Chi) surging through your body. It may run up to your head and back down your other leg, it may run down your other leg and then back up your spine and head before going down one or both arms. The reaction is different in each person, but I'm sure you'll feel it.

Contracting a muscle pushes blood out of the muscle and into the veins, helping to return used blood to the heart and lungs to be recharged. When the muscle relaxes, it absorbs freshly charged blood from the heart

and lungs. This fresh blood contains valuable electromagnetic energy from the heart, electromagnetic work potential from the positively charged oxygen in the blood cells, hormonal energy and chemical energy and work potential from your digested foods.

Exercising the muscles for each zone (1-6) delivers *beneficial energy* to the hormonal and organ systems, as well as to tissues related to the spinal segments in that particular zone. This system is the foundation for yoga, Tai Chi, Qigong and the Zone Exercises presented in this book.

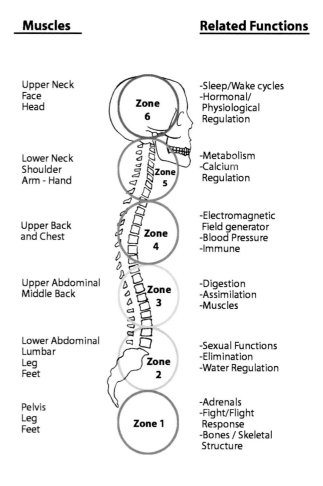

Muscles	Related Functions
Upper Neck Face Head	-Sleep/Wake cycles -Hormonal/ Physiological Regulation
Lower Neck Shoulder Arm - Hand	-Metabolism -Calcium Regulation
Upper Back and Chest	-Electromagnetic Field generator -Blood Pressure -Immune
Upper Abdominal Middle Back	-Digestion -Assimilation -Muscles
Lower Abdominal Lumbar Leg Feet	-Sexual Functions -Elimination -Water Regulation
Pelvis Leg Feet	-Adrenals -Fight/Flight Response -Bones / Skeletal Structure

Zone Exercises

Each system represented in your questionnaire is linked to a zone that will benefit that specific system (see your scoring graph on page 37). Review your graph and identify body systems where you scored in the medium to high range. You should perform one or more of the Zone Exercises for each of those zones. If you have multiple high zones and time is

Zone	Related Issues
Zone 1	Financial stress
Zone 2	Stress over relationships and sex
Zone 3	Personal power and self will, digestion
Zone 4	Stress over relationships and love
Zone 5	Communication
Zone 6	Mental congestion, lack of mental clarity or creativity

an issue, always start by performing exercises for the zones listed at the left of your scoring chart. Include additional zone exercises for systems to the right as time allows. If you don't see a zone exercise listed, such as for the Sleep/Wake Cycles column, this means there are no specific zone exercises to support that system directly. In this example you simply need to get to bed on time! To get the most from your Zone Exercises, consider the following tips:

1. The higher your score in any given category, the more important your Zone Exercises are to normalizing that body system. If time is an issue, always focus your energy on your stretches and Zone Exercises because those activities serve to balance your muscles and energy systems. This will provide more usable energy for your body than simply "working out." If you have time to do the entire program as presented, you'll get the most return on time invested, moving more rapidly toward better physical, emotional, mental and spiritual well-being!

2. There are several exercises demonstrated for each of the six zones. I suggest you try each of the exercises and choose the one that you feel is most effective. If you have more time you can do more than one Zone Exercise because they don't cause fatigue—they *energize!*

3. Zone Exercises can be done any time. If you feel tired or sluggish, perform a zone exercise and your energy levels will likely increase. Performed

before or after eating, Zone Exercises can improve digestion.

4. Practicing Zone Exercises will help you discover which ones work best for any given feeling, emotion and situation—both current issues or ones that may arise.

5. For anyone trying to cut down on sugar, caffeine or any other addictive substance, you may find Zone Exercises provide energy to compensate for the *fake*, or *empty* energy often provided by addictive substances.

6. Zone Exercises can help you unwind. By performing Zone Exercises, you bring more Chi into your body. If you have a hard time falling asleep or sleeping through the night, practice your Zone Exercises just before going to bed. Chi is intelligent—it knows when to speed up specific cells and/or body systems and when to slow them down! This is but one of many examples that the infinite intelligence of Mother Nature is at work.

When performing Zone Exercises, always remember that *the faster you move your body, the slower Chi energy moves and the slower you move your body, the faster Chi energy moves.* If you experiment with your Zone Exercises, you will soon experience this interesting phenomenon.

One way to determine how much effort to use with Zone Exercises is to perform them right after you eat. If you are working too hard, your digestion will feel compromised. If you are exercising at the correct level for a Zone Exercise, your digestion will feel improved.

Energy-building Exercises

Become as strong as an oak tree by doing nothing. I know, it sounds crazy. If you're feeling stressed to the point that you have no desire for exercise at all, your level of vitality is likely very low. Famous expert of Tai Chi and Qigong, Master Fong Ha, states in his book, *Yiquan and the Nature of Energy - The fine art of doing nothing and achieving everything* that, "aging can be seen ultimately as a decline in the life force or vitality, with death the end point of this decline, and since disciplines like Yiquan (standing meditation) work directly to cultivate vitality, they might well prove to be among the most valuable resources available to us as we strive for the longest, most vital lives possible." [3] I want you not only to read the words of the great Master Fong Ha, but also to use his valuable suggestion of cultivating vitality through stillness so that we can move you into other helpful exercises, further turning back the biological clock.

One of the best energizing exercises I learned from Master Fong Ha is the standing meditation, Yiquan. Chinese martial arts masters have developed amazing powers by using standing meditation as their primary form of exercise. Standing meditation is very simple to do and doesn't require equipment. You only need your body and can perform it anywhere.

Standing Meditation

To begin, stand with good posture; your knees unlocked, feet about hip width and parallel to each other, and your spine lengthened to comfortably make yourself as tall as you can. To achieve this position, gently draw your belly button toward your spine, tuck your chin slightly and relax the shoulders and arms, letting the shoulders roll back slightly (not drop forward). When in the correct position to perform your standing meditation your ear, shoulder, hip joint, knee and ankle should all line up when viewed from the side. You should be balanced on your feet. Further, your tongue should rest on the roof of your mouth just behind the front teeth (if you swallow, it will go where it belongs). Keep the tongue relaxed at all times. When in this position, you're prepared to get the most out of doing nothing because this is the best position to allow optimal flow of life force energy, often called Chi or Prana.

Once in the standing meditation position, you may perform the exercise of doing nothing in several ways:

1. Let your arms hang at your side completely relaxed

2. Pretend you are holding a soap bubble (or a Chi bubble) about the size of a basketball right in front of your lower abdomen/pelvis region. You should feel and imagine the Chi bubble being half in and half out of your body.

3. Change the size and location of the Chi bubble, moving it up and down the body to wherever you would like, always remembering to keep half the bubble in your body.

Breathe in through your nose and out through your nose or mouth. Your breathing should be deep, slow, rhythmical and relaxed, never forced. Just be sure that your belly expands as you breathe in, allowing your diaphragm room to drop down and pull air into the bottom of your lungs.

As you are doing nothing, your mind will want to wander. It will try to think about the stressors of your life. Try to be an observer, as though you were watching yourself from a distance. Each time your mind wanders away from this glorious chance to be quiet, to do nothing, take it by the hand and bring it back to that quiet place. Master Ha teaches people to count their breaths if they have a jumpy mind. This will give you something to focus on that is not stressful, and soon enough you will find yourself expanding, getting lighter, having deeper and more relaxed breathing and feeling energized!

If your body gets tired of standing while doing nothing, you can sit and continue the meditation, yet continue to stay aligned as before. When you feel rested, stand up again. Try to work yourself up to 30 minutes a day of doing nothing. An hour a day is even better! Most people find that after doing this exercise for 100 hours (over an extended period of time) there are some pleasurable and very noticeable changes in the body. Some of the changes people experience are:

• Improved sense of awareness

• Improved mental clarity

• Improved energy

• Improved athletic ability

• Disappearance of chronic ailments

• Tighter and more youthful looking skin

• Brighter eyes

• An increased ability to sense other people's feelings and thoughts

Why Do I Shake?

When you do nothing correctly, your body will increase its Chi reserves. Chi is life force energy and that energy contains all the wisdom and knowledge in the Universe. As your body collects Chi, it will find areas where you have blockages to Chi flow and will try to work through the resistance. You'll feel this as shaking in your body. It may be a leg, your lower back, your shoulder or arm, maybe even an internal organ(s). Don't let this scare you; it means your body is healing, getting stronger and more complete so your soul can express itself through a more perfect body. What greater reward could you ever expect from doing nothing?

Walking Meditation

A walking meditation is simply taking time out for yourself, time to get away from people and phones and break free from the stressors of everyday life to listen to your soul. As you walk, time your breathing to your steps. For example, inhale for four steps, hold your breath naturally for one step, and exhale for four steps. Adjust your effort so that you don't have to keep changing your breathing. It is a good idea to simply count your steps, emptying your mind of all things other than the step count and breathing until you've mastered the process and it becomes innate. A walking meditation should be no less than 15 minutes. It is best to walk in nature, where you can benefit from the natural earth energies, experience a variety of colors and appreciate life forms moving in their natural rhythm.

Slow Walking

Another great exercise I learned from Master Fong Ha, slow walking, is performed with the same consciousness described above for walking meditation, yet the goal is to walk as slowly as possible. As you perform slow walking, the key is to always be moving, but moving very slowly, like a cat sneaking up on a bird, yet staying very relaxed. With slow walking you should stay very much in touch with the now, the moment. The slower you go, the more Chi flow you will create and the better your balance will become. If you are an athletic person and want to take slow walking to another level of challenge, try slow walking across a park or reliable surface with your eyes closed! Slow walking can be very effective when performed for as little as ten minutes at a time.

Sample Zone Exercises

Refer to the following 13 pages for my favorite Zone Exercises. Each of these exercises will help channel energy to a specific zone of your body. Try them all and choose your favorites for your own Eat, Move and Be Healthy! program.

Walking is man's best medicine.

Hippocrates

Superman

- Start face down on the floor, or over a Swiss ball.

- Lift your left arm and right leg so that they are at about the same height.

- Your arm should be at a 45-degree angle from your head with your thumb pointed up.

- Hold this position for as long as you can with good form (up to 10 seconds) and switch sides.

Tempo	10 seconds hold/switch sides
Reps	5 each side

Qigong Toe-touch

- Stand with your feet together.

- Slide your hands down your legs, bending your knees.

- Place your hands directly over your toes, fingers aligned with toes.

- Inhale, raise your hips up and roll slightly back on to your heels until you feel a stretch in your hamstrings.

- Exhale and drop down again, rolling slightly forward toward the balls of your feet. You may slowly move your head and hips in a circle as you perform the exercise.

Tempo	natural breathing pace
Reps	10

Leg Raise

- Start face down on the floor or over a Swiss ball.

- Raise your legs up in the air.

- Bring your heels together, with your toes pointed outward.

- Tighten your hamstrings and glutes (butt muscles) and hold with good alignment for 10 seconds.

- Your head should not drop down or raise up.

Tempo	10 seconds hold/10 seconds relax
Reps	10

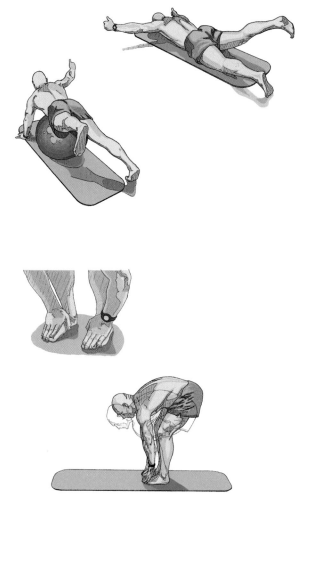
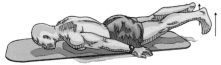
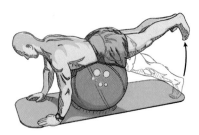

Hip Extension

- Start by sitting on a Swiss ball and roll back so that your upper back, shoulders and head rest on the ball.

- Pick your hips up so that your shoulders, hips and knees are in a straight line. Keep your shins vertical at all times.

- Slowly drop your pelvis straight down, as low as you comfortably can, then lift your hips back up to the ceiling. Keep your head and upper back on the ball.

- You should not roll forward or backwards on the ball as you perform the exercise (it is okay if the ball rolls slightly forward as you drop down, but your knees should not move in front of your feet).

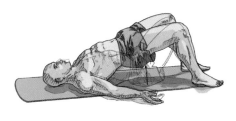

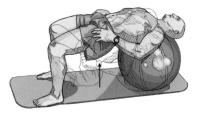

Tempo	10 seconds hold/10 seconds relax
Reps	5 each side

Wall Squat

- Stand with your back against a Swiss ball, supported by a wall.

- Inhale, then squat down as you exhale. Go only as low as you comfortably can.

- Keep your knees aligned with your second toe and do not let them drop in towards each other. You should not feel any discomfort in your knees.

- Stand up again slowly.

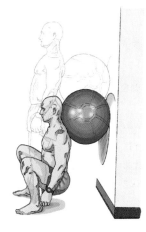

Tempo	slow
Reps	10

Breathing Squats

- Take a comfortable stance, wide enough to squat down between your legs. Place your arms at your sides or up in front of you.

- Inhale, then lower yourself down as you exhale. Go as low as you comfortably can, pause, then inhale as you return to standing.

- Repeat at the pace you naturally breathe. Breathe through your nose. If you need to exhale through your mouth, keep a little tension in your lips.

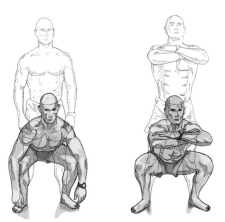

Tempo	4 seconds down/pause/4 seconds up
Reps	work up to 100

Feldenkrais Hip/Pelvis Integrator

- Lie on your back and bend your left leg, with your left arm at your side.

- Gently push onto your left foot so that you just barely lift your pelvis up.

- You should use as little effort as possible; imagine that you have a puppet string attached to the front of your pelvis, that it is lifting you up.

- Perform 10-20 repetitions, progressively rolling your pelvis over and lifting just one vertebra off the ground with each repetition. Lower the vertebrae one at a time in the opposite order.

- Make sure to relax. With each rep, allow your hips and chest to open up.

Tempo	slow
Reps	10 - 20 each side, or until you roll onto your side

Alternating Leg Drop

- Lie on your back.

- Bend your knees, keeping your feet together as you perform the exercise.

- Let your legs gently drop to the side, one at a time. Try to allow the energy of the lowering leg to assist the other leg as it is rises.

- Return to the start position one leg at a time.

Tempo	slow
Reps	10 each side

Leg Tuck

- Lie on your back with your knees bent.

- Inhale, then draw your legs into your chest as you exhale (you may open the legs to pull them in closer).

- Inhale again as you return your legs to the floor.

Tempo	slow with a natural pause between breaths
Reps	10

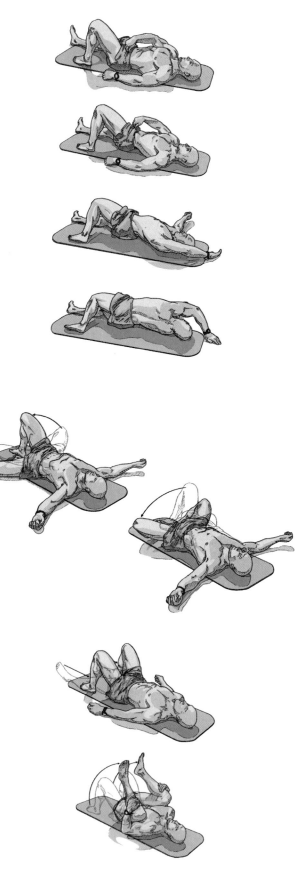

Pelvic Rock Exercises

Front to Back

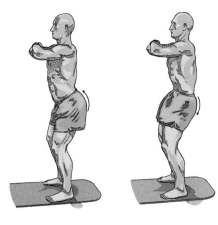

- Stand with soft knees, or sit upright on a Swiss ball.
- Inhale and rotate your pelvis forward (imagine that you have headlights on your butt and shine them up).
- Keep your trunk still as you move your pelvis.
- Exhale and rotate your pelvis back (shine the headlights down).

Tempo	breathing pace
Reps	10 each side

Side to Side

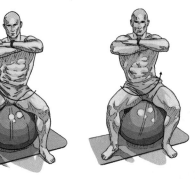

- Inhale and lift one hip up as you exhale, then return to the start position.
- Inhale and lift the other hip up as you exhale.
- Repeat going side-to-side.

Tempo	breathing pace
Reps	10 each side

Figure Eight

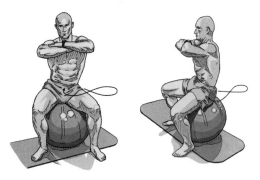

- Complete a figure eight, moving front-to-back and then side-to-side.
- Breathe as you did for the other pelvic rock exercises.

Tempo	breathing pace
Reps	10 each side

Horse Stance Dynamic

- On your hands and knees, place your wrists directly below the shoulders and your knees directly below the hips.

- Your legs should be parallel and elbows should remain turned back toward your thighs with your fingers directed forward.

- Inhale and raise your right arm up and out to a 45-degree angle and lift your left leg as high as you can without your pelvis swaying to the side.

- Exhale and tuck your elbow and knee in under your torso so that the elbow goes past the knee. Use your abdominals to pull you to the end of the movement.

- Repeat set on one side, rest and repeat on other side.

Tempo	breathing pace
Reps	10 each side

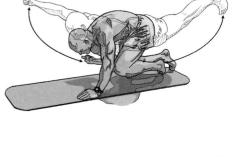

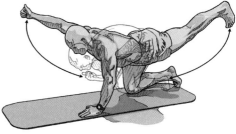

Piston Breathing

- Stand in a relaxed posture.

- Take a deep breath in, allowing your belly to expand.

- Exhale forcefully through your nose. (If you cannot breathe through your nose, exhale through your mouth while pursing your lips like a trumpet player).

Tempo	slow inhalation, pulsing exhalation
Reps	up to 100 pulses

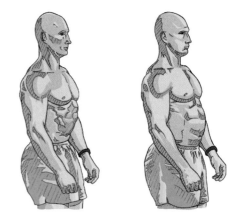

Swiss Ball Crunch

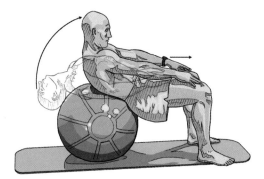

Caution: If you get dizzy when looking up at the sky or reaching into cupboards overhead, you may move a little more forward on the ball to perform this exercise. Stop this exercise immediately if you feel dizzy. This indicates a decrease in the blood supply to the brain and may be a symptom of vertebral artery occlusion. Consult your medical professional or C.H.E.K Practitioner.

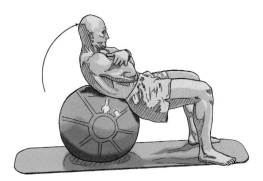

- Lie over a Swiss ball so that your back is comfortably on the ball. Your head should be extended back and touching the ball.

- Your tongue should be on the roof of your mouth.

- As you slowly crunch up, imagine rolling your spine from head to pelvis.

- On the way back, unwind from the low back to your head, one vertebra at a time.

- Exhale on the way up and inhale on the way back.

Arm positioning:

Beginner – arms reaching forward

Intermediate – arms across chest

Advanced – finger tips behind ears (do not support your head and neck with your hands)

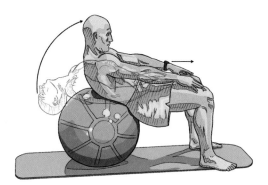

| Tempo | slow, breathing pace |
| Reps | up to 20 |

Energy Push

- Stand with your arms raised straight out in front of you.

- Inhale and bring your hands back in towards your body.

- Exhale and push your arms straight out with the intent of projecting energy from your core out of your arms and hands.

- Repeat, pushing to the center, front left, front right and back left and back right.

- As you push to the sides and back, keep your feet planted and turn your body towards the direction you are pushing.

- For the back position, only go as far as you comfortably can. Do not over-rotate your spine.

- The motion through the rib cage massages the organs of digestion.

Tempo	slow, breathing pace
Reps	20 total

Wood Chop

- Stand upright and bring your arms over your head as you inhale.

- Exhale as you come down, bending at the waist, as if you were chopping wood.

- There should be a natural pause at the end of the movement.

- Alternate your chopping; left, right and center.

Tempo	slow, breathing pace
Reps	21 total

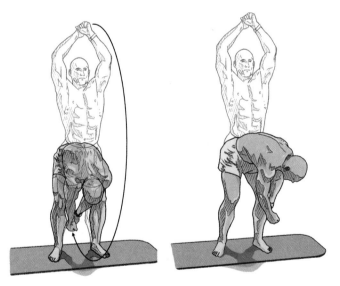

Zone 4

McKenzie Press-up

- Lie face down with your hands just outside the top of your shoulders.
- As you exhale, push yourself up, keeping your pelvis on the floor.
- Relax your back and butt.
- Inhale on the return.

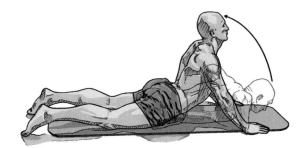

Tempo	slow, breathing pace
Reps	10

Feldenkrais Shoulder/Spine Integrator

Phase I
- Lie on your side with a foam roller, or towel just big enough to maintain good neck alignment, placed under your head. Your neck should be parallel with the floor.
- Your hips and knees should be at 90-degree angles, with your feet on top of each other.
- Place your top hand on your forehead and gently rotate your neck backwards as you inhale.
- Exhale as you return to the start position.
- Perform 10-20 reps, allowing your neck to rotate a little further and your arm drop a little closer to the floor each time.

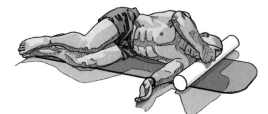

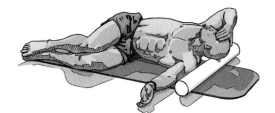

Phase II
- Assume the same starting position as Phase I, but place your arms out in front and on top of each other.
- Inhale as you slide the top hand across the bottom arm and your body.
- Exhale as you return, sliding as far forward as you comfortably can, allowing your top hand and wrist to glide over your bottom hand.

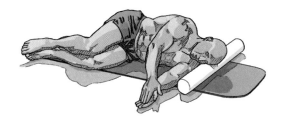

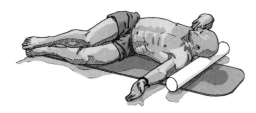

Tempo	slow
Reps	10 - 20 each side

Prone Cobra

- Lie face down with your arms at your sides.

- As you inhale, pick your chest off the floor while simultaneously squeezing your shoulder blades together and rotating your arms out so that your palms face away from your body.

- Keep your head and neck in neutral alignment, with your toes on the floor.

- You should feel the muscles between your shoulder blades doing the work. If you feel stress in your low back, squeeze your butt cheeks together prior to lifting your torso.

- Hold until you need to breathe out, and exhale as you lower your torso to the floor.

Tempo	slow, breathing pace
Reps	10 - 20

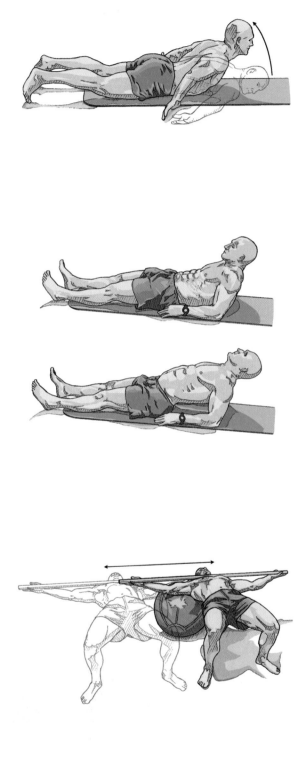

The Fish

- Lie back, resting on your arms.

- Inhale, pick your chest up as high as you can.

Tempo	10 seconds and relax
Reps	10

Lateral Ball Roll

- From a sitting position on a Swiss ball, roll back so that your head, shoulders and upper back are supported by the ball.

- Lift your hips up so that they are in line with your knees and shoulders.

- Place your tongue on the roof of your mouth.

- Hold your body in perfect alignment (hips and arms should stay parallel to the floor) and shuffle your feet as you roll across the ball to one side.

- Pause, then return back to the center.

- Move only as far to the side as you comfortably can, while holding perfect alignment. You may find that you can only move an inch or two; that is fine.

Tempo	hold end position for 3 seconds
Reps	5 each side

Zone 5

Neck Ball Exercises

- Stand next to a wall or post.
- Use 50% effort for the following exercises.

Tempo	breathing pace
Reps	10 each side

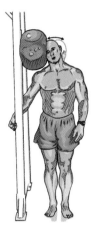

Neck side bend

- Place the side of your face slightly under the ball.
- Bend your head into the ball as you exhale.

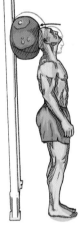

Neck extension

- Place the back of your head against the ball.
- You may hold onto the doorway for support.
- Press your head into the ball as you exhale.

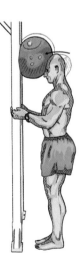

Neck flexion

- Face ball.
- Place your tongue on the roof of your mouth.
- Push your head into the ball as you exhale.

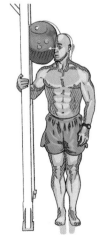

Neck rotation

- Place the side of your head behind the apex of the ball.
- Turn your head into the ball as you inhale and back out as you exhale.

Neck Rotations

- Let your head drop down naturally as you exhale.

- Rotate it around slowly, letting it follow your natural range of motion barrier, inhale as you begin moving to the side and back.

- Spend extra time in tight zones; imagine that you are breathing through the tight muscles.

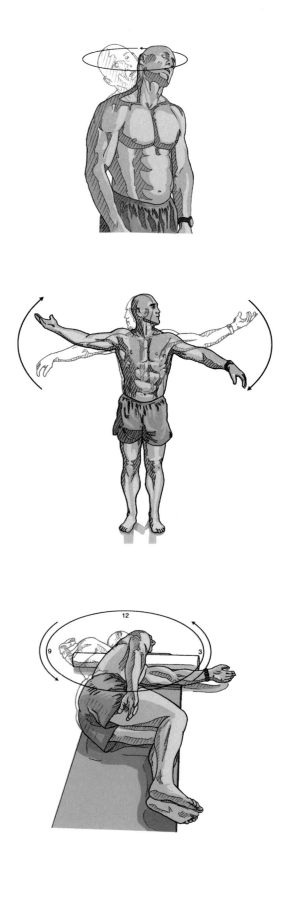

Tempo	slow, breathing pace
Reps	up to 20 each direction

Thoracic Mobilization

- Hold arms straight out to the side, stay relaxed.

- Turn your right arm up and left arm down.

- As you look down the left arm, slightly contract the right arm as you turn the palm up and inhale at the same time.

- When you naturally want to exhale, turn your head to the other side and reverse arm positions, repeating to the opposite side.

Tempo	breathing pace
Reps	10 each side

Shoulder Clocks

- Stand or lie down on your side with your knees bent.

- Visualize that your shoulder is in the middle of a clock.

- Elevate your shoulder toward your ear (12 o'clock), then roll your shoulder either forward (1, 2, 3 o'clock) or backward (11, 10, 9 o'clock) around the clock. Inhale as you move through the back half of the clock (7 - 12 o'clock) and exhale as you move through the front half of the clock (1 - 6 o'clock).

- Keep your head looking forward and hand relaxed.

Tempo	breathing pace
Reps	10 circles each direction

Zone 6

Alternate Nostril Breathing

- Plug one nostril with a finger or your thumb.
- Breathe in—your chest should rise in the last 1/3 of your breath only.
- Breathe out through your nostril, keeping the other one plugged.
- Try to breathe in and out for the same amount of time; i.e. 5 seconds in and 5 seconds out.
- Alternate nostrils with each complete breath or with each inhalation.

Tempo	slow
Reps	10 times each side

This exercise balances the left and right sides of your brain and the autonomic nervous system.

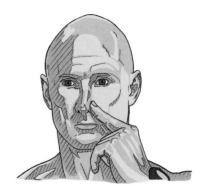

Eye Rolling

- Look to the left and inhale as you roll your eyes around in a circle.
- Start breathing out as your eyes look downward and inhale as they move upward.
- You may find one direction is harder or that your head wants to move in one direction; work in that direction more.

Tempo	breathing pace
Reps	5 - 10 each direction

Precaution: If you get a headache from this exercise, consult an optometrist.

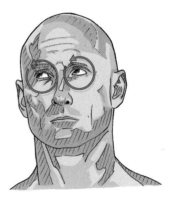

Cross Crawl

- Raise your arms up.
- Pick up your left leg and bring your right elbow to the left knee as you exhale.
- Alternate sides.

Tempo	breathing pace
Reps	10 - 20 each side

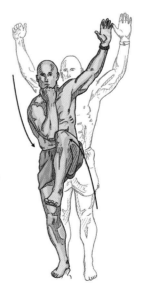

Face Energizer

- Breathe in and look up toward the ceiling.

- Open your mouth and eyes wide and stick your tongue out.

- Exhale and look down, contracting your face muscles as you sigh a big sigh of relief.

Tempo	slow
Reps	10

This exercise helps improve your energy if you feel tired.

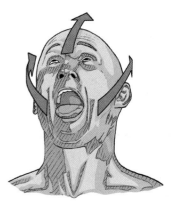

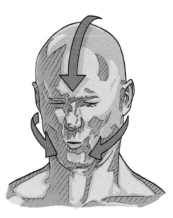

Scalp Shifting

- Contract your scalp muscles as you inhale and relax your scalp as you exhale.

- Looking up with your eyes as you contract your scalp muscles improves the energy flow.

Tempo	2 seconds up and back, 2 seconds down and in
Reps	10

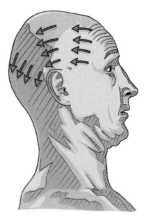

Sifu Fong Ha

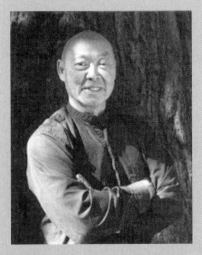

Sifu Fong Ha has been practicing Chinese internal arts since his childhood and has studied with many renowned teachers. He began his studies of Yang-style Taijiquan in 1953 with Tung Yin Chieh, and continued with Yang Sau-Chung, the eldest son of Yang Cheng-fu. His training in the Internal System of Martial Arts, Yiquan, was with Master Han Sing-Yuan, a disciple of Master Wang Hsin-Chai, the founder of the Yiquan, also known as Dachenquan.

One of the few I Ch'uan teachers in the West, Fong Ha is well known for his power, graciousness and cosmopolitan charm. With humor and insight, he encourages students to be true to themselves, to recognize their inner strengths, develop at their own pace and actualize their potentials. He directs the Integral Chuan Institute in Berkeley, California and teaches nationally and internationally. He is the author of *Yiquan and the Nature of Energy: The fine art of doing nothing and achieving everything*.

Sifu Fong Ha has been teaching Ta Chi Chuan and Qigong in the Bay Area since 1968 while serving as a Public School teacher with San Francisco Unified School District. After his retirement from the School System, he now devotes his time in teaching and sharing his arts for cultivating vital energy and maintaining good health. You can reach him via his website: www.fongha.com.

Approach

Just as the bud of a flower contains within it the innate form of the perfect flower, so do we all contain within ourselves the innate form of our own perfection. Under the proper conditions of sun, water and nutrients, the bud unfolds to reveal the flower. Likewise under the proper conditions of our practice, that which is perfect within us—physically, mentally and spiritually—begins to unfold.

Essence

Chi Kung (Qigong) practice is expressed in four fundamental disciplines:

- Sitting meditation
- Standing meditation (Wu Chi Chi Kung or Wuji Qigong)
- Intention practice (I Ch'uan or yiquan)
- Tai Chi Ch'uan

We begin with sitting and standing meditation. Qigong, literally "practice of vital energy," helps us break through a lifetime of old habits and programmed patterns of behavior and movement, allowing what is essential in us to come forth. This practice cultivates Chi, breaks down blocks to the free flow of Chi throughout the body and integrates the upper and lower body.

I Ch'uan (or "intention practice") develops our ability to direct chi through focusing the intention. In the broader sense, this practice develops our ability to focus the mind for improved concentration, creativity and productivity.

From stillness, we begin to move. Practice of the 108 moves of the Tai Chi Ch'uan long form further develops Chi, builds strength in movement, stamina and the ability to relax in strength. At the highest level of practice, the movements of the form become informed or filled by Chi.

To Your Health

It's difficult to be healthy in an unhealthy environment, and unfortunately we live in an unhealthy environment. Through the diligent practice of Qigong, we cultivate our Chi, which then begins to flow freely throughout the body, strengthening the weak points and reinforcing the strong points, and providing a defense against the insults of air pollution, toxins in our foods and water and the stresses of our fast-paced lives.

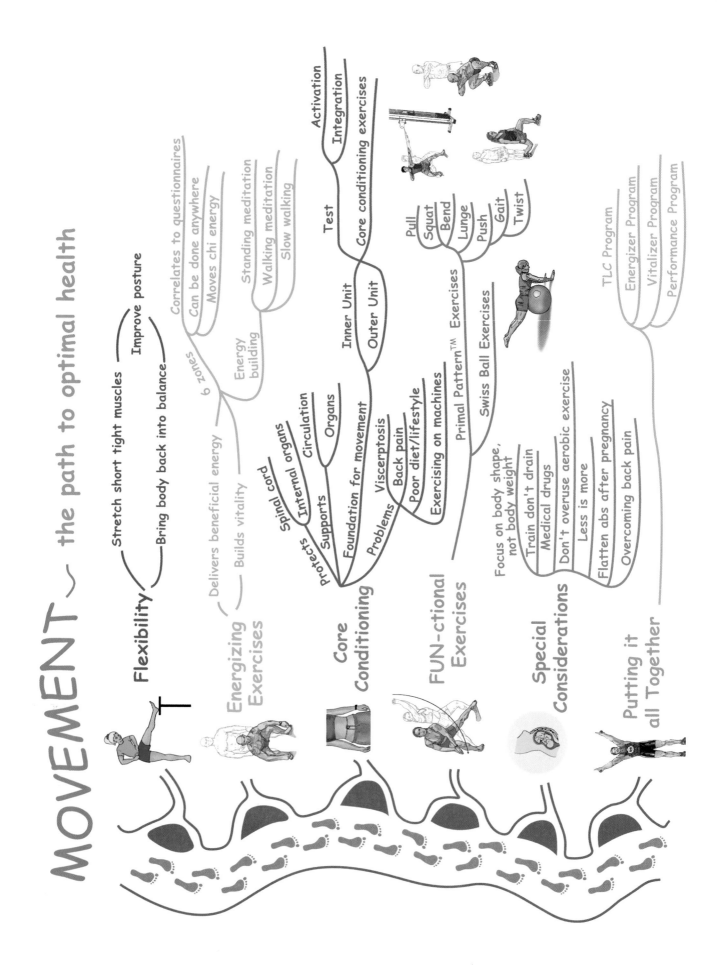

MOVEMENT ~ the path to optimal health

Flexibility
- Stretch short tight muscles
  - Improve posture
  - Bring body back into balance

Energizing Exercises
- Delivers beneficial energy
  - Builds vitality
- 6 zones
  - Correlates to questionnaires
  - Can be done anywhere
  - Moves chi energy
- Energy building
  - Standing meditation
  - Walking meditation
  - Slow walking

Core Conditioning
- Spinal cord
  - Protects
  - Internal organs
  - Circulation
  - Supports
  - Organs
- Foundation for movement
  - Problems
    - Viscerptosis
    - Back pain
    - Poor diet/lifestyle
    - Exercising on machines
- Inner Unit
- Outer Unit
  - Test
  - Activation
  - Integration
  - Core conditioning exercises

FUN-ctional Exercises
- Primal Pattern™ Exercises
  - Pull
  - Squat
  - Bend
  - Lunge
  - Push
  - Gait
  - Twist
- Swiss Ball Exercises

Special Considerations
- Focus on body shape, not body weight
- Train don't drain
- Medical drugs
- Don't overuse aerobic exercise
- Less is more
- Flatten abs after pregnancy
- Overcoming back pain

Putting it all Together
- TLC Program
- Energizer Program
- Vitalizer Program
- Performance Program

GETTING TO THE CORE

The core is your entire torso, including internal organs. Many people think the extremities perform most tasks and that the core is simply along for the ride. In truth, the extremities rely on the core for stabilization and force production. You can think of your core as an action center. The core is very complex and serves many vital functions that contribute to your overall health. Let's take a look at key core functions in order to appreciate the importance of this area of your body and better understand why I have placed so much emphasis on it.

Core Functions

Protection of your central nervous system and internal organs

The core provides a protective shield for your spinal cord and internal organs. The bony spinal column houses the spinal cord (part of your nervous system), while the rib cage and powerful outer abdominal muscles act as a shield to protect your internal organs from external blows or invasion. The shield function is one of the reasons Nature has developed our rectus abdominis muscle in short muscular blocks, giving it the beloved washboard look.

Support for your internal organs

The core houses all internal organs with the exception of those vital organs in the head, such as the brain and eyes (Figure 1). When the body moves and is exercised correctly, the internal organs are mobilized. This natural mobilization helps keep your organs from adhering together, improves fluid flow through the organs and is very helpful to maintaining normal bowel habits. When key core

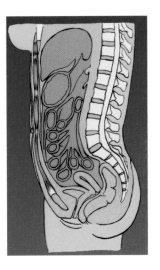

Figure 1: The core houses most of your internal organs, providing both protection and support for these vital organs.

muscles stop functioning correctly, support for your internal organs is diminished and their function is challenged.

Circulatory support

Behind the abdominal organs, along the spine, lies the largest artery in the body, the *abdominal aorta*, and the largest vein in the body, the *inferior vena cava*. When the body moves correctly and is properly exercised, pressure changes occur in the core that assists the heart and extremity muscles to circulate blood and lymphatic fluid throughout the body. If for any reason the core stops functioning correctly, the heart not only has to work harder, but the fluids flowing through the core become relatively stagnant. If your core function diminishes and you can't effectively move fluids through your organs, the chances of fungal and parasite infections, constipation and disease increases, while your energy levels progressively decrease.

Foundation for movement

The core is your body's foundation for movement. If the core does not function properly, you'll most likely experience extremity and spinal pain, as well as increased chances of injury.

How the Core Works

Based on purpose, the core can be divided into two functional units—the *Inner* and *Outer Units*. Though these two systems always work together, it's helpful to divide the core muscles into functional groups to better understand an otherwise *very complex system.*

The inner unit

The inner unit of the core consists of four major muscle groups that work as a system (Figure 2). The major inner unit muscles are the deep muscles running along the spine (multifidus), the muscles of the pelvic floor, the deepest abdominal muscle (transversus abdominis [TVA]) and the large breathing muscle (diaphragm). Two other muscles, the internal oblique and large latissimus dorsi, also play a part in inner unit function.

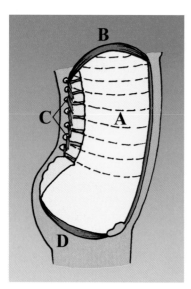

Figure 2: The Inner Unit.
A. TVA B. Diaphragm
C. Multifidus D. Pelvic Floor

The inner unit muscles are unique because they function together like a well-tuned crew of rowers. Their primary job with regard to movement is to stiffen the spine, rib cage and pelvic girdle so that the head, arms and legs have a stable working foun-

dation. Current research indicates that if your body functions correctly, the inner unit muscles "turn on" about 30 milliseconds before arm movement and about 110 milliseconds before leg movement. This happens regardless of the direction or speed of limb motion.[1]

"You can't fire a cannon from a canoe" is an old saying that describes the importance of inner unit function to the stability of your body. Stabilization begins in the core during functional movements and migrates into the periphery. If your inner unit stops functioning correctly, you can't effectively stabilize your core or extremities and you're much more likely to be injured, particularly in the lower back, where there's a lot of load on the spine. In other words, lack of inner unit functionality makes you the unstable canoe, and moving your arms or legs quickly equates to firing the cannon, which wouldn't be a good idea—unless you like swimming with your canoe. If your body works correctly and can stabilize, movement of your arms and legs takes place from a more stable platform, which would be like firing a cannon from a battle ship.

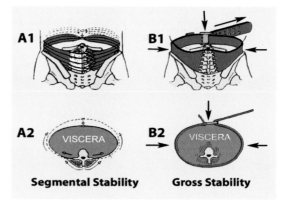

Figure 3: The TVA, your natural weight belt, offers more effective stabilization of the core, especially the spine, than a weight belt.

Improved stability is created for the spine and lower extremities through the action of the transversus abdominis (TVA) on the lower back and pelvis. As you can see in Figure 3 (A1 & A2), when the belly button is naturally drawn inward by TVA contraction during efforts to stabilize, the two halves of the pelvis are drawn toward each other like a nutcracker. When the TVA contracts, the large sheet of connective tissue (thoracolumbar fascia) that attaches to the bony prominences of the lumbar spine are pulled upon from both sides, resulting in increased stability on both sides of the spine at once. Unfortunately, many people mistakenly believe that wearing a weight belt or lumbar corset will increase spinal stability. Weight belts and corsets are generally wide in the back, which reduces the natural range of motion of the lumbar spine. Restricting upper lumbar motion with a tight belt often exaggerates lower lumbar motion in compensation, usually at the lowest vertebral level (L5/S1). This area is already the most commonly injured segment of the lower back. As you can see in Figure 3 (B1 & B2), regardless of how tight the belt, there is no way to create multi-dimensional stability of the spine because without inner unit contraction there is no stabilizing force on the spine. Therefore, any benefits gained by the belt may soon be lost due to injury and pain. This is why I always tell my clients, "Don't buy a girdle—build one!"

The deep abdominal wall (TVA) is ideally suited to perform the girdle-like supportive functions that allow you to have a flat stomach. The dreaded *paunch belly* is but one of the many ill effects of a dysfunctional abdominal wall. There are several reasons for paunch bellies and the more advanced condition, *visceroptosis* (visceral = organs, ptosis (toe-sis) = drooping). (Figure 5)

Factors That Can Disrupt Abdominal Muscle Function

Organs talk to muscles

Internal organs borrow their pain-sensitive nerve fibers from the muscular system. This means that when an organ is in pain, the brain can't determine if it's the muscle or the organ that hurts. The brain only knows which segment of the spine (as illustrated by a piano key on the keyboard in Figure 4) the pain message came from. In return, the brain then tells all the tissues and organs on that nerve channel to behave like they're in pain. Since pain always weakens muscles, the abdominal muscles generally lose tone and don't respond to exercise like a muscle that doesn't think it's in pain!

While this may sound like a radical concept, you're probably more familiar with this phenomenon than you realize. For example, when someone is about to have a heart attack, they don't feel pain in their heart, but rather on the left side of their chest and in the left arm muscles. Many women have pain in their back and sometimes down their legs during their menstrual period, not just in the area of their female organs. Further, people often suffer from back pain when they're constipated and find that a laxative or enema eliminates the pain. Organs talk to muscles all the time—we just have to learn to listen.

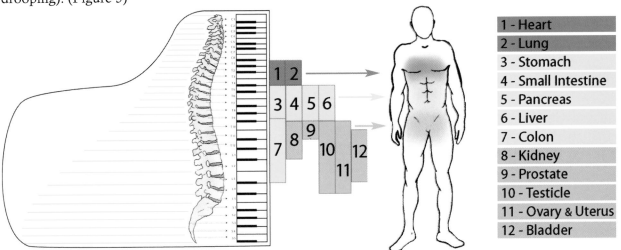

1 -	Heart
2 -	Lung
3 -	Stomach
4 -	Small Intestine
5 -	Pancreas
6 -	Liver
7 -	Colon
8 -	Kidney
9 -	Prostate
10 -	Testicle
11 -	Ovary & Uterus
12 -	Bladder

Figure 4: Your body has many different reflex pathways. The segments of your spine are like the keys of a piano. Different organs, muscles, etc., will send messages to different segments of the spine and vice versa. If you have pain in your lower back, those pain signals may be sent to your digestive organs and abdominals as well. You may not necessarily feel pain in these areas, but the organs and muscles will behave like they are in pain and not function as they should. This may result in impaired digestion or abdominal weakness.

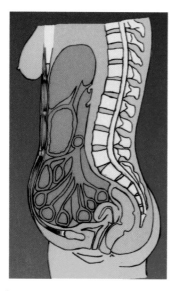

Figure 5: Visceroptosis is when the organs, or viscera, drop or fall down from their optimal position.

Visceroptosis

Visceroptosis is a common problem, particularly among females. When the body's natural girdle (particularly the TVA) becomes defective, it can no longer support the internal organs. Constipation can cause the large transverse colon to become enlarged and heavy. If the abdominal wall is not able to provide support, the colon, liver and stomach begin to droop, putting abnormal pressure on the rest of the digestive tract and the underlying uterus and bladder. This can lead to increased menstrual pain, incontinence and prostate-related problems.

Diet/lifestyle

Consuming foods and/or drinks that you're allergic or intolerant to will affect your abdominal function. Anything that causes inflammation of an internal organ that communicates through the nervous system and controls an abdominal muscle will cause the muscle to weaken and/or be non-responsive to exercise. Other causes of inflammation in the organs that communicate with your abdominal muscles are stress, alcohol consumption, medical drugs, food additives, preservatives and colorings. There is also suspicion growing among holistic-minded scientists and healthcare professionals that eating irradiated foods and foods that have been heated by microwave ovens cause inflammation in your digestive organs.

Back pain

Nerves that feed the joints of the spine are branches of the nerves that feed the muscles around the spine. Therefore, anything that causes pain in the spine between the area near the bottom of your sternum (chest bone) and the bottom of your spine can stop the muscles from working correctly. It's also important to realize that this works both ways: If a muscle is in pain, those messages are sent to the related organ(s), resulting in the organ(s) behaving as if it were in pain.

Dirty machine tricks

I can't tell you how many clients I've had who just couldn't flatten their abdominal wall despite regular visits to the gym for months—or even years. Many sought help with back pain, sacroiliac joint problems, or pain in the hip, knee or ankle, while others were just frustrated because they couldn't get rid of their paunch belly. In many cases, these clients had logged hundreds of hours exercising on conventional gym machines (ab crunch machines, leg presses, hamstring curl machines, knee extension, butt blaster machines, etc.), looked great on the outside—to the untrained eye—but could not eliminate their paunch.

This happens, in part, because your nervous system, in its effort to stabilize the spine, doesn't want to do any more work to activate the deep abdominal muscles than it has to. After all, how much stabilization do you need when you're *bolted to the floor* and wearing a seat belt! Your brain only activates the muscles in direct relation to the demand. The machine's resistance challenges the outer unit (bigger muscles designed to move the body) while doing a great job of stabilizing the load with large bolts, pins and rails. The result is a massive recruitment of the big muscles with relatively little, if any, significant contraction of the smaller stabilizer muscles crossing the working joints.

The dirty trick is that though some of your muscles get stronger on the machines, your stabilizer system does not get equally as strong. You probably won't be able to lift anything close to the same weight

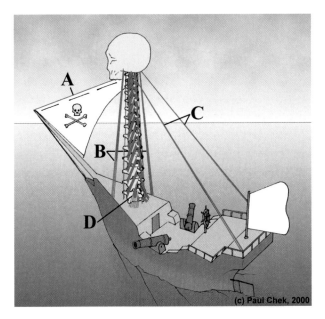

(c) Paul Chek, 2000

Figure 6:
The mast of this pirate ship represents your spine.
A. Rectus Abdominis (six-pack muscle)
B. Internal and External Obliques (muscles along the sides of your torso)
C. Erector Spinae (larger muscles along spine)
D. Segmental Stabilizers (smaller inner unit muscles of the spine)

with a barbell or dumbbells that you can lift on a machine. If you can lift the same amount, your form will most likely be poor due to lack of support from your under-trained stabilizer muscles. The appearance of new, bigger muscles from working out on the machines may provide false confidence—until you try to pick up the equivalent free weight, a squirming child or a heavy power tool. In any of these cases, you're likely to get hurt because you can't stabilize your spine or the extremity joints being used. Though the body has a number of neurological stopgaps to prevent such an injury, in many instances the person with an unbalanced muscular system can generate enough force in a short enough time that the nervous system can't react. The result is injury. This is but one of many reasons I suggest that you do **not** use gym machines. Instead, stick to free weights and other forms of functional exercise.

Note: I consider dumbbells, barbells and cable machines such as the lat. pull down, low row and cable cross over machines to be "free weights" because they allow unrestricted motion in any direction.

The outer unit

The Outer Unit is comprised of those muscles that are best designed to *move* the body. These muscles are generally larger than those in the inner unit, usually cross multiple joints and are easily seen on the surface of the body. Bodybuilders have likely focused on training these muscles because they're visible and are generally larger than the inner unit (stabilizer) muscles.

Outer unit muscles are like the engine in your car, and the inner unit muscles are like the suspension system and the bolts that hold the frame together and the wheels on; *it doesn't really matter how strong your engine is if your frame breaks or your wheels fall off!*

To better understand how the inner and outer units interact, follow along as I walk you through Figure 6. Imagine your body is a pirate ship. If the mast were comprised of 24 mobile segments like the human spine, you'd need a series of little muscles to hold them together so the mast could stand upright. Now consider that the large guy lines holding up the mast of the pirate ship are the large outer unit muscles. If you tighten the big outer unit muscles through exercise without proportionately tightening and strengthening the little inner unit muscles along the spine, the mast (spine) would eventually collapse.

Guy-wire A represents your rectus abdominis. If you perform too many crunches and sit-ups relative to extension exercises, your mast (spine) will begin to bend forward. This is why so many so-called "fit people" have such poor posture.

Testing and Integration of Your Inner and Outer Units

To find out if your inner unit is functioning correctly and to determine where you should start with your core conditioning exercises, complete the following tests. If you do not pass any of the tests, you will need to practice either the test or the other recommended exercises. These exercises will help you regain proper core function. Once you can easily perform the test exercises correctly you are ready to move onto the more advanced core conditioning exercises.

Core Function Tests

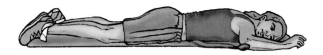

1. TVA Activation Test

- Lie face down, with a blood pressure cuff placed under your belly button.

- Exhale then inflate the cuff to 40mmHg.

- Relax your body and draw your belly button upward, off the cuff.

- Do not let yourself cheat by pressing on the floor with your shoulders, knees or feet, or by tucking your tail under—simply draw your belly button in.

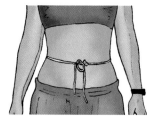

The goal is to decrease the pressure in the cuff by at least 10mmHg. If you cannot do that, you will need to practice the 4-Point Tummy Vacuum Exercise (page 126). Try this test each week until you're successfully able to pass it.

2. Forward Bend Test

- Cut a section of string long enough to tie around your waist. Stand upright, take a deep breath and draw your belly button inward. With your belly button drawn, tie the string around your waist. It should feel tight if you let your stomach hang out.

- Place an object in front of you (a weight—one that you can pick-up comfortably, but is not too light, is ideal). Now bend over and pick-up the object. Repeat a few times and notice what happens around the string.

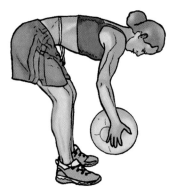

If you feel the string around your waist tightening or staying the same, your TVA is most likely not activating. You should feel the string loosen as you bend forward and your TVA turns on to stabilize the spine as you bend and lift the weight. If you did not pass this test, practice the 4-Point Tummy Vacuum and progress to the Swiss ball exercises on pages 132-135.

As your performance improves with the lower abdominal exercises, you should practice wearing the string around your waist in the house or even at work. This will serve as a reminder to properly activate your TVA before picking up or moving any object. When this becomes automatic, you can stop using the string.

Core Function Tests

3. Lower Abdominal Coordination Test

• Lie on your back with your knees fully bent.

• Place one hand under your lower back (or both if more comfortable), then bring your feet off of the floor.

• Tilt your pelvis backward and flatten your back against your fingers.

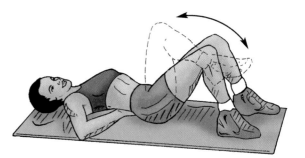

• Hold pressure, keeping the bony prominences of your spine on your fingers as you lower your feet to the ground.

• Pay attention to the bones of the spine as they press your fingers, not the muscles, for accurate testing.

If you cannot maintain the pressure of your spine on your fingers as you lower your feet to the ground, you've lost the ability to coordinate pelvic stabilization along with leg movement. This is a common cause of low back pain. However, you can retrain your abdominal muscles by performing Lower Abdominal 1, 2 and 3 on pages 126 and 127.

4-Point Tummy Vacuum

- Assume a kneeling position with your hips over your knees and your shoulders over your hands. With your spine in neutral alignment, take a deep breath in and let your belly drop toward the floor.

- Exhale and draw your belly button in toward your spine, while keeping your back in the start position.

- Hold (with the TVA activated) for as long as you comfortably can.

- When you need to breathe in, relax your abdominal wall as you inhale and repeat the exercise for 10 reps.

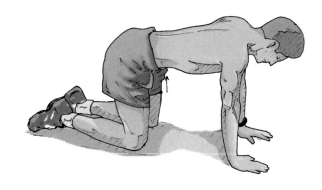

Lower Abdominal 1

- Lie on the ground with your knees bent and feet flat on the floor.

- Place a blood pressure cuff under your low back, directly underneath your belly button.

- Pump the blood pressure cuff to 40mmHg.

- Exhale, draw your belly button in toward your spine and gently increase pressure on the blood pressure cuff by rotating your tailbone toward the ceiling until the blood pressure cuff reads 70mmHg.

- Hold this position for as long as is comfortable, up to 10 seconds, then rest for 10 seconds.

- Repeat this 10 times.

- While performing this exercise, try to relax the entire body while holding the needle at 70mmHg; this includes your jaw, neck, shoulders, trunk and legs.

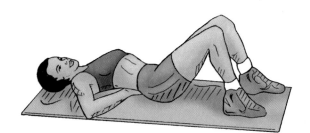

Lower Abdominal 2

- Lie on the ground with your knees bent and feet flat on the floor.

- Place a blood pressure cuff under your low back, directly underneath your belly button.

- Pump the blood pressure cuff to 40mmHg.

- Exhale, draw your belly button in toward your spine and gently increase pressure on the blood pressure cuff by rotating your tailbone toward the ceiling until the blood pressure cuff reads 70mmHg.

- Raise one foot off the ground until your thigh is perpendicular to the floor, keeping the needle of the blood pressure cuff at 70mmHg.

- Place the foot back on the ground and perform the same movement with the other leg.

- Alternate legs, performing 12-20 reps.

- If you have difficulty keeping the needle on 70mmHg, try using smaller leg movements.

- When it becomes easier to perform this exercise, straighten the lifting leg for an increased challenge.

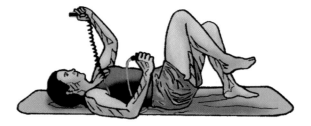

Lower Abdominal 3

- Lie on the ground with your knees bent and feet flat on the floor.

- Place a blood pressure cuff under your low back, directly underneath your belly button.

- Pump the blood pressure cuff to 40mmHg.

- With your knees bent, raise both legs off the ground until your thighs are perpendicular to the floor. The blood pressure cuff should read 70mmHg.

- Exhale, draw your belly button in toward your spine and slowly lower your one leg to the ground while keeping the needle on 70mmHg.

- Raise your legs back to the starting position and perform 12-20 repetitions.

- If you have difficulty keeping the needle on 70mmHg, try using smaller leg movements.

- When it becomes easier to perform this exercise, straighten your leg for an increased challenge, or lower both legs at the same time.

- Remember to keep your body relaxed.

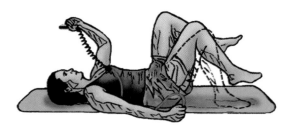

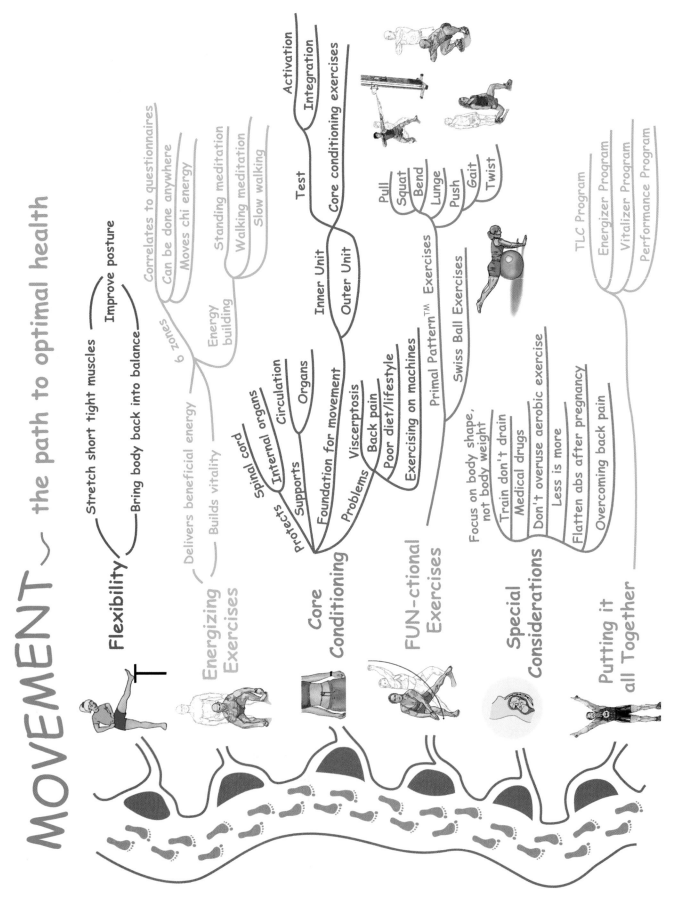

MOVEMENT ~ the path to optimal health

Flexibility
- Stretch short tight muscles — Improve posture
- Bring body back into balance

Energizing Exercises
- Delivers beneficial energy
- Builds vitality
  - 6 zones
    - Correlates to questionnaires
    - Can be done anywhere
    - Moves chi energy
  - Energy building
    - Standing meditation
    - Walking meditation
    - Slow walking

Core Conditioning
- Protects
  - Spinal cord
  - Internal organs
- Supports
  - Circulation
  - Organs
- Foundation for movement
- Problems
  - Viscerptosis
  - Back pain
  - Poor diet/lifestyle
  - Exercising on machines
- Inner Unit
- Outer Unit
  - Test
  - Core conditioning exercises
    - Activation
    - Integration

FUN-ctional Exercises
- Primal Pattern™ Exercises
  - Pull
  - Squat
  - Bend
  - Lunge
  - Push
  - Gait
  - Twist
- Swiss Ball Exercises

Special Considerations
- Focus on body shape, not body weight
- Train don't drain
- Medical drugs
- Don't overuse aerobic exercise
- Less is more
- Flatten abs after pregnancy
- Overcoming back pain

Putting it all Together
- TLC Program
- Energizer Program
- Vitalizer Program
- Performance Program

Chapter 8

FUN-CTIONAL EXERCISES

The term "functional exercise" has, unfortunately, fallen prey to the same abuse as the term "natural" and is quickly losing its meaning in the exercise industry. I interpret functional exercise to mean any exercise that works to achieve a chosen goal or objective. If you found that you were unable to achieve optimal performance in the Prone TVA activation test, Forward Bend Test or the Lower Ab Coordination Test (Chapter 6), your first objective should be to restore function to the abdominal wall. (See pages 124 through 127) By assuring that your brain is communicating properly with your inner unit and that your inner and outer units work synergistically together, you can safely move into the Primal Pattern™ exercises which will serve as the foundation for your future exercise programs.

Primal Pattern™ Movements

Once your inner and outer units are functioning correctly, it's time to discover *Primal Pattern™ Movements*. Primal Pattern Movements are the seven key movements that I feel were necessary for survival in our developmental environment. In other words, if you couldn't correctly perform these seven movement patterns quickly and effectively without thinking about what your body was doing, you probably wouldn't survive in the wild. Even though our lifestyle is very different from our developmental ancestors, these seven movement patterns are still key to performing daily tasks and staying injury free.

Squat: Early man had to squat to move heavy objects, build shelter and eat. Today, we still have to squat to sit on the toilet or a chair and get in and out of cars. Many of us continue to lift heavy objects on the job or in the gym.

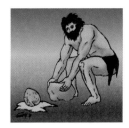

Bend: In order to build shelter, prepare food and lift objects, early man would have used a bend pattern. Today, the bend pattern is most often used by construction workers, nurses, parents (picking up their kids) or golfers (addressing the ball). Like all Primal Pattern Movements, bending is still required in our daily activities, and, if you can't do it correctly, your chances of injury escalate.

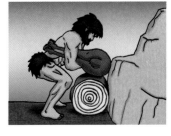

Lunge: Lunging was an essential Primal Pattern for traversing rough terrain. Today, you can see the lunge pattern used in most sports and even in the work place. While throwing, an athlete's failure to lunge correctly often results in shoulder injuries due to compensation. In the non-athlete, failure to lunge correctly greatly increases your chances of falling.

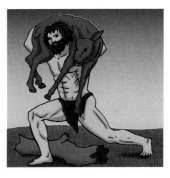

Falls causing hip fractures are one of the leading causes of death among the elderly. These incidents can often be avoided by mastering the lunge pattern.

Push: Pushing would have been a key pattern in moving heavy objects to build shelter or to clear land, and it may have been a successful tactic during fights. Anyone who has worked on a farm has had to herd animals into pens 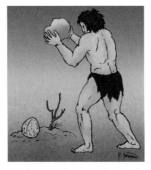 or shoots, load them onto trucks and occasionally push a sheep, horse, cow or pig. If you're pushing a loaded trolley that abruptly stops, for example, your pushing and stabilizing muscles had better be coordinated, or, you are likely to injure your back.

Pull: Once downed, a game animal isn't going to follow you home! Our ancestors would have had to pull heavy loads, like animals, to a safe 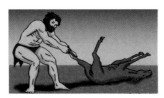 place. With the development of watercraft, rowing was a key movement for some tribes. Today, the pull pattern is seen in many sports and household activities.

Twist: Twisting may well be the most important of all the Primal Pattern Movements because it's an integral part of most functional activities. Twisting is rarely a pattern in itself but is a catalyst pattern that has great influence on the efficiency of any Primal Pattern. For example, twisting is an essential part of 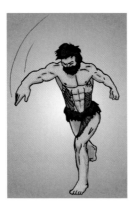 throwing, which was key for hunting and protection. The most common source of back injuries today is a movement that combines twisting and bending. Since twisting movements of the spine are integral to almost every movement performed in a functional environment, it's safe to say that if you can't twist correctly, *you must learn to do so because injury is lurking.*

Gait: Walking, jogging and sprinting are variations of what is technically called gait. Each of us has a walking gait, a jogging gait and a sprinting gait. As developmental beings, we generally used the most economical means of hunting and gathering because food wasn't always readily available. With a kill on his back, early man had to walk home through rough terrain. When it was important to communicate messages over long distances during times of battle or emergency, jogging was often employed (B in figure below), while running from a tiger or enemy may well have required all out sprinting (C in figure below). Today, all but those who are bed or wheelchair bound continue to walk, while a small segment of the population jogs and a smaller segment of the population (mostly athletes) still sprints. Though we won't cover exercises that target gait, your program contains numerous exercises that will contribute to your ability to perform all variations of gait more efficiently. An exercise such as the Supine Lateral Ball Roll will increase the stability of your pelvis and core, which will likely improve your gait and decrease your chance of injury.

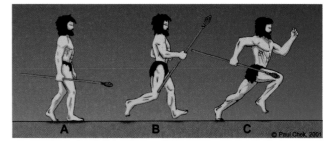

Many adults today lack good balance or motor skills because they didn't develop correctly as babies. When a baby is rushed through the reptilian (tummy crawling) and mammalian (dog crawling) phases and encouraged to walk too soon, inner and outer unit muscles don't properly learn to work together. To restore the ability to move correctly, you should include one or more Swiss ball exercises into your program. These Swiss ball exercises will stimulate and activate all the inner and outer unit muscles in preparation for Primal Pattern exercises.

One Chunk at a Time

Chunking describes how our nervous system learns portions of a movement. As we master one "chunk," we begin to learn and master the next chunk, until we have a new motor program. The process a baby goes through in order to learn how to walk is a common example of chunking.[1]

For another example of chunking, look at the throwing sequence below. The movement begins with a lunge as the first chunk (A), which accelerates the trunk, winding up the muscles that rotate so they store energy, much like the rubber tubes on a sling shot store energy when you stretch them. The twist movement is stacked atop the lunge as the second chunk of the throw pattern (B). Finally, like the tail of a whip, you see the arm coming through to push, or accelerate, the ball as the final chunk of the throw pattern (C). The inability to perform any given Primal Pattern, or chunk, will overload other body segments that must compensate to accomplish the motor task when multiple chunks or patterns must be used together.

Years of clinical observation and research have made me increasingly aware of the importance of improving Primal Pattern movement skills. After twenty years of conditioning athletes and rehabilitating orthopedic injuries, I am convinced that anyone with a lack of Primal Pattern movement is at much greater risk of injury due to motor skill deficiency. Implementing Primal Pattern training techniques will increase your ability to move efficiently and reduce your chance of injury.

On the following pages, you will find a variety of functional exercises to begin your exercise program. See Chapter 10 for sample programs and directions on putting together your own program.

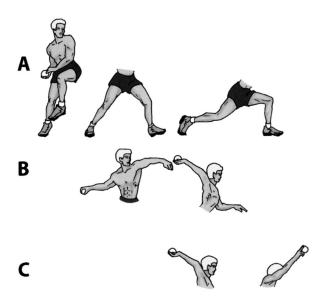

The throwing motion can be broken down into a series of Primal Patterns.
A. Lunge
B. Throw
C. Push.

Swiss Ball Exercises

Back Extension

- Lie face down over a Swiss ball.

- Keep your toes on the ground and lift your torso up.

- As you inhale, extend up, rotate your arms outward—draw your shoulder blades together and turn your palms outward.

- It is important to maintain good alignment: chin tucked and head in line with your spine.

- Slowly return to the starting position as you exhale.

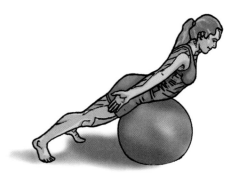

Reverse Hyperextension

- Lie face down over a Swiss ball with your hands on the floor.

- Your back and head should be in line.

- Inhale, then keep your legs straight as you raise them up as far as you comfortably can.

- Make sure your butt muscles are working, not just your back.

- Lower your legs back to the starting position as you exhale.

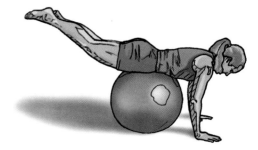

Swiss Ball Push-up

- Roll out over a Swiss ball into the plank position with your feet or shins on the ball (the farther the ball is from your torso, the harder the exercise will be).

- Place your hands below your shoulders with a comfortable width.

- Keep your spine and head in alignment; do not let your head drop forward or your lower back sag down. Draw your belly button inward, then drop your chest toward the ground, holding good alignment. Push back to the start position, maintaining perfect form.

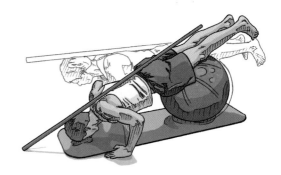

Swiss Ball Exercises

Forward Ball Roll

- Start by kneeling in front of a Swiss ball with your forearms just behind the apex of the ball. The angle at your hips and shoulders should be the same (imagine being able to place a box in the space between the back of your arms and your thighs).

- Gently draw the belly button inward and hold good alignment of your back and head.

- Roll forward, moving your legs and arms equally, so that the angles at the shoulders and hips remain equal. As you roll farther out, progressively increase the effort used to draw your belly button inward.

- Stop at the point just before you lose form. You will feel your low back drop down when your form breaks. You should stop just before this point.

- For beginners, go to the finish position and hold for 3 seconds, then return to the start position. Your tempo should be 3 seconds out, 3 seconds hold, 3 seconds return.

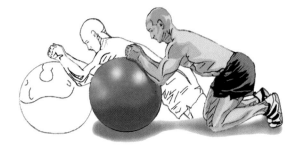

Lateral Ball Roll

- Begin by sitting on a Swiss ball. Roll down the ball so that your head, shoulder blades and upper back are comfortably supported by the ball, and raise your hips so your body is level.

- Place your tongue on the roof of your mouth and hold your body in perfect alignment. Begin shuffling your feet as you slowly roll to one side; when you reach the point where you feel like you will lose your perfect alignment or your balance on the ball, stop, hold for one second, then slowly return back to the starting position.

- Always keep your shoulders level, as shown.

- Keep your feet in alignment with your body except for the shuffling necessary to roll laterally.

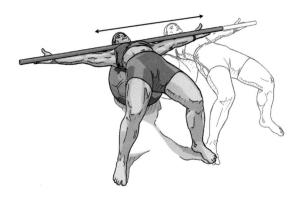

Swiss Ball Exercises

Twister-feet on Ball

- Start in a push-up position, with your feet on a Swiss ball and your hands on the floor; position your feet so you can grasp the ball with your feet and legs.

- Holding your spine in perfect alignment, draw your belly button gently in toward your spine.

- Slowly begin twisting your lower body to both sides, going as far as you can without losing perfect form.

- As you become more adept at performing this exercise, speeding up the tempo will make the exercise more challenging.

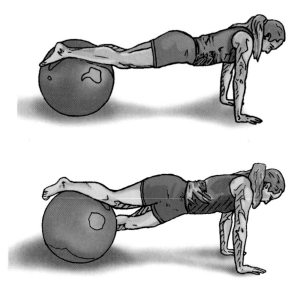

Swiss Ball Side Flexion

- Sit on a Swiss ball with your feet at the junction of a wall and the floor.

- Slowly rotate over the ball so one of your hips is squarely on top of the ball and your feet are securely anchored against the wall; the upper thigh of the top leg should be in line with your body.

- While lying sideways over the ball with your arms at your sides, slowly raise yourself sideways until your body is perpendicular to the floor; reverse the motion until you are once again at the starting position. Visualize curling up sideways one vertebra at a time, starting with your head.

- Increase the difficulty by placing your arms across your chest or raised above your head.

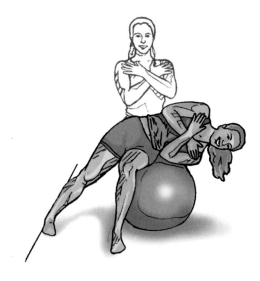

Swiss Ball Exercises

Russian Twist

- Roll back onto the ball so that your head, shoulders and upper back are supported by the ball.

- Lift your hips up so that they are in line with your knees and shoulders.

- Clasp your hands and raise your arms so that they point straight up toward the sky (holding a weight will make the exercise more challenging).

- Place your tongue on the roof of your mouth.

- Rotate the ball under you, going from side-to-side.

- Keep your head straight and look up at the ceiling; do not let your hips drop downward.

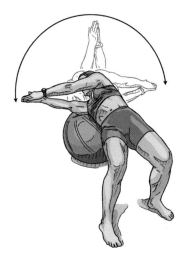

Jackknife

- Start by getting into a push-up position with your feet on a Swiss ball and your hands on the floor.

- Holding your spine in perfect alignment, draw your belly button gently in toward your spine.

- While maintaining neutral spinal alignment throughout the movement, draw your knees toward your chest, hold, then return to the start position.

- Your butt should not rise up in the air; only lift your hips as high as needed to bend your knees underneath you, keeping your butt as low as possible.

- This exercise can be made easier by placing the ball closer to your body; for example, on your shins.

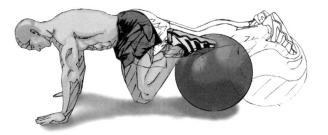

Primal Pattern™ Exercises

Included on the following pages are a variety of Primal Pattern Exercises for you to choose from when designing your own program. The level of each exercise is indicated by the symbols below.

E = ENERGIZER LEVEL   V = VITALIZER LEVEL   P = PERFORMANCE LEVEL

Choose only the exercises that are at your current exercise level or easier. Remember, your exercise level is based on your overall total score from your questionnaires. See Chapter 2 for the questionnaires and score chart.

See page 249 for a list of equipment resources.

Squat Exercises

Wall Squat

- Place a Swiss ball between your lower back and a wall.

- Take a comfortable stance, arms at your sides. You should be standing up straight, not leaning back onto the ball.

- Inhale and then lower yourself down into a squat as you exhale. Go as low as you comfortably can, then inhale as you return to standing.

- Breathe through your nose if you can. If you need to exhale through your mouth, purse your lips to keep a little tension in them.

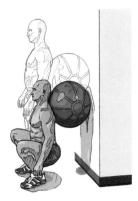

Breathing Squat

- Take a comfortable stance that is wide enough for you to squat down between your legs. Place your arms at your sides or up in front of you for a more advanced version.

- Inhale and then lower yourself down as you exhale. Go as low as you comfortably can, then inhale as you return to standing.

- Keep your torso upright and your weight between the balls of your feet and your heels.

- Breathe through your nose if you can. If you need to exhale through your mouth, purse your lips to keep a little tension in them.

- The pace at which you lower and raise yourself should perfectly match your breathing rate. Your breathing rhythm should stay the same throughout the exercise. If your breathing speeds up, reduce the depth.

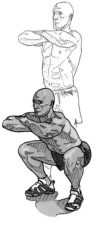

E = ENERGIZER LEVEL	V = VITALIZER LEVEL	P = PERFORMANCE LEVEL

Squat Exercises

Squat with Support   E

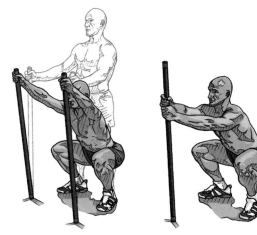

- Perform the above breathing squat while holding onto one or two supports. I recommend using a broom handle, Body Bar™ or dowel rod. These will provide you with enough assistance, yet are still unstable and will make the exercise more functional than if you used a stable object such as a doorway for support.

- Remember, only squat down as far as you comfortably can.

- As your strength increases, reduce the use of the support(s).

Overhead Squat   V   P

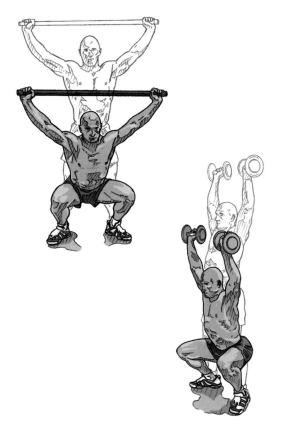

- Take a comfortable stance that is wide enough for you to squat down between your legs. Hold a bar or dumbbells (performance level only) straight above your head.

- Inhale and draw your belly button inward.

- Drop down into a comfortable squat. A wider stance is often needed for this version of the squat.

- Exhale through pursed lips as you stand up.

- Keep the weight above your head for the entire set.

Note: The breathing pattern is different for this version of the squat. Since you are now using additional weight, you will need to activate your inner unit more to stabilize—this is best done by keeping air in your diaphragm and drawing your belly button in as you descend into the squat. As you exhale and return to standing, it is important to keep your lips tight as you breathe out.

E = ENERGIZER LEVEL   V = VITALIZER LEVEL   P = PERFORMANCE LEVEL

Squat Exercises

Single Arm Overhead Squat P

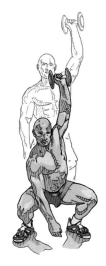

- Take a comfortable stance that is wide enough for you to squat down between your legs. Hold one dumbbell straight above your head.

- Inhale and draw your belly button inward.

- Drop down into a comfortable squat. Keep your torso as vertical as possible. Do not lean to one side.

- Exhale through pursed lips as you return to standing.

- Keep the weight above your head for the entire set, alternating arms each set.

Single Leg Squat P

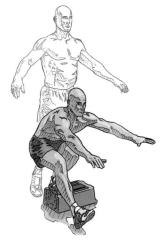

- Stand on the edge of a step or solid box.

- Hold one leg off the ground as you drop into a squat position, keeping your torso as upright as possible.

- The middle of the knee of your supporting leg should stay in alignment with your second toe during the exercise.

- When you return to standing, still on just one leg, think of pushing the ground away from you.

E = ENERGIZER LEVEL	V = VITALIZER LEVEL	P = PERFORMANCE LEVEL

Bend Exercises

Static Bend $\boxed{\text{E}}$

- From a standing position with your feet shoulder width apart, bend forward so that your hands rest just above your knees.

- Keep your head and spine in a neutral position.

- Hold that position for 30 – 60 seconds or for as long as you can with correct form.

- If you can hold this position for over 3 ½ minutes, progress to the kneeling bend.

Kneeling Bend $\boxed{\text{E}}$

- Kneel on a mat or towel to cushion your knees.

- From an upright position, breathe in, draw your belly button inward, then bend forward until your forehead touches the mat, or as far as you comfortably can.

- Make sure your belly button is still drawn in, then return to the start position as you breathe out through pursed lips.

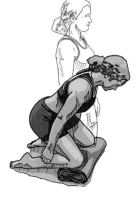

Seated Bend Pull $\boxed{\text{E}}$ $\boxed{\text{V}}$

- Sit on a Swiss ball and hold a cable or elastic cord out in front of you.

- Exhale and bend forward, keeping a natural curve in your low back; do not let your back round as you bend forward.

- As you inhale, return to the starting position and bring your arms up toward your chest in a rowing motion. Do not shrug your shoulders.

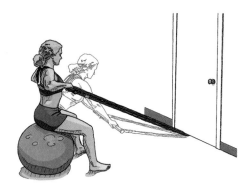

$\boxed{\text{E}}$ = ENERGIZER LEVEL $\boxed{\text{V}}$ = VITALIZER LEVEL $\boxed{\text{P}}$ = PERFORMANCE LEVEL

Bend Exercises

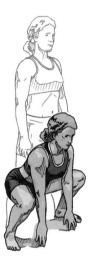

Deadlift

- Begin in a sumo stance (feet a bit wider than shoulder width and turned out slightly; you should be able to comfortably squat down far enough to touch your hands to the ground).

- If you are doing the bodyweight version, start with your arms at your sides and let them fall in between your legs as you drop down.

- If you are using weights, hold your weight (bar or dumbbell) in front of your thighs and look forward, head and chest held high.

- Take a deep diaphragmatic breath and pull your belly button in toward your spine.

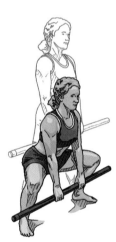

- Bend forward slightly until the weight is just above your knee. Keep a natural curve in your low back. If you were to pinch a bit of skin at the level of your low back, you should be able to hold it as you bend forward from the hips.

- As the weight passes your knees, use your legs to lower your body down as far as you can comfortably go. Do not lean forward any more or round your back, and keep your weight equal between the balls of your feet and your heels.

- Imagine pushing the ground away from you as you stand back up. As you return to standing, keep your torso upright and maintain the curve in your low back. You should feel your butt and hamstring muscles working with this exercise.

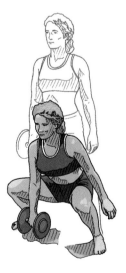

E = ENERGIZER LEVEL	V = VITALIZER LEVEL	P = PERFORMANCE LEVEL

Bend Exercises

Deadlift Row

- Take a wide stance and hold your weight (cable, elastic cord, bar or dumbbells) out in front of you with one or two hands. Perform a deadlift as described above.

- As you return to standing, bring your arms up toward your chest in a rowing motion. Do not shrug your shoulders.

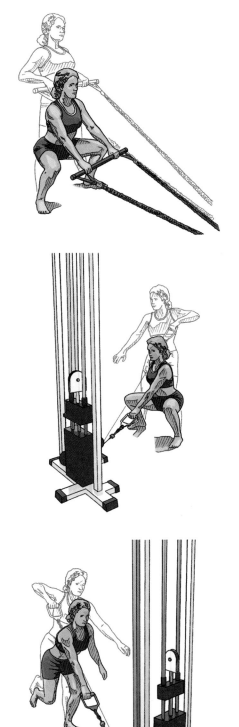

Deadlift Single Arm Row P

- Perform the exercise as described above with a single arm.

Single Leg Deadlift with Row P

- Perform the exercise on only one leg, with a single arm row. With this version, make sure that your knee does not drop inward; the middle of your knee cap should stay in line with your second toe. Using the opposing arm and leg is easier than using the same side arm and leg.

| E = ENERGIZER LEVEL | V = VITALIZER LEVEL | P = PERFORMANCE LEVEL |

Lunge Exercises

Static Lunge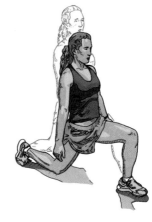

- Begin standing with your feet together.

- You may hold weights in your hands or a bar across your back to make the exercise more challenging.

- Draw your belly button inward.

- Step forward so that your back thigh and front shin are perpendicular to the floor when you drop down.

- Keep a good upright posture and drop down so that your knee just touches the floor, then come back up. Your ear, shoulder, hip and knee should all be in a line when you reach the end position.

Static Lunge with Support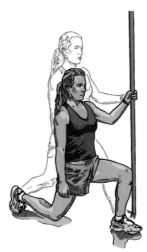

Perform the above static lunge while holding onto one or two supports. I recommend using a broom handle, Body Bar® or dowel rod. These will provide you with enough assistance, yet you are still unstable and will make the exercise more functional than if you used a stable object such as a doorway for support.

Walking Lunge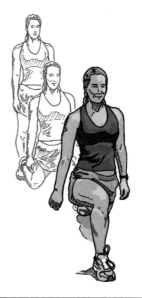

- Begin with a forward lunge.

- Remember to draw your belly button inward just prior to stepping forward.

- Instead of pushing off with your front foot and returning to the start position, push off with your back foot and step straight into a second lunge.

- Continue in a straight line.

E = ENERGIZER LEVEL   V = VITALIZER LEVEL   P = PERFORMANCE LEVEL

Lunge Exercises

Multi-directional Lunge

You will be lunging in 5 different directions with each leg. To help visualize where to step, picture standing in the middle of a clock. Begin each step standing with good posture and facing in the same direction. Initiate each movement by drawing your belly button inward and keep an upright posture; do not lean forward, to the side or backwards.

1. Front Lunge: $\boxed{V}$ $\boxed{P}$

Step to the 12 o'clock position (straight forward). Your front shin should be straight and perpendicular to the floor and your back knee should just touch the floor.

2. Front 45° Lunge: $\boxed{P}$

Step half way between the 12 and 3 o'clock, or the 12 and 9 o'clock positions (45° to the front). Keep your head and eyes forward, shoulders and pelvis square to the front, and allow the trailing leg to pivot naturally as you drop into the lunge. A common mistake is to turn the whole body 45° and lunge, which is no different than a front lunge.

3. Lateral Lunge: $\boxed{P}$

Step out to the side (3 or 9 o'clock position). Keep both feet facing forward and bend the leg you are stepping with.

4. Back 45° Lunge: $\boxed{P}$

Step back half way between the 3 and 6 o'clock, or the 6 and 9 o'clock positions. Keep your body facing forward, but step back with your foot facing inward at about 45°. Drop your back knee down so that it just touches the floor, then return to standing.

5. Back Lunge: $\boxed{V}$ $\boxed{P}$

Step straight back (6 o'clock position), into the same position as a front center lunge. Remember, your front shin should be straight and perpendicular to the floor and your back knee should just touch the floor.

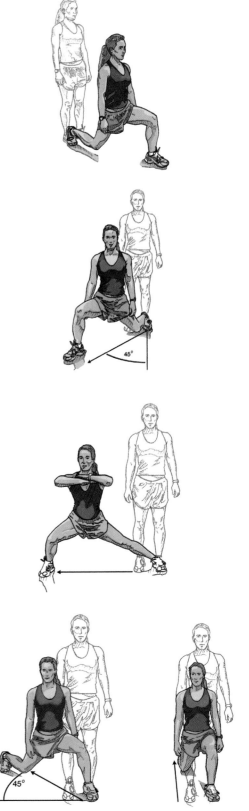

$\boxed{E}$ = Energizer Level $\boxed{V}$ = Vitalizer Level $\boxed{P}$ = Performance Level

8

Lunge Exercises

Multi-directional Lunge with Twist

As with the multi-directional lunge, you will be lunging in 5 different directions with each leg. With this version of the exercise, you will be adding a twist to each lunge movement. To help visualize where to step, picture standing in the middle of a clock. Begin each step standing with good posture and facing in the same direction. Initiate each movement by drawing your belly button inward and keep an upright posture; do not lean forward, to the side or backwards. For the twist motion, hold a light weight (medicine ball or dumbbell) to one side. As you lunge, bring the weight over your head, to the other side. You always want the weight to go over your front leg.

1. Front Lunge: Begin holding the weight on the side that will be your back leg; the weight will end up over the leg you step with.
2. Front 45° Lunge: Start with the weight on the side of your back leg. Keep your head and eyes forward as you twist.
3. Lateral Lunge: Begin with the weight opposite the side you are stepping toward.
4. Back 45° Lunge: Hold the weight to the side of the leg that you are stepping back with and bring the weight over the front leg as you lunge back.
5. Back Lunge: Again, hold the weight to the side of the leg that you are stepping back with.

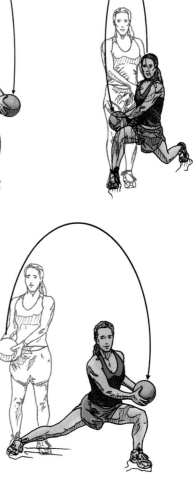

Lunge with Overhead Press

The overhead press may be added to the multi-directional lunge exercise.

- Hold a dumbbell in one had and start with the weight lowered to your shoulder. As you move into the lunge, press the weight above your head.

- This version of the exercise increases the demand placed on your core. Make sure to hold your torso straight; do not lean to one side.

- Lower the weight as you return to standing.

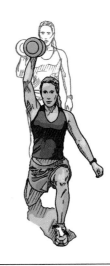

E = ENERGIZER LEVEL	V = VITALIZER LEVEL	P = PERFORMANCE LEVEL

Pull Exercises

Seated Cable Pull □E

- Sit upright on a Swiss ball and face a cable column that has been adjusted to shoulder height. Take a stable stance on the ball.

- Grab the cable handle, using the arm on the same side as the rear leg.

- Initiating the movement with your trunk, gently draw your belly button in toward your spine and simultaneously rotate your trunk toward the back leg while pulling the cable away from the column.

- Keep the forearm in exact alignment with the cable throughout the movement; do not let your elbow drop below or rise above the line of the cable. Reach along the cable with your opposite arm.

- Reverse this movement until you reach the starting position and repeat.

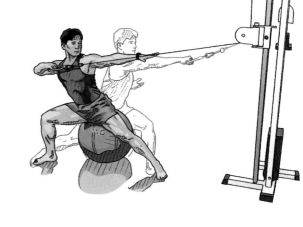

Single Arm Cable Pull □E □V

- Stand facing a cable column that has been adjusted to shoulder height.

- Take a split stance, with one leg forward and the other behind you; your knees should be soft and unlocked.

- Grab the cable handle, using the arm on the same side as the rear leg.

- Initiate the movement with your trunk, gently draw your belly button in toward your spine and simultaneously rotate your trunk toward the rear leg while pulling the cable toward your shoulder.

- Keep the forearm in exact alignment with the cable throughout the movement; do not let your elbow drop below or rise above the line of the cable. Reach along the cable with your opposite arm as you pull.

- Reverse this movement until you reach the starting position.

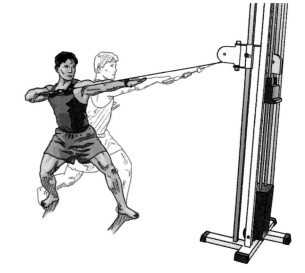

□E = Energizer Level	□V = Vitalizer Level	□P = Performance Level

Pull Exercises

Note: If you have trouble performing the single arm cable pull motion, try breaking the movement into three parts and practice them separately as shown below.

- First practice just the leg movement. Hold the cable handle out in front of you, with your torso opened to the side and shift your weight from one leg to the other.

- Next add a twist to this motion. Begin facing the cable, and, as you shift your weight to the back foot, turn your torso toward the back leg.

- Once you feel comfortable with each of these movements, integrate them together and add the pulling motion with your arm to perform the single arm cable pull. Think of sequencing your movements from the ground up.

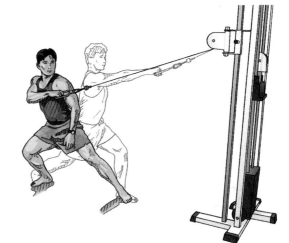

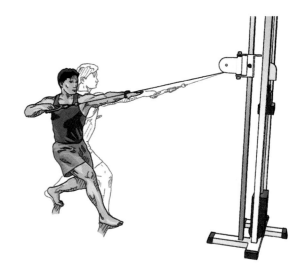

P

Ipsilateral Cable Pull

Perform the single arm cable pull as described above, but stand so that your front leg is now on the same side as the arm that is holding the cable.

| E | = Energizer Level | V | = Vitalizer Level | P | = Performance Level |

Pull Exercises

Single Leg Cable Pull

- Stand facing a cable column or resistance band that has been adjusted to shoulder height.

- Stand on only one leg. The exercise will be easier if you stand on the leg opposite the arm you are pulling with. For a greater challenge, stand on the same side leg.

- Initiating the movement with your trunk, gently draw your belly button toward your spine and simultaneously rotate your trunk away from the stance leg while pulling the cable toward your shoulder.

- Keep the forearm in exact alignment with the cable throughout the movement; do not let your elbow drop below or rise above the line of the cable. Reach along the cable with your free arm.

- Reverse this movement until you reach the starting position and repeat this movement.

Single Leg Bosu Cable Pull

Perform the single leg cable pull as described above, but now stand on a Bosu Ball (either side up). This will create an unstable environment and will result in a much more challenging exercise.

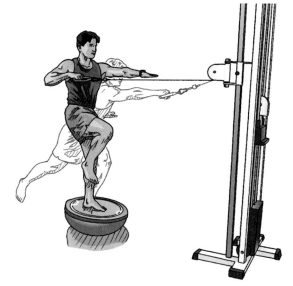

| E | = Energizer Level | V | = Vitalizer Level | P | = Performance Level |

Twist Exercises

Twist with Bodyweight 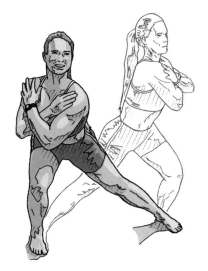 E

- Stand in a wide stance, with your toes turned outward up to 30°.

- Hold your arms up in front of you and keep your torso upright as you perform the exercise.

- Shift your weight to one side (about 70% of your weight should go to that side and about 30% should remain on the other leg).

- As you shift your weight, turn your torso so that your shoulders face sideways, but keep your head and eyes facing forward. Rotate only as far as you can comfortably turn while keeping an upright posture; do not lean forward as you twist.

- Return to the start position and repeat the movement to the other side. The motion should be continuous; do not stop in the middle.

Lateral Ball Roll E V P

- From a sitting position on a Swiss ball, roll back so that your head and shoulders are supported by the ball.

- Lift your hips up so that they are in line with your knees and shoulders.

- Place your tongue on the roof of your mouth.

- Hold your body in perfect alignment (hips and arms should stay parallel to the floor) and shuffle your feet as you roll to one side.

- Pause and return back to the center.

- Move only as far to the side as you comfortably can while holding perfect alignment. You may find that you can only move an inch or two; that is fine.

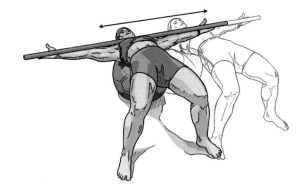

E = ENERGIZER LEVEL   V = VITALIZER LEVEL   P = PERFORMANCE LEVEL

Twist Exercises

Swiss Ball Russian Twist

- From a sitting position, roll back onto a Swiss ball so that your head and shoulders are supported by the ball.

- Lift your hips up so that they are in line with your knees and shoulders.

- Clasp your hands and raise your arms so that they point straight up toward the sky.

- To make the exercise more challenging, hold a weight.

- Place your tongue on the roof of your mouth.

- Rotate the ball under you as you move your arms from side to side.

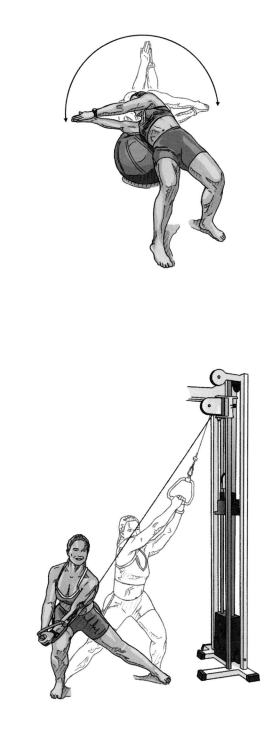

Wood Chop

- Face sideways to a cable column (as shown) and take a stable stance slightly wider than shoulder width.

- Grasp the handle with the hand furthest from the cable column and place the other hand over it.

- Start with 70% of your weight on the leg closest to the cable.

- Draw your belly button in toward your spine and initiate the movement by bending your legs, pushing away from the weight stack and rotating your trunk away from the cable column while simultaneously pulling the handle downward across your body. The movement ends when your hands are just above or slightly outside your foot.

- Inhale as your arms go up and exhale through pursed lips as you bring your arms down and across your body. When lifting a load under which you can only do 12 or fewer reps, you may need to hold your breath through the initial part of the movement and then release your breath through pursed lips after passing the hardest part of the movement.

- Perform on each side.

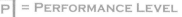

E = ENERGIZER LEVEL	V = VITALIZER LEVEL	P = PERFORMANCE LEVEL

Twist Exercises

Wood Chop with Bodyweight

Perform the exercise as described below but without the cable. Instead, imagine holding onto a handle, and duplicate the chopping motion by bringing your arms across your body as you shift your weight from one leg to the other. Perform on each side.

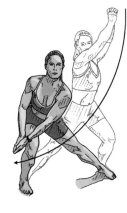

Single Leg Wood Chop

- Face sideways to a cable column and stand on one leg. This version of the exercise will be easier if you stand on your outside leg; for more of a challenge, stand on the leg near the cable column.

- Grasp the handle with the hand furthest from the cable column and place the other hand over it.

- Draw your belly button in toward your spine and initiate the movement by rotating your trunk away from the cable column while simultaneously pulling the handle downward across your body; the movement ends when your hands are above or just outside the foot you are standing on.

- Perform on each side.

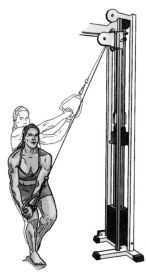

Single Arm Single Leg Wood Chop

- This version of the exercise will be easier if you stand on your outside leg; for more of a challenge, stand on the leg near the cable column.

- Grasp the handle with the hand closest to the cable column.

- Draw your belly button in toward your spine and initiate the movement by rotating your trunk away from the cable column while simultaneously pulling the handle downward across your body; the movement ends when your hand is slightly outside the foot you are standing on.

- Perform on each side.

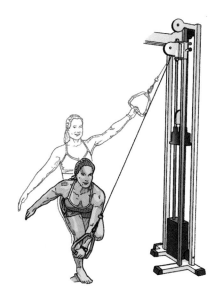

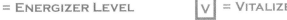

E = ENERGIZER LEVEL   V = VITALIZER LEVEL   P = PERFORMANCE LEVEL

Push Exercises

Wall Push-up $\quad$ E

- Stand about two feet away from a wall.

- Place your hands on the wall about chest width apart at shoulder level.

- Draw your belly button in, keep your body straight and drop your weight towards the wall.

- Push into the wall to return to the starting position, again keeping your body in perfect alignment.

- When you can perform more than 20 reps with perfect form, move your feet farther away from the wall, or progress to the Swiss ball push-up.

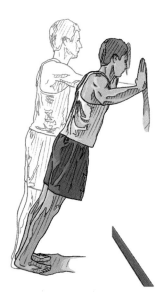

Swiss Ball Push-up $\quad$ E V

- Roll out over a Swiss ball into the plank position, with your feet or shins on the ball (the farther the ball is from your torso, the harder the exercise will be).

- Place your hands so that they are at the level of your shoulders and a comfortable width apart.

- Keep your spine and head in alignment. Do not let your head drop forward or your lower back sag down or hunch up. Bring your belly button inward and drop your chest toward the ground, holding good alignment. Return to the start position, maintaining perfect form.

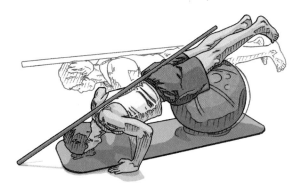

E = Energizer Level	V = Vitalizer Level	P = Performance Level

Push Exercises

Push-up

- Lie face down on the floor with your hands placed comfortably at shoulder level.

- Draw your belly button inward. Exhale through pursed lips, push yourself up to a plank position.

- Keep your spine and head in alignment, and do not let your head drop forward as you perform the exercise.

- Inhale as you lower yourself down so that your nose just touches the ground, keeping perfect alignment, and repeat.

- If you cannot perform the exercise with perfect form from your toes, complete the exercise as described above from your knees.

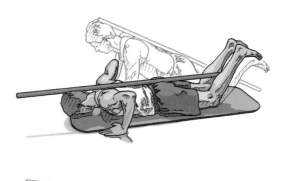

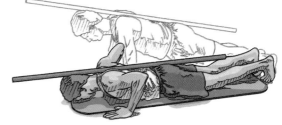

Explosive Push-up with Clap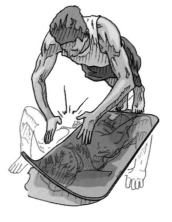

- Lie face down on the floor with your hands placed comfortably at shoulder level.

- Keep your spine and head in alignment. Do not let your head drop forward as you explode upward. Think of pushing the ground away from you.

- The aim is to push yourself up high enough that you can complete a clap before returning to the ground.

- Inhale and hold your breath as you push explosively up. Breathe between reps.

- Perform only as many reps as you can with good form and without your speed dropping. Your set should not last longer than 12 seconds.

Push Exercises

Seated Cable Push

- Sit upright on a Swiss ball and face a cable column that has been adjusted to shoulder height. Take a stable stance on the ball.

- Grab the cable handle using the arm on the same side as the rear leg.

- Gently draw your belly button in toward your spine and initiate the movement with your back leg and trunk, rotating your trunk toward the forward leg while pushing the cable out in front of your shoulder.

- Keep the forearm in exact alignment with the cable throughout the movement. Do not let your elbow drop below or rise above the line of the cable.

- Move your free arm in the opposite direction.

- Reverse this movement until you reach the starting position and repeat this movement.

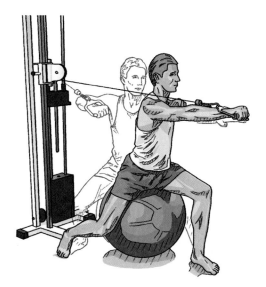

Single Arm Cable Push V P

- Stand facing a cable column that has been adjusted to shoulder height.

- Take a split stance with one leg forward and the other behind you; your knees should be soft and unlocked.

- Grab the cable handle, using the arm on the same side as the rear leg.

- Draw your belly button in and initiate the movement with your back leg and trunk and simultaneously rotate your trunk toward the forward leg while pushing the cable out in front of your shoulder.

- Keep the forearm in exact alignment with the cable throughout the movement. Do not let your elbow drop below or rise above the line of the cable. Reverse this movement with your free arm.

- Reverse this movement until you reach the starting position and repeat this movement.

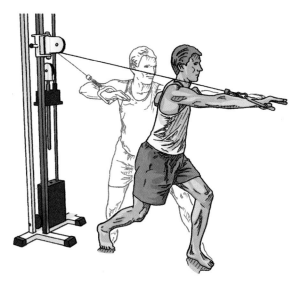

| E = ENERGIZER LEVEL | V = VITALIZER LEVEL | P = PERFORMANCE LEVEL |

Push Exercises

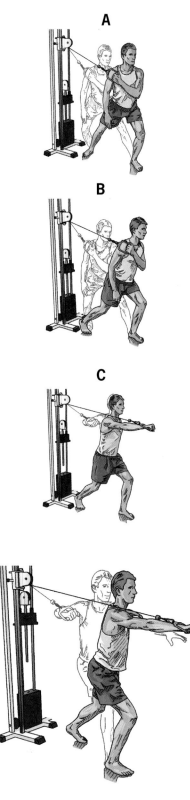

Note: If you have trouble performing this motion, try breaking the movement into three parts and practice them separately as shown below.

A. First practice just the leg movement. Hold the cable handle at your shoulder, draw your belly button toward the spine and shift your weight from one leg to the other.

B. Next, add a twist to this motion. As you shift your weight to the front foot, turn and face forward.

C. The final segment to practice is the arm motion. Stand in a split stance, facing forward. Hold your torso still and just push forward with your arm. You will need to use a lighter weight for this motion.

Once you feel comfortable with each of these movements, integrate them all together to perform the single arm cable push in sequence (A + B + C).

Ipsilateral Cable Push ⬚ P

Perform the single arm cable push as described above, but stand so that your front leg is now on the same side as the arm that is doing the push.

| E | = ENERGIZER LEVEL | V | = VITALIZER LEVEL | P | = PERFORMANCE LEVEL |

Push Exercises

Single Leg Cable Push [P]

- Stand facing a cable column or resistance band that has been adjusted to shoulder height.

- Stand on only one leg. The exercise will be easier if you stand on the leg opposite the arm you are pushing with. For a greater challenge, stand on the same side leg.

- Draw your belly button inward and initiate the movement with your trunk and front leg and simultaneously rotate your trunk toward the forward leg while pushing the cable out in front of your shoulder.

- Keep the forearm in exact alignment with the cable throughout the movement. Do not let your elbow drop below or rise above the line of the cable. Reverse this movement with your free arm.

- Reverse this movement until you reach the starting position and repeat this movement.

Single Leg Bosu Cable Push [P]

Perform the single leg cable push as described above, but now stand on a Bosu Ball (either end up). This will create an unstable environment and will result in a much more challenging exercise.

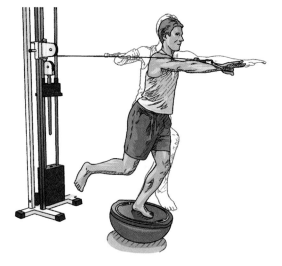

[E] = ENERGIZER LEVEL	[V] = VITALIZER LEVEL	[P] = PERFORMANCE LEVEL

Case History
Don Bodenbach of "The Nature of Health"
AM 1000 KCEO, San Diego, CA, a client of
Paul Chek

I met Paul Chek through a doctor friend of mine. I told Paul about a goal I had to dunk a basketball. I have played basketball most of my life and have never slam dunked before, but for whatever reason, I decided that I should give it a try at six feet tall, 45 years old and definitely a white man. I had discussed this idea with several of my long time basketball friends, trainers and medical professionals who understand the game. I certainly got encouragement and pats on the back, but it was clear that no one thought it was more than a pipe dream. Paul, on the other hand, not only explained exactly what I would need to do in terms of training to reach my goal, he had no doubt that I could do it. I knew Paul was well respected for his abilities to rehabilitate and train people of all kinds, including professional athletes, so his confidence in me really put some wind in my sails. I expected a training program specific to the jumping movement and not much else. Instead, I was thoroughly evaluated physically for structural strengths and weaknesses and, surprisingly, for my dietary habits. For the past 10 years I have been interviewing the world's top experts in the field of natural medicine on my weekly radio show in San Diego. I felt I had a pretty good handle on diet and supplementation. After spending just a small amount of time with Paul, I knew I was dealing with someone who has extraordinary knowledge and insights into human health. So I decided to pay attention to what he had to say and to follow his advice on training and diet. The results have been phenomenal. Within five months my vertical jump increased seven inches, which is unheard of for someone my age. My weight went from a thin 168 pounds to a muscular 183 pounds. I have been underweight my entire life, and despite many attempts to gain weight over the years, nothing had worked. Paul's dietary advice and metabolic typing made all the difference. My body responded incredibly well to the eating plan he outlined for me. My level of energy and vitality improved dramatically, which gave me the stamina to endure the workouts and allowed me to recover effectively. I have since been able to consistently spike a volleyball and have made a dunk in practice with a basketball. Not only have I accomplished my goals, but my life has improved in so many ways. After interviewing over a thousand experts in all walks of natural and alternative medicine, I know that Paul Chek is a rare and exceptional person who walks his talk. He is a true inspiration for me, by example and through his knowledge. You bring the desire, Paul Chek will take care of the rest.

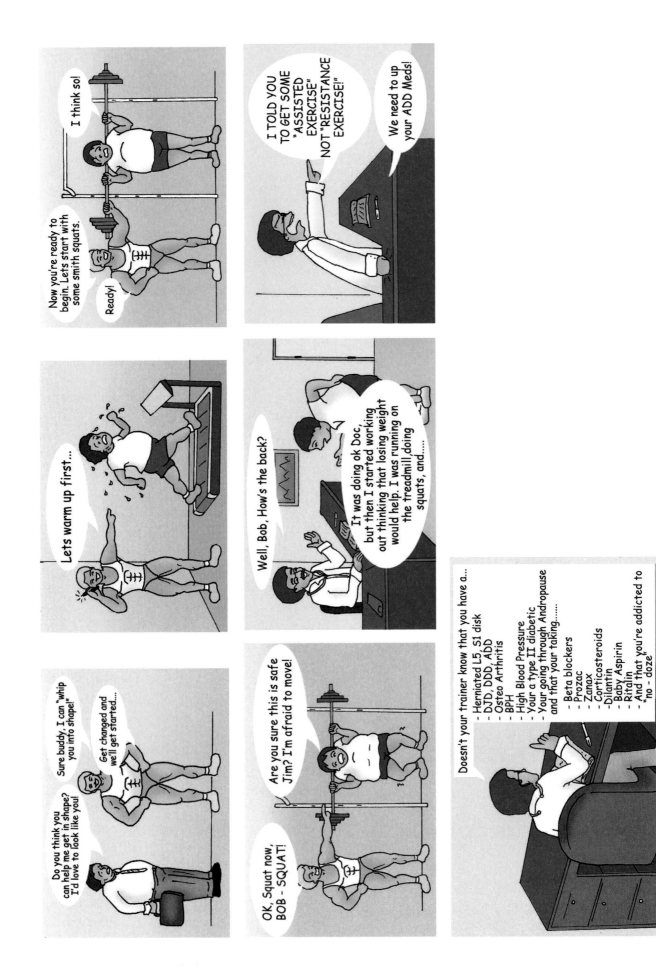

Chapter 9

SPECIAL CONSIDERATIONS

Numerous statistics and references available today indicate that levels of disease, dysfunction, drug dependence and obesity are at an all time high. People's activity levels are at an all time low, with only about 3% of women and 8% of men participating in regularly scheduled exercise.[1] For those who do make the effort, the combined effect of sedentary living, over-consumption of medical drugs, fast and processed foods, and elevated levels of environmental toxicity can introduce risk when taking on a new exercise program. To get the most from your exercise program and to avoid injury it's extremely important to understand how to train properly. In addition to consulting your physician before embarking on an exercise program (and listening carefully to what they say, as Bob found out on the previous page), the following considerations will save confusion down the road.

Throw Your Scales Away!

I mean it! The scale doesn't tell you how much *fat* you've lost nor how much *muscle* you've gained—both of which are vital to your health. Numerous patients and clients have told me that they gave up on exercise programs because they were gaining *weight*. When asked to describe their program, it was obvious they were adding much needed muscles, which are more dense than fat, *thus the weight gain*. Then, when they thought they were gaining fat, they made a common mistake—they *cut calories*!

Cutting calories is generally a disastrous thing (Chapter 13). The body's response to caloric restriction is to decrease the number of enzymes in the body that burn fat and increase the number of enzymes that store fat. The body soon begins altering hormone output and slowing your metabolic rate so you can survive with the reduced fuel level. The harder you exercise, the more stress you put on a starving body and the slower your metabolism becomes. This happens because the thyroid continues to down-regulate your metabolism to keep you alive. If you eat according to your metabolic type, you won't be as likely to over-eat, as it is hard to over-eat when you consume adequate amounts of fat.

Dieters, be aware that if you follow the program outlined in this book you might gain weight, and may get slightly bigger before you get lighter and smaller. In short, this happens because you've got to convince your physiology that you won't ever starve yourself again. The more you've skipped meals or been on a diet and the longer you've been eating incorrectly for your metabolic type, the more likely it is you'll go through a period of weight gain. Generally, clients in this category gain between six and 12 pounds in the first eight weeks of eating and training correctly. Then, like magic, they start dropping pounds and shrinking at a rate that is often faster than seems normal.

Muscle is the most metabolically active tissue in your body. Increasing the number of active muscle cells improves your ability to burn up that unwanted fat. Once past the initial phase of reprogramming your physiology, you'll look and feel better each week. Focus on how well your clothes are fitting instead of on your weight. Your body wants to be healthy and fit. It's literally *designed to be so*. Mother Nature makes no mistakes.

No Pain – No Gain!

Don't believe it! Next time someone tells you that, tell them Paul Chek says, "Pain = No Gain." Your "Eat, Move and Be Healthy" program is all about training *smarter*, not *harder*. Our goal is to **train**, not **drain**. Your body gets stronger **at rest**, not when you're exercising. Exercise is merely the stimulus that triggers the growth and repair response that builds more muscle, increases metabolism and makes you stronger.

Your "Eat, Move and Be Healthy" program focuses on *compound exercises.* Such exercises use more muscles, so they burn more calories—which will in turn increase your metabolic rate. Many Swiss ball and Primal Pattern™ exercises use practically every muscle in your body at once. This is the best way to elevate your metabolism and burn off unwanted fat.

About Medical Drugs

If you're currently on at least one medical drug, you should always have your doctor approve participation in your exercise program. Also, consider the following precautions about medical drugs while on this program:

1. As your body begins to feel, look and function better on your "Eat, Move and Be Healthy program," the same doses of medication may begin to produce more pronounced side effects. This is because the healthier you become, the less your body generally needs of any given drug. If you notice unusual symptoms, consult your doctor about reducing your dose or stopping the drug(s) all together.

2. Some drugs are addictive and should be eliminated over time. Don't go cold turkey with medical drugs without your doctor's guidance.

3. Many drugs, such as beta-blockers, affect heart rate and blood pressure—sometimes making it difficult for you to elevate your heart rate even during exercise. You need to know the side effects of any drug you're taking so as to understand why you feel a given way as your body's physiological functioning improves. I recommend referring to the book *Drug Facts and Comparisons* to get the truth on side effects.[2] You can also consult Mosby's Drug Consult CD for a comprehensive listing of side effects.[3] Knowing the side effect of a drug is very important. I've known people to give up on a good diet and exercise program because they thought the diet or exercise was causing unwanted symptoms. However, when I researched the symptoms and cross-reactions of drug combinations, I discovered that they were actually due to the drug(s). Never exercise on pain medications. You can't feel what you're doing to your body and may get hurt.

Can Crunches Burn Fat off the Midsection?

Anyone with basic training in physiology knows you can't spot reduce with exercises. In other words, working the muscles in a targeted section of the body will not reduce the fat there. Still, so-called experts continue to fill the airwaves with this false message. It's simply not true. If it were, there'd be a hell of a lot of people with six packs because there are millions of people doing their 100 + sit-ups or crunches a day and have more of a *washtub* than a *washboard* to show for it!

Don't Overuse Aerobic Exercise

Many people are obsessed with aerobic exercise these days. While a certain level of cardiovascular activity is healthy, you don't need to beat yourself up with a daily running regiment, or by going to step-class five times a week. Though some people stay fit and trim on an aerobic-based fitness program, one size doesn't fit all. Two main problems arise with excessive cardio training: muscular imbalances and related injury, and poor results.

Have you noticed runners who look as if they're in severe pain as they run down the road? If your body isn't balanced, repetitive movements such as running or aerobics are going to constantly stress the weak areas, further worsening the situation.

You don't need aerobic activity three times a week for 30 minutes to be fit. Consider how fit and beautiful sprinters and other track-and-field athletes look. It's sacrilegious for a sprinter to do aerobic exercise.

Chunky Aerobics Instructor Syndrome (CAIS) is a term I learned from strength coach Charles Poliquin. Poliquin found that his athletes and clients quickly adapted to aerobic exercise but soon found they were unable to keep body fat off with aerobics alone. His research led him to conclude that the body adapts to any given stimulus very quickly, and for the best results, he needed to change the program for his athletes frequently.

Not too long after Poliquin told me about the CAIS I remember reading a report on the findings of a study on body fat percentages, that backed up Poliquin's observations. The researchers found that professional female aerobics instructors who averaged three hours of teaching daily maintained a body fat of 22 - 24% while female step instructors had roughly 19% body fat. These body fat percentages may seem low compared to anyone with a Budwiser tumor over their belt line, but consider that the average Olympic athlete hovers around 13% body fat for females and 8% for males, and many of them train less than three hours a day.

Go to any gym for proof of CAIS. There you'll find women who have logged thousands of miles on their favorite treadmill or who have worn out three sets of pedals on their favorite stepper, yet their body shape never seems to improve. If you don't find them on the machines, you can usually find them in the snack bar buying another bottle of fluorescent blue sugar water and some designer performance bar.

So what's the answer? Keep your body guessing. There are many effective ways to keep lean and not over utilize aerobics. Here are some options:

Mix your training schedule by alternating resistance training days with aerobics days.
Rest a day in between, or after, these two training days. You can also add aerobics training to the end of a resistance-training workout. I especially recommend this for females who fear bulking up with resistance training, because aerobic training causes the release of *glucocorticoids*, which are *stress hormones!* Stress hormones are catabolic, which means they are tissue destructive and will prohibit formation of additional muscle tissue. This is one of the reasons many distance runners look like they've just escaped a Gulag work crew where their biggest meal was four and a half pinto beans and scent of beet-root. As little as 15 - 30 minutes of aerobic training a day will do the trick on resistance training days, and thirty minutes is acceptable as a workout with most aerobic activities. More is often just *longer*, not necessarily *better.*

Mix your aerobic activities regularly.
- Perform 3 - 5 minutes of an aerobic activity and then immediately jump to a different machine or another form of aerobics. Continue switching this for about 30 minutes. Athletes in better condition can train longer, as needed.

- Change the type of aerobic activity for each workout. For best results, choose activities that your body hasn't adapted to. Try something new!

- Perform a given aerobic workout, alternating days with resistance training or sports training/participation. Do this for no longer than two weeks if you're more of a *cat* type (get bored easily) and three weeks if you are a *salamander* type (enjoy repetitive activities).

- Change the movement, change the exercise. In other words, if you try doing the activity backwards and sideways while juggling, your motor system is challenged enough so that you won't adapt to the exercise so quickly. Try running backwards for a quarter mile out of every mile you run and you'll likely feel a significant difference.

- Use interval training. This is why elite endurance athletes are lean, while gym rats who abuse aerobics look like poster children for Syndrome-X. When you mix 30 seconds to 3 minutes of intense effort (periods of 80 - 90%+ at maximum effort) with 30 seconds to 5 minutes of rest between efforts, the metabolic adaptations are similar in effect to resistance training but without the muscle mass development. Sprinters often develop muscle mass by using 10 to 100 meter sprints with 1 to 5 minutes rest and no other training. This type of training can be effective if done once a week initially, progressing to 2 - 3 times a week for the intermediate and advanced exercisers.

Circuit weight training.

Circuit training with free-weights is an excellent way to build your heart and lung capacity while building improved muscle tone and increasing your metabolic rate. There are many sorts of circuits, such as the sample programs in this book. Some additional options are:

- A circuit of 12 - 18 exercises (30 reps of each exercise with 60 - 90 seconds rest between circuits). Perform one to two circuits.

- Go for 30 minutes to 1 hour as fast as you can—with good form—through 10 - 14 exercises. This can include cardio-machines, weights, calisthenics and even sporting activities like hitting a heavy bag.

- Use five resistance training exercises sequenced from the most complex to least complex, focusing primarily on big functional exercises like squats, lunging, rowing, cable pushing, chin-ups, etc. Take 60 - 90 seconds of rest between circuits and build up to 4 circuits.

Less Is More!

Yes, you read correctly, less is more! When I was the trainer of the U.S. Army Boxing Team, I told athletes that it was always better to under-train than to over-train. This is because the under-trained fighters always had reserves, but the over-trained fighters lacked staying power for the long, hard sparring sessions and fights. In addition, over-training suppresses the immune system, resulting in infections and chronic fatigue.

Don't stress over your exercise program. If you aren't enjoying your training, find something that you can enjoy. The secret is to make it a *life style change*. If you try to go about your exercise program like a sprinter, you're sure to burn out. Go about it as though your goal was to make the most beautiful body in the world, from the inside out. Remember, it's a lifetime project and missing a session now and then is just fine. Be consistent, enjoy yourself; the joy of doing it will have more health benefits than stressing over the day you missed.

Flattening Your Abs After Pregnancy

Today, many women have distended abdominal muscles years after having children. Sadly, this is unnecessary. The abdominal muscles go through a unique lengthening process when a woman becomes pregnant. As the fetus grows, there's increased stretch placed on the abdominal wall from the inside. This stretch force causes the body to add functional units called *sarcomeres* to the abdominal muscles, making them progressively longer (Figure 1).

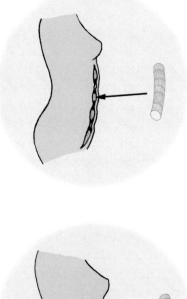

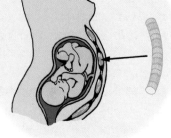

Figure 1: Abdominal wall muscles

After childbirth, the stretch force is reduced and the sarcomeres begin reducing in number. Normally, the muscles should return to normal length. Unfortunately, this natural rebounding process may not occur if the woman becomes pregnant again too soon, gains excess weight or has a cesarean section.

If the female becomes pregnant again before her body has fully restored itself to normal muscle length/tension ratio, posture and body weight, there's a greater chance with each additional child that the body may not *remember* what it should be like. I've noticed that female clients who have had more than two children in a two-year period or less have a higher incidence of abdominal wall dysfunction.

In some American Indian tribes, it was forbidden for a brave to get a female pregnant more often than once every three years. The elders knew from experience that this weakened the women so much that it was a threat to the survival of the tribe.

Some women use pregnancy as an excuse to eat everything in sight. In no time, their torso looks more like a self-storage unit with everything but the roll-up doors. It's important to remember that *you get fat from the inside out!* Your abdominal muscles don't differentiate between stretch from a fetus and stretch from fat. Either will induce a stretch force, keeping the muscles long and resulting in an unattractive abdominal wall, not to mention increasing your chances of back pain.

Cesarean sections can cause a lot of problems for females. I've rehabilitated numerous females with low back pain that developed within 3 - 6 months after having a cesarean section. When the doctor cuts through the abdominal wall, the muscles are wounded. There are three layers of muscle comprising the abdominal wall, and when the layers of muscle are sewn back together scarring occurs, leaving significant adhesions and causing dysfunction in the abdominal wall.

Where there's scaring and adhesions, muscle fibers, as well as independent layers of muscle, lose their ability to slide across one another effectively. The

resulting pain *always causes inhibition (weakness) in muscles*. Women soon learn to avoid contracting the painful muscles and develop faulty muscle recruitment patterns. This directly destabilizes the back and indirectly destabilizes the entire body.

Damage to the pelvic floor is a common occurrence during pregnancy. The muscles can become damaged from the stretch pressure due to the expanding womb or from an episiotomy. There may also be damage to nerves, leaving the pelvic floor disabled to varying degrees. Because the pelvic floor, deep abdominal, deep back and diaphragm muscles all work as part of a system (Chapter 6), when the muscles of the pelvic floor are damaged, the result may be the inability to properly use the abdominal wall muscles. After about 6 - 12 months, a woman with this dysfunction will typically have what I call a *Heart Bottom Syndrome* (Figure 2).

When the pelvic floor becomes dysfunctional, the smaller portion of the butt muscles (gluteus maximus fibers located by the pelvic floor), become hyperactive as they assist in stabilizing the pelvis and its contents. This leads to atrophy of the larger butt muscles and prominence of the gluteus medius muscles (butt muscles on the sides).

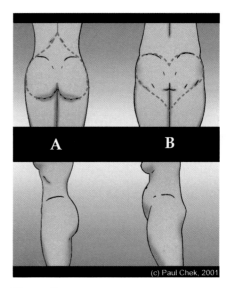

Figure 2:
A: A functional bottom
B: A dysfunctional bottom with Heart Bottom Syndrome

If you think you have Heart Bottom Syndrome, I highly recommend consulting a C.H.E.K Practitioner or a physical therapist skilled in restoration of pelvic floor and abdominal wall dysfunction. It's important to understand that Heart Bottom Syndrome places you at far greater risk of orthopedic and visceral injury when exercising and performing daily tasks because you cannot effectively stabilize your spine.

My approach

To restore abdominal muscles to their optimal length, follow this protocol:

1. Eat correctly for your metabolic type (Chapter 3).

2. Eat high-quality foods and drink adequate water (Chapter 4).

3. Perform the core function tests and corresponding corrective exercises on pages 124 - 127.

If you've followed this protocol for four weeks and don't see improvement, consult a C.H.E.K Practitioner for a comprehensive assessment.

Overcoming Back Pain During Exercise

Since back pain during exercise is common today, trainers should be taught to identify "red flags," which are indicators that the body is at greater risk of injury. Once recognized, modifications to correct the situation should be initiated immediately. In order to help you avoid potential injury, carefully consider the following common causes of back pain when exercising:

Muscle imbalances: When a muscle becomes short and tight, the antagonist (opposite) muscle(s) often becomes long and weak. This creates an imbalance in the body. To quickly determine if this is the case, simply try stretching any tight muscle in the region where you're feeling discomfort. If this helps your performance, you're probably balancing your muscles. If the relief is only short-term, you may need to stretch the tight muscles between each set while resting. The body often *learns* these faulty recruitment patterns. You'll have to repeatedly stretch the tight muscle(s) until it relearns the

correct recruitment sequence. If this doesn't work, you'll need the help of a skilled C.H.E.K Practitioner or rehabilitation professional trained in assessment of the musculoskeletal and visceral systems.

Bulging discs: It's estimated that up to 70% of the population has an undiagnosed bulging disc in the neck or back. Yet, many of these people have no pain—*a fact that perplexes the medical community.*[4]

A key indicator of a disc bulge is that flexion (forward bending) of the spine, (such as when doing an abdominal crunch or sit-up) will increase the bulge, moving it toward a pain sensitive nerve root or the spinal cord. If your pain begins in the region of the spine and progressively migrates down and away from your spine to include or be felt somewhere away from your spine, such as the hip, shoulder or arm, *you may have a disc bulge compromising nerve tissue or the cord.* It would be wise to discontinue flexion exercises until a qualified medical professional or a C.H.E.K Practitioner helps you determine if you have a disc injury. This may include an MRI.

Faulty recruitment of muscles: Faulty recruitment of muscles may be due to muscle imbalance, pain, inactivity and/or poor training. Faulty recruitment of muscles around joints exposes the joint involved to excessive compression, torsion and shear—the primary enemy of joints. If unchecked by the muscular system, compression, torsion and shear often lead to inflammation, pain and injury.

Pain in any muscle or joint can cause this same scenario. For example, if you injure one of your sacroiliac joints in a fall from a bike, the pain will generally cause the gluteus medius muscles (lateral butt muscles) to shut down. If this goes unattended for any period of time, the body will adapt by using other muscles in efforts to stabilize the region. In time, this places enough stress on the body so that either the joint you injured, the muscles that are now over-working, or other joints being incorrectly stabilized because of the faulty recruitment, become painful. If you can't track your problem to a given incident, it could be any number of related issues. If this sounds remotely familiar, get a professional assessment. Performing any exercise that hurts only makes things worse—possibly much worse.

As you can see, there are many reasons why people experience pain while exercising, including just downright doing too much! Please remember that your goal is to *train, not drain* the body and that there is *no* reward for training in pain. Pain is an indicator that damage is being done, not that damage is about to be done. If you don't know why you're hurting, find someone who can help you. Pain is the most powerful reprogramming agent in the human body. In short order, you'll train the system to function incorrectly, and even the best therapists in the world may not be able to help you.

If you've had a physician assess you and have been given the go-ahead to exercise yet still have low back pain (or pain elsewhere), follow the stretch assessments and core assessment protocols in this book. You may find that body pains go away within as little as a week or two as a result of improved core function and eating the right foods for you.

It's not what you are that holds you back, it's what you think you are not.

Denis Waitley

Always bear in mind that your own resolution to succeed is more important than any other thing.

Abraham Lincoln

Chapter 10

PUTTING IT ALL TOGETHER

I hope you're excited about starting your new exercise program. If not, don't worry. I've developed something for everyone, because exercise should never introduce stress into your life. If you don't like to exercise, read on to learn more about a "no workout" routine. Now, let's look at how to implement the plan that's right for you, using Chapter 2 as your guide.

Regardless of the level of exercise you've chosen, you'll no doubt find yourself pressed for time on occasion. In order to ensure you perform the most important part of your routine always prioritize your workout in the following order:

1. No Workout Routine
2. Energy Building Exercises (Chapter 6)
3. Stretching (Chapter 5)
4. Restore Core Function (Chapter 7)
5. Functional Exercises (Chapter 8)

Remember, exercise places stress on the body. If you don't cultivate enough energy through proper eating, water consumption, sleeping and energy-building exercises, a traditional approach to exercise will do nothing but break you down. Simply restoring energy balance and flow through the body (Chapter 8), along with eating and drinking correctly (Chapters 3 and 4), will take you a long way toward health and vitality.

Fitness fanatics

If you're an active person who regularly exercises and taking time to do zone exercises just seems *tooo slooow* for you, please consider the following:

If your exercise routine is so intense that you could not comfortably perform it with a stomach full of food, your hormonal and nervous system produces a stress response, activating your sympathetic nervous system. While this may feel "right" in the short term, you may be addicted to the endorphin release from this form of exercising. Though exercise is not a bad thing to be addicted to, problems will arise if you suffer from nagging injuries or if the total score from your questionnaires is above 260.

If your total score for all questionnaires is 260 or above, no matter how much you like exercising, you're probably doing more harm than good with high intensity exercises. Your primary goal at this point should be to lower your total score to below 150! When your score is below 150, your body will respond more favorably to high intensity exercise. You must remember that being fit and being healthy are not necessarily synonymous! This is why many elite athletes die at an early age.

You can balance your energy systems quite effectively by stretching the tight muscles identified in the stretching tests outlined in Chapter 5. If you don't want to perform zone exercises or active meditations as a means of energy balancing, at least make sure you stretch.

You may want to stretch to balance your energy systems and develop your own program based on the guidelines in this chapter. However, make sure the exercises you develop match the program scheme indicated by your total score. Those scoring above 260 should choose exercises in line with the Energizer program, while those scoring 150-260, should choose the Vitalizer program.

You may decide to use stretches to balance your energy systems and use outdoor activities, or sports participation and practice as your exercise. Just be aware that if your exercise intensity is taking more out of your body than your eating and resting plan are putting back in, your scores will not go down in the next four weeks. In fact, I've seen over-zealous athletes elevate their scores by working too hard to become fit and ending up unhealthy. The balanced athlete is a healthy athlete!

If you're pressed for time and can only perform one or two exercises, choose the exercises that most suit your needs. For example, if your lower abdominal muscles protrude and you scored high in the digestion or detoxification system health questionnaires, you'll get more mileage from performing an exercise such as the 4-point TVA than you will the bent over row. The 4-point TVA activates your natural body pumps, aiding your digestion, elimination and activating the lazy TVA. If you have time only to stretch or do zone exercises, choose the activity that will provide the most benefit to your body at that time. If your body feels tight and restricted, stretching will be most helpful, while if your questionnaire scores are high in one or more categories, performing your zone exercise(s) will be most beneficial.

Ugh, even the thought of a zone exercise is a drag!
If you honestly don't have the get-up and go to perform one zone exercise without feeling stressed, that's okay. However, you do need to work on getting your energy up. The energy exercises on pages 104 - 116 will help revitalize you.

Perhaps you're one of the people with an excessively hectic schedule and trying to fit extra activities will stress you even more. You must realize, however, that *if you're truly dedicated to improving your health you need to make changes and create time for yourself each day.* Besides an improved drinking and eating plan, your solution can be found in two places—the parking lot and the stairs.

Park your car toward the rear of the parking lot wherever you go. In some shopping centers, this could mean walking as much as a quarter mile round trip, not including distances inside the building. This simple plan can equate to a mile a day!

Promise yourself not to take the elevator or escalator unless you have to carry something heavy. If you work in a high rise office building and have to travel between floors throughout the day, this little plan alone could significantly increase your metabolic rate, moving you ever closer to your desired body shape. Also realize that as your metabolic rate increases, your ability to metabolize toxins, move fluids through your body and eliminate waste also improves.

How to Build Your Own Program

Your "Eat, Move and Be Healthy" program is very flexible—you can do as much or as little as you want. The main goal is to improve your health and vitality. Undoubtedly, the various levels of stress, fitness and vitality among readers will require tremendous versatility in program design. In order to effectively accommodate each of your needs, it's important to follow the instructions below for optimal results.

Exercise intensity
If you haven't already completed your questionnaires and graphed your scores, do so now. Your total score is very important, as it determines which program intensity is right for you.

The intensity zones are as follows:

0-150 = High vitality body that can handle stressors up to the Performance Program (page 184).

151-259 = Moderately stressed body that should exercise at Vitalizer Program intensity or lower (page 178).

260 or > = High stress zone, indicating that any exercise program of greater intensity than the Energizer is likely to further stress your body and prevent you from attaining health and vitality (page 175). If you are in this zone and don't exercise at all, or are experiencing discomfort somewhere in your body, you should start with the "Tender Loving Care" (TLC) program (pages 172).

Exercise selection

Sample programs are provided for each of the intensity levels described above. After 6 - 8 weeks, you'll need to modify your program in order to stimulate your body and progress to the next level. And, of course, you may decide to design your own program from the start. The first step toward modifying or building a program is choosing the right exercises for your needs. The colored boxes by each exercise on pages 137 - 156 identify the difficulty level or levels of the exercise. You will notice that some exercises have multiple levels of difficulty. Such exercises can be made more difficult by performing the more advanced variations, adding more weight or increasing the speed.

When you select new exercises for your program, always begin your routine by placing your most challenging exercises at the beginning. For example, a multidirectional lunge is more complex and thus more demanding of the nervous system than a squat and should be performed before the squat in most cases. An exception to this rule is when you have a harder time performing a less complex exercise than you do a more complex exercise. For example, perhaps squats are difficult for you due to a previous back injury or weakness, yet you find the multidirectional lunge easy because you have a background in tennis. If so, put the exercise that is most challenging for you first in your program.

Any of the corrective or isolating exercises, such as the Lower Abdominal exercises or the 4-Point TVA, should always be last in the order of exercises when more complex movements, such as Primal Pattern™ exercises, are being used.

I use five exercises in the sample programs primarily because when performed in a circuit format, you can finish the program, including stretching beforehand, in under an hour. Performing more exercises generally requires more time and makes your strength development more diffuse.

Should I use the circuit or station format?

The sample programs are all in a circuit format. This means that you'll perform one set of each exercise back to back, then rest for the designated time and repeat the circuit. Doing so enables you to complete your entire workout, including stretching, within an hour. Since you'll be doing a lot of "work" in a short period of time, circuit training is effective for increasing your metabolic rate.

Station training is ideal if you don't have the strength or endurance to go from one exercise to the next without resting or if you want increased strength in a given Primal Pattern. For example, if you're a tennis player who wants to develop a more explosive lunge pattern, you'll benefit from altering your workout structure so that your lunge sets are done back to back, with a rest period between each set. This will cause a greater level of fatigue in the nervous system and muscles involved in the lunge pattern, making you become stronger in the lunge pattern more quickly than by using a circuit workout.

Program Variables

To design your own exercise routine using the exercises and principles of your *Eat, Move and Be Healthy* program, you'll need a basic understanding of acute exercise variables; rest, intensity, repetitions (reps), tempo and sets. The following section will explain how to use each of these variables correctly so you can achieve the desired outcome.

Rest

> **Rest:** The amount of time taken to rest between exercises or a circuit of exercises.

If you're attempting to increase muscle mass or elevate your metabolic rate, keep rest periods short, between 60 to 90 seconds. This rule applies to both station training and circuit training because the longer you rest, the more your metabolic rate slows and the less work volume you complete in a given time period.

However, if you cannot recover from successive exercises during circuit workouts or station training workouts, increase rest periods. The key concern is your exercise form! If form deteriorates because you're trying to do more than you can handle, the chance of injury escalates. Take as much time as you need to rest so that you can complete your next set with good form. If you need more than five minutes of rest in a station format, stop the exercise and move to the next. This would be a signal that your body is too fatigued to continue. If you begin a circuit format with a one minute rest and feel that you're just too fatigued to perform with good form when you start your next circuit, increase your rest time. You may need to do this with each circuit. I often use an *ascending rest period*, which means that I increase the rest by a given increment, such as 30 seconds each circuit, to accommodate fatigue yet maintain good form.

When performing more advanced programs, such as the Performance program, you may need to increase the rest between circuits because the exercises are complex enough that the nervous system may not recover during a shorter rest period. If the exercise is fairly intense, the nervous system takes about 5 - 6 times longer to recover than the muscular system. This is why people in the gym or in sports training often feel like they've rested long enough after a minute or two, but when they go back to performing the exercise or drill, they can't perform well. They're at risk of injury because the nervous system needs time to recover.

Intensity

Intensity: A measure of applied strength relative to maximum strength.

Intensity is generally recorded as a percentage of your one-rep max (the maximum amount of weight that you could lift). To simplify this concept, I'll use a "safety rep range" for the programs in this book. You'll see indicators such as "-2" in the Intensity Column. This indicates that once you've completed the prescribed number of repetitions in the Reps Column, you should always feel as if you can complete an additional rep or two, as indicated. For example, if the program calls for 10 reps and the intensity is "-2", you should choose a level of resistance that allows 12 reps to be performed with perfect form, but only complete the 10 reps recommended.

The more advanced exercisers, who are already in pretty good shape, can use this rule to apply to the first set or circuit only. This is because as you fatigue, you'll get to the point where you can only perform 10 reps with good form anyway, while those with less conditioning may fatigue so rapidly that they have to reduce the load/resistance of each set or circuit to maintain perfect form and stay in the given rep range. If you cannot perform the prescribed number of reps, decrease the weight or select an easier version of the exercise. On the other hand, if you feel like you could perform several more reps after you complete the set, you should increase the intensity by adding more weight or progressing the exercise.

Reps

Reps: The number of times you repeat a given exercise or movement in a set.

Repetition (reps) is the number of times you repeat a given exercise or movement in a set (one round of the exercise). Generally, if you want to add muscle mass, you should perform 8 – 12 repetitions. For strength, with some endurance, you should work in a 12 - 20 rep range. As you go beyond 20 repetitions in a set, you're progressively increasing endurance and will therefore develop less strength or muscle mass.

Tempo

Tempo: The pace at which you execute an exercise.

Tempo is the pace at which you execute the exercise. The programs included in this book will use the following tempos:

Slow = A 1 - 2 - 3 count in each direction: 1 - 2 - 3 down, pause, and 1 - 2 - 3 up.

Moderate = A 1 - 2 count or moving at a natural pace for that movement; not fast and not slow.

Fast = Completion of each phase of the movement in one second or less; but not as fast as you possibly can or explosively.

Sets

> **Sets:** The completion of the prescribed number or reps for a given exercise.

A set is the completion of the prescribed number of repetitions for a given exercise. If you have an exercise that is performed on each side—a single arm cable row, for example—perform the given number of reps on each side of your body. As a reminder, the reps will be written as "8 - 12 each."

You'll often notice two numbers in the Sets Column, such as 1 - 4. This means you should begin your exercise program by performing only one set of the exercise. As you progress from workout to workout, you can increase the number of sets as you feel you can tolerate it. You'll know to increase the number of sets when you begin your next workout and are not sore from your last training session. You should always feel as if you can do better than the previous workout; otherwise, don't increase the number of sets.

Periodization

Periodization is a system of applying the principles of work and rest. Your sample programs are periodized using a method called undulation. Undulation means that some days will be harder, while others are easier. The weeks will also undulate. Your program should get progressively harder for the first few weeks, followed by an easy week at the end of that phase in order to let your body recover.

If you build your own program, simply follow the periodization scheme used for the sample programs to achieve optimal results. Just be sure not to start at an advanced level. For example, don't start your exercise program by using the scheme I've applied to the fourth week because it's likely to be too demanding on your body as a new program. Test your body by starting at week one and move forward from there to the point that feels right, giving you adequate stress and recovery for your current level of conditioning.

A periodization schedule is given for each of the sample programs. Colored bars representing the different exercises are used for each day. Yellow represents stretching for all of the programs and should be done daily. The colors indicate which exercises of your program should be done on a given day. Follow the variables in the table as shown for each exercise. The full program is set up in a circuit format. If you are not performing all of the exercises, just circuit the ones you are doing for that day.

On each day, perform only the activities that relate to the color shown and always perform them in the order of the color presentation. Stretching is recommended every day. You may perform additional Zone Exercises on any day.

If you would like a full assessment and personalized program, consult a C.H.E.K Practitioner (see www.chekinstitute.com for one near you).

Using the sample programs

To make things easy for you, four sample programs (one for each intensity level) are provided on the following pages. Each program contains four to five exercises. Follow the variables given in the table for each exercise.

The column with different color blocks is your periodization schedule. Note that there are blocks for each day of the week for four weeks. Each block (labeled: S, A, B or C) corresponds to the exercises you are to perform each day. The boxes are color-coded to match the boxes to the left containing a picture of the exercise(s) for that block. You will do your stretches every day. For some days, you will only do your stretching and one or two other exercises, while on other days, you will perform all the exercises. A brief description of each exercise is also provided. Good luck and have fun!

TLC Program

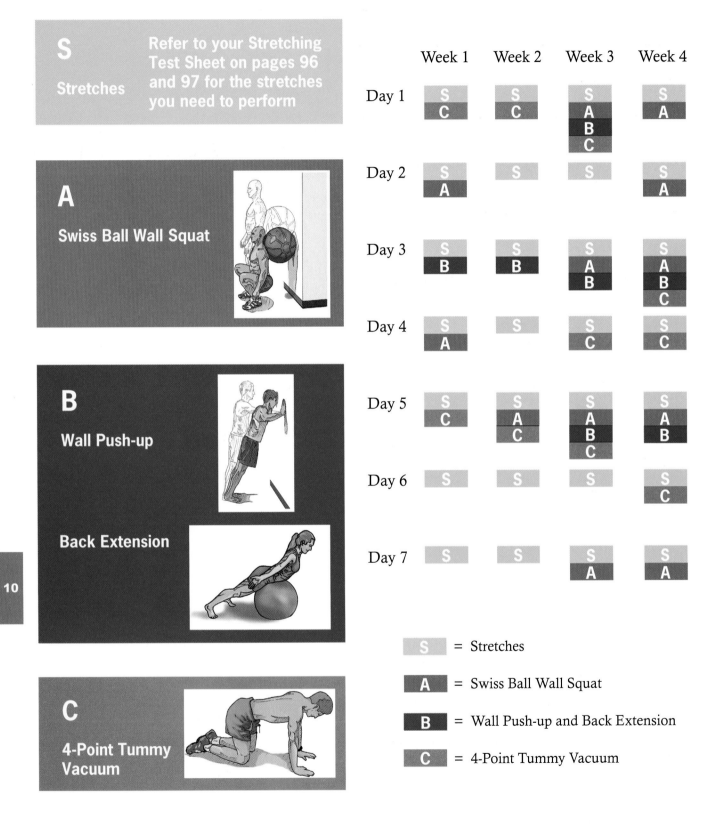

S — Stretches
Refer to your Stretching Test Sheet on pages 96 and 97 for the stretches you need to perform

A — Swiss Ball Wall Squat

B — Wall Push-up / Back Extension

C — 4-Point Tummy Vacuum

	Week 1	Week 2	Week 3	Week 4
Day 1	S / C	S / C	S / A / B / C	S / A
Day 2	S / A	S	S	S / A
Day 3	S / B	S / B	S / A / B	S / A / B / C
Day 4	S / A	S	S / C	S / C
Day 5	S / C	S / A / C	S / A / B / C	S / A / B
Day 6	S	S	S	S / C
Day 7	S	S	S / A	S / A

- **S** = Stretches
- **A** = Swiss Ball Wall Squat
- **B** = Wall Push-up and Back Extension
- **C** = 4-Point Tummy Vacuum

10

TLC Program

Exercise	Rest	Intensity	Reps	Tempo	Sets
SB Wall Squat	↓	-2 reps	5 - 20	Breathing	1 - 3
Wall Push-up	↓	-2 reps	5 - 20	Slow	1 - 3
Back Extension	↓	-2 reps	1 - 8	Hold 30 seconds Rest 15 seconds	1 - 3
4-Point Tummy Vacuum	1 - 3 minutes ↓		10	Hold 10 seconds	1 - 3

Wall Squat

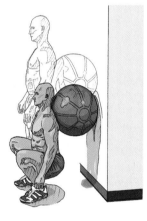

- Place a Swiss ball between your lower back and a wall.

- Take a comfortable stance with your arms at your sides. You should be standing up straight, not leaning back onto the ball.

- Inhale and then lower yourself down into a squat as you exhale. Go as low as you comfortably can and inhale as you return to standing.

- Perform 10 reps at the pace you naturally breathe.

- Breathe through your nose if you can; if you need to exhale through your mouth, keep a little tension in our lips.

Wall Push-up

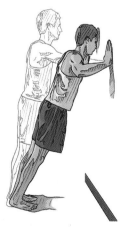

- Stand about two feet away from a wall.

- Place your hands on the wall about chest width apart at shoulder level.

- Keep your body straight, draw your belly button in and drop your weight towards the wall.

- Push into the wall to return to the starting position, again keeping your body in perfect alignment.

Back Extension

- Lie face down over a Swiss ball.

- Keep your toes on the ground and lift your torso up.

- Inhale as you extend up, rotate your arms outward—draw your shoulders blades together and turn your palms outward.

- It is important to maintain good alignment—chin tucked and head in line with back as you exhale.

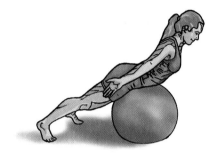

4-Point Tummy Vacuum

- Assume a kneeling position with your hips over your knees and your shoulders over your hands.

- With your spine in neutral alignment, take a deep breath in and let your belly drop toward the floor.

- Exhale and draw your belly button in toward your spine while keeping your back in the start position.

- Hold for as long as you comfortably can.

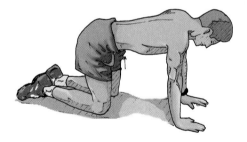

10

Energizer Program

S
Stretches
Refer to your Stretching Test Sheet on pages 96 and 97 for the stretches you need to perform

A
Static Lunge

B
Bent Over Row

Russian Twist

C
Reverse Hyperextension

4-Point Tummy Vacuum

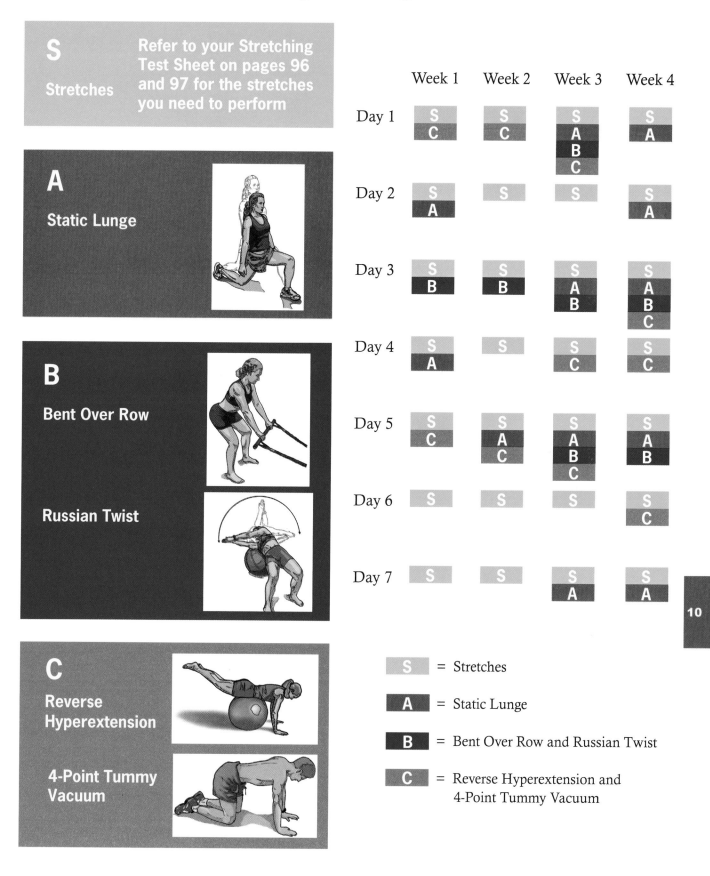

	Week 1	Week 2	Week 3	Week 4
Day 1	S / C	S / C	S / A / B / C	S / A
Day 2	S / A	S	S	S / A
Day 3	S / B	S / B	S / A / B	S / A / B / C
Day 4	S / A	S	S / C	S / C
Day 5	S / C	S / A / C	S / A / B / C	S / A / B
Day 6	S	S	S	S / C
Day 7	S	S	S / A	S / A

S = Stretches

A = Static Lunge

B = Bent Over Row and Russian Twist

C = Reverse Hyperextension and 4-Point Tummy Vacuum

10

Energizer Program

Exercise	Rest	Intensity	Reps	Tempo	Sets
Static Lunge	↓	-2 reps	1 - 10	Slow	1 - 3
Bent Over Row	↓	-2 reps	10	Slow	1 - 3
Russian Twist	↓	-2 reps	10	Moderate	1 - 3
Reverse Hyperextension	↓	-1 rep	10	Slow	1 - 3
4-Point Tummy Vacuum	1 - 3 minutes ↓		10	Hold 10 seconds	1 - 3

Static Lunge

- Begin standing with your feet together.

- You may hold weights in your hands or a bar across your back to make the exercise more challenging.

- Step forward so that your back thigh and front shin are perpendicular to the floor when you drop down.

- Keep a good upright posture and drop down so that your knee just touches the floor, then come back up. Your ear, shoulder, hip and knee should all be in a line when you reach the end position.

- Repeat all reps on one leg and then switch legs.

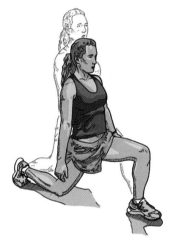

Bent Over Row

- Holding weights, cable handle or tubing in your hands, bend forward so that your hands rest just above your knees.

- Keep your head and spine in neutral as shown.

- As you draw the weights up to your side, imagine that you are a puppet and your elbows are being lifted toward the sky by strings.

- Keep the elbows up, do not pull them back toward your hips; keep your shoulders relaxed, not shrugged.

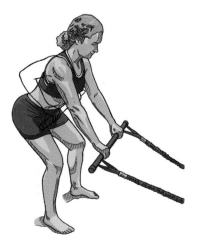

Energizer Program

Swiss Ball Russian Twist

- From a sitting position, roll back onto a Swiss ball so that your head, shoulders and upper back are supported by the ball.
- Lift your hips up so that they are in line with your knees and shoulders.
- Clasp your hands and raise your arms so that they point straight up toward the sky (holding a weight will make the exercise more challenging).
- Place your tongue on the roof of your mouth.
- Rotate over the ball, going from side-to-side.
- Do not let your hips drop downward.

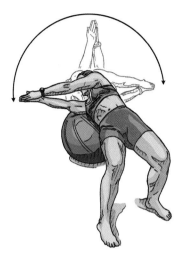

Reverse Hyperextension

- Lie face down over a Swiss ball with your hands on the floor.
- Your back and head should be in line.
- Keeping your legs straight, raise them up as far as you comfortably can.
- Lower your legs back to the starting position.

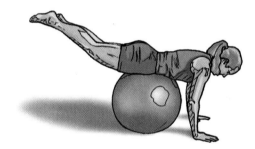

4-Point Tummy Vacuum

- Assume a kneeling position with your hips over your knees and your shoulders over your hands.
- With your spine in neutral alignment, take a deep breath in and let your belly drop toward the floor.
- Exhale and draw your belly button in toward your spine while keeping your back in the start position.
- Hold for as long as you comfortably can.
- Repeat 10 times on your natural breathing pattern.

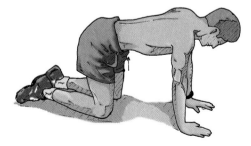

Vitalizer Program

S

Stretches — Refer to your Stretching Test Sheet on pages 96 and 97 for the stretches you need to perform

A — Multi-directional Lunge

B
- Single Arm Cable Push
- Single Arm Cable Pull

C
- Lateral Ball Roll
- Forward Ball Roll

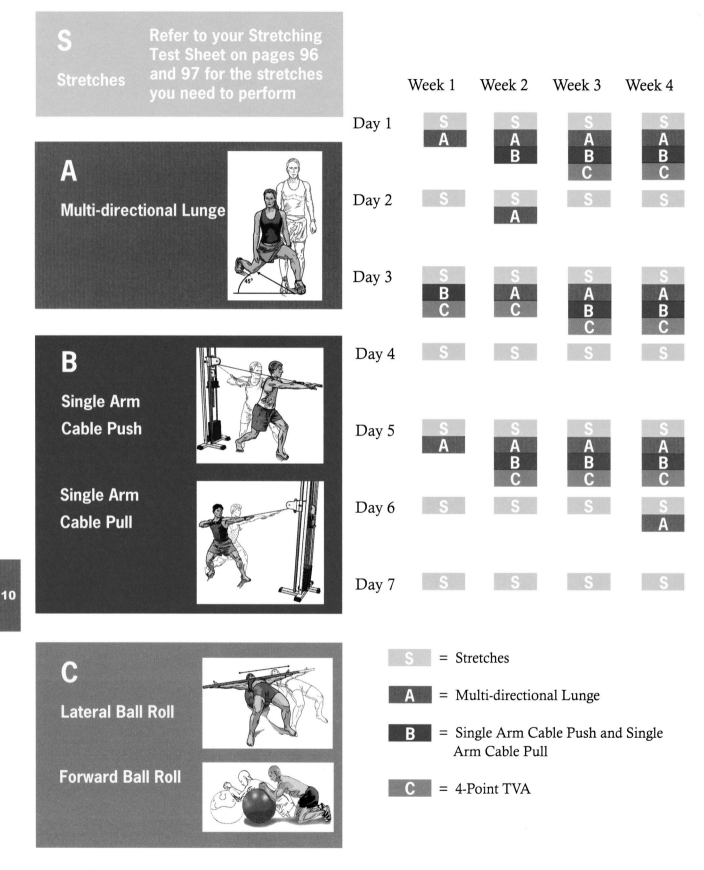

	Week 1	Week 2	Week 3	Week 4
Day 1	S A	S A B	S A B C	S A B C
Day 2	S	S A	S	S
Day 3	S B C	S A C	S A B C	S A B C
Day 4	S	S	S	S
Day 5	S A	S A B C	S A B C	S A B C
Day 6	S	S	S	S A
Day 7	S	S	S	S

S = Stretches

A = Multi-directional Lunge

B = Single Arm Cable Push and Single Arm Cable Pull

C = 4-Point TVA

Vitalizer Program

Exercise	Rest	Intensity	Reps	Tempo	Sets
Single Arm Cable Push	↓	-2 reps	10 each	Moderate	1 - 4
Single Arm Cable Pull	↓	-2 reps	10 each	Slow	1 - 4
Multi-directional Lunge	↓	-1 rep	1 - 2 each	Moderate	1 - 4
Lateral Ball Roll	↓	-1 rep	4 - 8 each	Hold 3 seconds	1 - 3
Forward Ball Roll	1 - 3 minutes ↓		10	Slow	1 - 3

Single Arm Cable Push

- Stand facing a cable column that has been adjusted to shoulder height.

- Take a split stance with one leg forward and the other behind you; your knees should be soft and unlocked.

- Grab the cable handle, using the arm on the same side as the rear leg.

- Initiate the movement with your trunk; gently draw your belly button in toward your spine and simultaneously rotate your trunk toward the forward leg while pushing the cable out in front of your shoulder.

- Keep the forearm in exact alignment with the cable throughout the movement. Do not let your elbow drop below or rise above the line of the cable.

- Reverse this movement until you reach the starting position and repeat this movement.

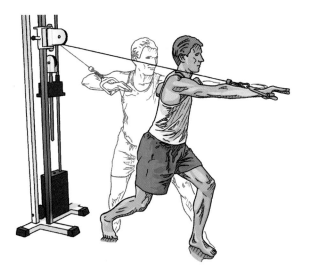

10

Vitalizer Program

Single Arm Cable Pull

- Stand facing a cable column that has been adjusted to shoulder height.

- Take a split stance with one leg forward and the other behind you; your knees should be soft and unlocked.

- Grab the cable handle, using the arm on the same side as the rear leg.

- Initiating the movement with your trunk, gently draw your belly button in toward your spine and simultaneously rotate your trunk toward the rear leg while pulling the cable toward your shoulder.

- Keep the forearm in exact alignment with the cable throughout the movement. Do not let your elbow drop below or rise above the line of the cable.

- Reverse this movement until you reach the starting position.

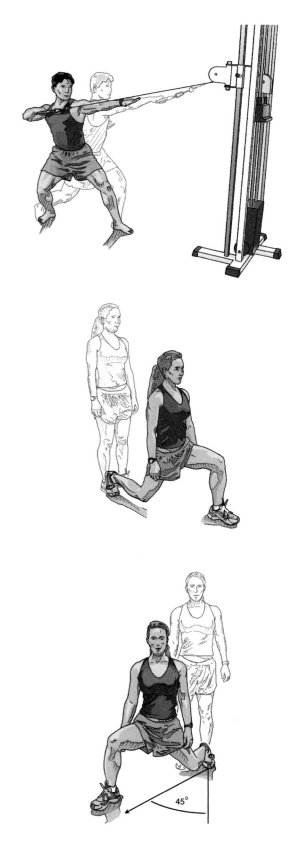

Multi-directional Lunge

You will be lunging in 5 different directions with each leg. To help visualize where to step, picture standing in the middle of a clock. Begin each step standing with good posture and facing in the same direction. Initiate each movement by drawing your belly button inward and keeping an upright posture. Do not lean forward, to the side or backwards.

1. Front Lunge:
Step to the 12 o'clock position (straight forward). Your front shin should be straight and perpendicular to the floor and your back knee should just touch the floor.

2. Front 45° Lunge:
Step half way between the 12 and 3 o'clock, or the 12 and 9 o'clock positions (45° to the front). Keep your head and eyes forward, shoulders and pelvis square to the front, and allow the trailing leg to pivot naturally as you drop into the lunge. A common mistake is to turn the whole body 45° and lunge, which is no different than a front lunge.

Vitalizer Program

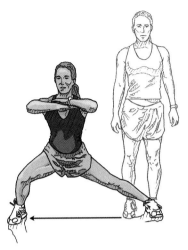

3. Lateral Lunge:

Step out to the side (3 or 9 o'clock position). Keep both feet facing forward and bend the leg you are stepping with.

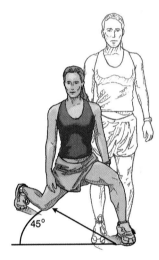

4. Back 45° Lunge:

Step back half way between the 3 and 6 o'clock or the 6 and 9 o'clock positions. Keep your body facing forward, but step back with your foot facing inward at about 45°. Drop your back knee down so that it just touches the floor, then return to standing.

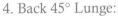

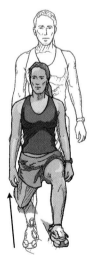

5. Back Lunge:

Step straight back (6 o'clock position), into the same position as a front center lunge. Remember, Your front shin should be straight and perpendicular to the floor and your back knee should just touch the floor.

Vitalizer Program

Lateral Ball Roll

- From a sitting position on a Swiss ball, roll back so that your head and shoulders are supported by the ball.

- Lift your hips up so that they are in line with your knees and shoulders.

- Place your tongue on the roof of your mouth.

- Hold your body in perfect alignment (hips and arms should stay parallel to the floor) and shuffle your feet as you roll to one side.

- Pause, then return to the center.

- Move only as far to the side as you comfortably can while holding perfect alignment. You may find that you can only move an inch or two; that is fine.

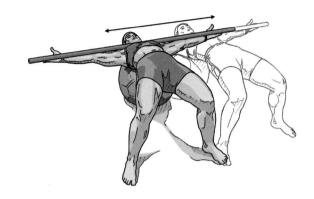

Forward Ball Roll

- Start kneeling in front of a Swiss ball with your forearms just behind the apex of the ball. The angle at your hips and shoulders should be the same (imagine being able to place a box in the space between the back of your arms and your thighs).

- Draw your belly button inward and hold good alignment of your back and head.

- Roll forward, moving your legs and arms equally, so that the angles at the shoulders and hips remain equal.

- Stop at the point just before you lose form (you will feel your low back drop down when your form breaks).

- Your tempo should be 3 seconds out, up to 3 seconds hold, and 3 seconds return.

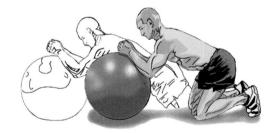

Performance Program

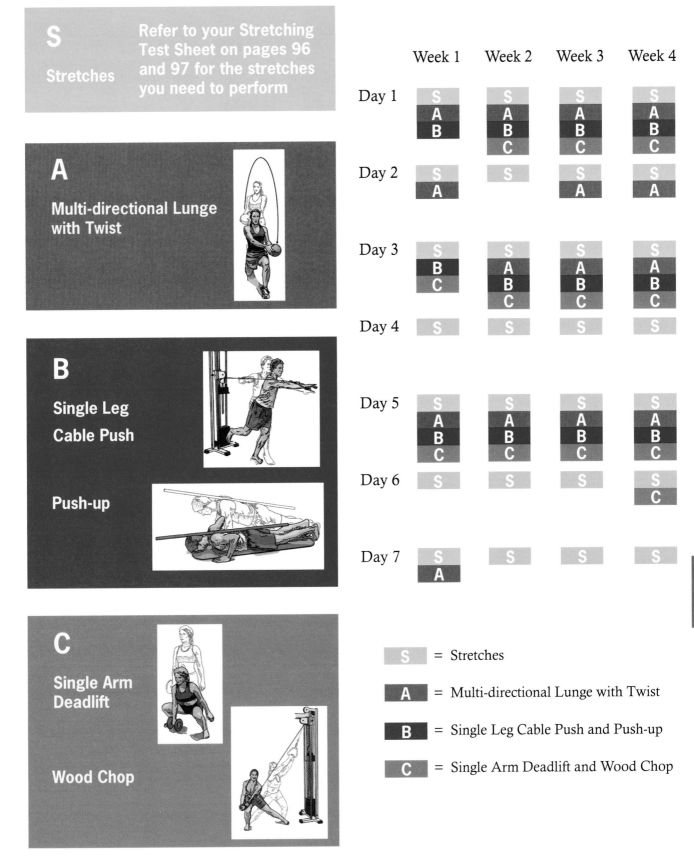

S Stretches — Refer to your Stretching Test Sheet on pages 96 and 97 for the stretches you need to perform

A Multi-directional Lunge with Twist

B Single Leg Cable Push
Push-up

C Single Arm Deadlift
Wood Chop

	Week 1	Week 2	Week 3	Week 4
Day 1	S A B	S A B C	S A B C	S A B C
Day 2	S A	S	S A	S A
Day 3	S B C	S A B C	S A B C	S A B C
Day 4	S	S	S	S
Day 5	S A B C	S A B C	S A B C	S A B C
Day 6	S	S	S	S C
Day 7	S A	S	S	S

S = Stretches
A = Multi-directional Lunge with Twist
B = Single Leg Cable Push and Push-up
C = Single Arm Deadlift and Wood Chop

Performance Program

Exercise	Rest	Intensity	Reps	Tempo	Sets
Multi-directional Lunge with Twist	↓	-2 reps	1 - 3 each	Moderate	1 - 4
Single Leg Cable Push	↓	-2 reps	10 each	Moderate	1 - 4
Push-up	↓	-2 reps	10	Slow	1 - 4
Single Arm Deadlift	↓	-2 reps	10 each	Slow	1 - 4
Wood Chop	1 - 3 minutes ↓		10 each	Moderate	1 - 4

Multi-directional Lunge with Twist

As with the multi-directional lunge, you will be lunging in 5 different directions with each leg. With this version of the exercise, you will be adding a twist to each lunge movement. To help visualize where to step, picture standing in the middle of a clock. Begin each step standing with good posture and facing in the same direction. Initiate each movement by drawing your belly button inward and keeping an upright posture, do not lean forward, to the side or backwards. For the twist motion, hold a light weight (medicine ball or dumbbell) to one side. As you lunge, bring the weight over your head, to the other side. You always want to weight to go over your front leg.

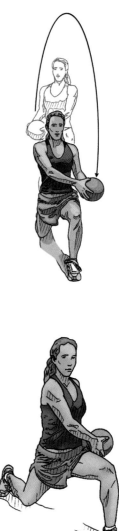

1. Front Lunge:
Step to the 12 o'clock position (straight forward). Your front shin should be straight and perpendicular to the floor and your back knee should just touch the floor. Begin by holding the weight on the side that will be your back leg, so when you twist, the weight will end up over the leg you step with.

2. Front 45° Lunge:
Step half way between the 12 and 3 o'clock, or the 12 and 9 o'clock positions (45° to the front). Again, start with the weight on the side of your back leg. Keep your head and eyes forward as you twist.

Performance Program

3. Lateral Lunge:

Step out to the side (3 or 9 o'clock position). Keep both feet facing forward and bend the leg you are stepping with. Start with the weight opposite to the side you are stepping towards.

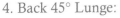

4. Back 45° Lunge:

Step back half way between the 3 and 6 o'clock or the 6 and 9 o'clock positions. Keep your body facing forward, but step back with your foot facing inward at about 45°. Drop your back knee down so that it just touches the floor. Now, hold the weight to the side of the leg that you are stepping back with and bring the weight over the front leg as you lunge back.

5. Back Lunge:

Step straight back (6 o'clock position), into the same position as a front center lunge. Again, hold the weight to the side of the leg that you are stepping back with.

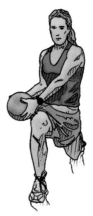

Single Leg Cable Push

- Stand facing a cable column that has been adjusted to shoulder height.

- Stand on only one leg. The exercise will be easier if you stand on the leg opposite the arm you are pushing with. For a greater challenge, stand on the same side leg.

- Initiating the movement with your trunk, gently draw your belly button in toward your spine and simultaneously rotate your trunk toward the forward leg while pushing the cable out in front of your shoulder.

- Keep the forearm in exact alignment with the cable throughout the movement. Do not let your elbow drop below or rise above the line of the cable.

- Reverse this movement until you reach the starting position and repeat this movement.

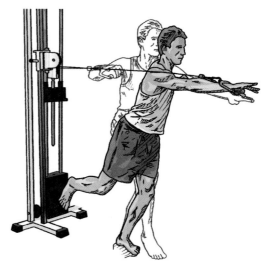

Push-up

- Lie face down on the floor with your hands placed comfortably at shoulder level.

- Keep your spine and head in alignment; do not let your head drop forward as you push yourself up to a plank position.

- Lower yourself down so that your nose just touches the ground, keeping perfect alignment, and repeat.

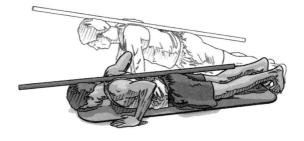

Performance Program

Single Arm Deadlift

- Begin in a sumo stance (feet a bit wider than shoulder width apart and turned out slightly; you should be able to comfortably squat all the way down).

- Hold a dumbbell in one hand (in front of the leg) and look forward, with your head and chest held up.

- Take a deep diaphragmatic breath and pull your belly button in toward your spine.

- Bend forward slightly until the dumbbell is just above your knee. Keep a natural curve in your low back. If you were to pinch a bit of skin at the level of your low back, you should be able to hold it as you bend forward.

- Keeping your torso at that position, drop your body down as far as you can comfortably go. Do not lean forward or round your back.

- Imagine pushing the ground away from you as you stand back up. As you return to standing, keep your torso upright and the curve in your low back. You should feel your glut and hamstring muscles working with this exercise.

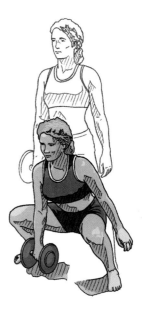

Wood Chop

- Face sideways to a cable column and take a stable stance slightly wider than shoulder width.

- Grasp the handle with the hand furthest from the cable column and place the other hand over it.

- Draw your belly button in toward your spine and initiate the movement by rotating your trunk away from the cable column while simultaneously pulling the handle downward across your body; the movement ends when your hands reach the hip furthest from the cable.

- Once you have become proficient at this movement, move to the advanced level of the exercise, which includes a weight-shift on each leg; begin the movement with 70% of your weight on the leg closest to the cable and while bringing the handle across your body, gradually shift your weight so 70% is on the other leg by the end of the movement.

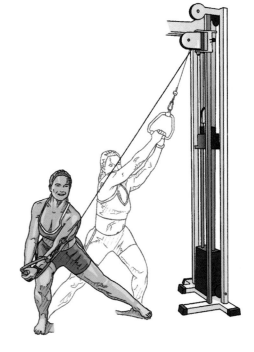

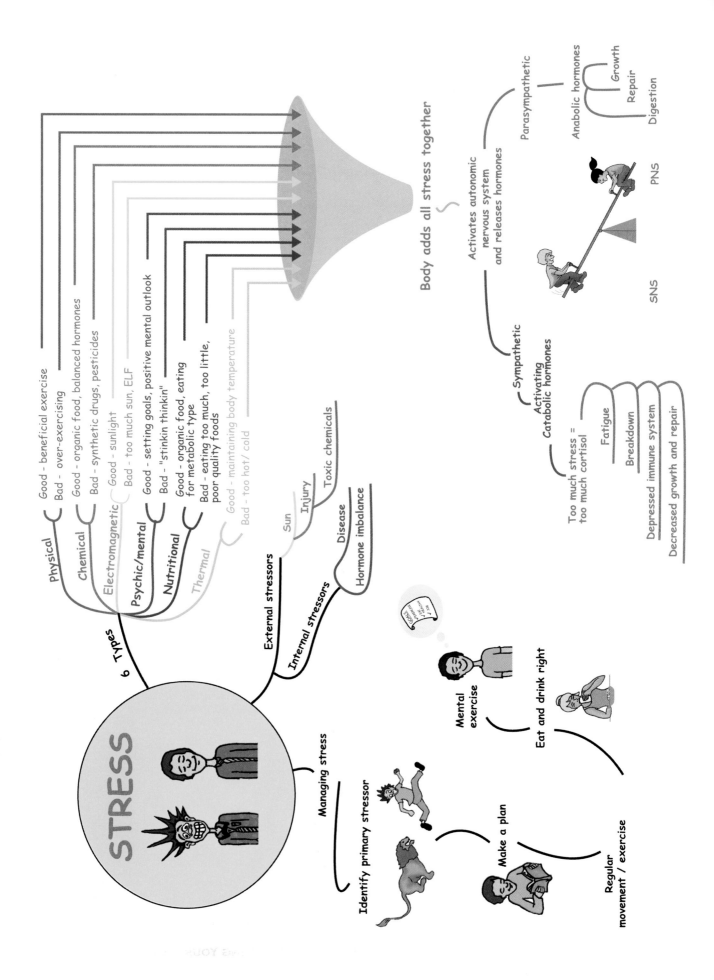

Chapter 11

Is Stress Affecting Your Health?

Stress is very often the root of many people's problems, whether they recognize it or not. You'll often hear that someone is "under too much stress." You, too, may feel this way. But what exactly is stress? How can some withstand more stress than others? Is stress always a bad thing? Let's take a look.

A Typical Day

You've been so busy preparing for tomorrow's meeting that you didn't realize the hour. It's approaching midnight and you're bushed. You need to wind down, so you watch television for a while. At 1:04 a.m. you're finally relaxed enough to go to sleep. But you suddenly wake in a sweat and note the time—3:14 a.m. After a quick trip to the bathroom, you hop back into bed. But you can't get back to sleep. Tomorrow's busy schedule races through your mind. Forty minutes later you're still lying there, counting backwards from one hundred, trying to fall asleep. The next thing you know, the alarm clock is ringing off the nightstand. You can't believe it's already 6:00 a.m.—you feel like you just got to sleep. Just ten more minutes... Beep! Beep! Beep! You have to pry your eyes open to see the clock. It's 6:10 a.m. and you don't dare hit the snooze button again. You head for the kitchen in search of coffee, knocking on the kids' doors as you pass. Before the water can even begin to drip through the coffee filter, your brain is trying to figure out how to get the kids up, fed and off to school, take your shower, get dressed, finish off that last report and get on the road before the traffic jam starts.

Finally, the kids are off to school. You're dressed and ready to go when you realize you haven't eaten. No worry, you grab another coffee and a bagel from the cafe on your way to the office. Work is crazy, as usual. Your co-worker is sick, so you offer to work through lunch to cover his clients. Between meetings, while eating an apple and sipping your fourth cup of coffee, you realize you forgot to pay the bills last weekend. Then your daughter calls to remind you that she has soccer practice tonight.

It's 5:06 p.m. and you can't wait to get home. But you first must drop off clothes at the cleaners, shop for groceries, work your way through traffic to pick up your daughter at soccer and your son from daycare. Now it's almost seven o'clock and you cook dinner while trying to prepare for tomorrow's meeting and help the kids with homework, and of course, get those bills paid. After dinner, exhausted, looking at a pile of dishes and a cluttered kitchen, you wonder how long you'll have to work like this. You have a final cup of coffee, clean up and get back to preparing your reports for tomorrow. It's only Monday, but you could swear it's at least Thursday.

Does this sound like you? Or perhaps you're thinking that this would be a relaxing day compared to yours. Even if your day isn't this chaotic, we all experience some degree of stress.

What Is Stress?

You probably think of stress as inherently bad, but this isn't always the case. Just as bones and muscles need physical exercise to stay strong, we also need certain amounts of stress to stay healthy. A complete lack of stress would not be a good thing! There are six major types of stress, each of which can have "good" or "bad" effects.

1. Physical stress

2. Chemical stress

3. Electromagnetic stress

4. Psychic or Mental stress

5. Nutritional stress

6. Thermal stress

1. Physical stress

The Good: Physical stress in the form of movement or exercise is very beneficial. The actual stress comes from loading the muscles and bones of our body under the influence of gravity. Astronauts in space need regular exercise in order to counteract the loss of bone and muscle mass that occurs under zero gravity conditions.

Adequate movement and exercise also helps us to maintain an optimal **metabolic rate**, keeping us from becoming overweight. Considering that only about 8% of men and 3% of women exercise regularly, and that about 60% of Americans are overweight at present, you can see that we are in great need of more of this good stressor.[1]

> **Metabolic Rate:** The rate at which all physical and chemical processes take place within your body.

The Bad: Over-exercising can be every bit as bad as not exercising enough. While under-exercising can contribute to becoming fat and sluggish inside, over-exercising can cause immune system suppression.[2] This can lead to increased incidence of upper respiratory infection, chronic fatigue and a number of other maladies. Extreme exercise for athletes is often linked to poor performance and increased incidence of injury.

Another form of adverse physical stress is poor posture. Posture has a significant influence on breathing, muscle function, joint health, circulation and internal organ support. When the body structure is not in balance, the rest of the system follows.

2. Chemical stress

The Good: Our bodies are full of chemicals—naturally produced chemicals that are essential for health. The work of producing these key chemicals is a necessary stress for the body. For example, when your body systems are working correctly, exercise results in chemical adaptations in the form of hormonal changes that alter your biochemistry to increase protein synthesis, energy production and myriad other chemical reactions. The action of sunlight on the skin results in the production of Vitamin D and the regulation of the hormones melatonin and cortisol—both chemical reactions. Plant and animal foods (preferably organically raised) are made up of organic chemicals—vitamins, enzymes, proteins and fats that we need to survive.

The Bad: Today we are bombarded with thousands upon thousands of chemicals that were not around one hundred years ago. Many of these chemicals are synthetic, and our bodies do not have mechanisms to neutralize them. Synthetically manufactured medical drugs, such as aspirin, are among the most common forms of unfavorable chemical stress. Other examples of dangerous chemical stressors are agricultural chemicals such as pesticides, herbicides, fungicides and certain fertilizers. These chemicals are often made from the same formulas used to make biological weapons, yet nearly two billion pounds of these chemicals are sprayed on our foods each year in the U.S. alone.[3] Many health problems have been linked to this form of chemical stress.

3. Electromagnetic stress

The Good: Certainly, my favorite form of electromagnetic stress is sunlight. Without sunlight, we wouldn't be alive. I'd say that qualifies sunlight as a good electromagnetic stress! The electromagnetic field of the earth is also a good form of this kind of stress. This invisible field helps control the rhythm of our hormones and other physiological functions. A common example of the earth's electromagnetic effects can be experienced when weather patterns change. At the onset of a thunderstorm, many people feel changes in their joints, muscles and even their moods.

The Bad: The most obvious form of bad electromagnetic stress is over-exposure to sunlight, resulting in sunburn. In Australia and New Zealand, the ultraviolet rays are poorly filtered by the thin ozone layer. This means you can begin to burn in under 12 minutes on a summer day. Most people know that overexposure to radiation such as medical x-rays can also be harmful to your health. Often overlooked is the *extremely low frequency* (ELF) pollution emitted by electronic devices such as computers, cell phones, microwave ovens, electric motors, your TV and even an electric blanket. Many of these forms of stress are insidious, causing dysfunction in your hormonal and autonomic nervous systems.

4. Psychic or Mental stress

The Good: Thinking and using your mind productively represents good psychic or mental stress. Having a plan or setting goals in your life and doing the work to achieve them is also a positive form of this stress. Other examples include overcoming adversity to become a stronger, better person. Without psychic stress, our minds would not develop fully.

The Bad: A common form of bad psychic stress is focusing on things that you don't want in life instead of what you do want—what I call "Stinking Thinking." Other forms of psychic stress include verbal abuse from others, studying so much that your mental faculties begin to diminish, and challenging religious or spiritual beliefs that are imposed upon you — even if self imposed. Being rushed or taking on more work or responsibility than you can manage will also produce unhealthy psychic stress.

5. Nutritional Stress

The Good: Eating in accordance with your metabolic type (Chapter 3), eating organic foods (Chapter 4) and not over- or under-eating are all representative of good nutritional stress. In these instances, the term stress is used to indicate the stress of digestion, assimilation and metabolizing of foods. For example, your body must be stressed with the challenge of extracting the nutrition from your food or it will become lazy, much like a person's muscles become lazy if you put them in a sling or cast and don't use them.

The Bad: Eating too much, too little or eating the wrong food proportions for your metabolic type are unhealthy forms of nutritional stress. Consuming foods with toxins such as pesticides, herbicides, food preservatives, colorings, thickeners, emulsifiers and the like can be very stressful to the body as well. In my opinion, this type of stress from food is responsible for a large percentage of disease today.

6. Thermal stress

The Good: Maintaining your body temperature at 98.6°F (32°C) is the most obvious of the good thermal stressors. When it's hot or cold outside, the thermoregulatory system is stressed in order to keep your internal temperature constant. It's good to stress this system now and again to maintain its dynamic capacity.

The Bad: Anything that burns you is a form of adverse thermal stress! In addition, the opposite thermal stress would be anything that brings your body temperature too low for an extended period of time.

What Stress Does to Your Body

The six types of stress described above can be broken down into two groups, **internal** and **external**.

External stressors

External stressors are things that stress the body from the outside, such as sunlight, physical pain (caused by injury or other external forces) emotional trauma and toxic chemical exposure.

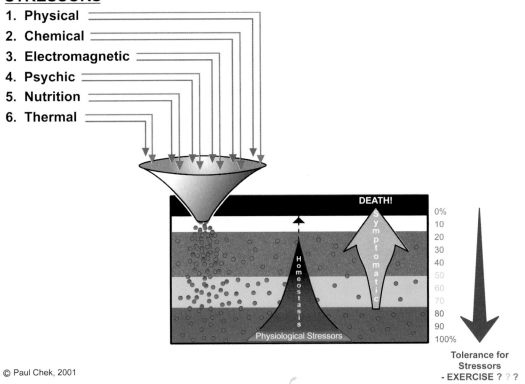

STRESSORS
1. Physical
2. Chemical
3. Electromagnetic
4. Psychic
5. Nutrition
6. Thermal

© Paul Chek, 2001

Figure 1: All stressors are funneled together within your body and processed by your nervous system. The green arrows represent good stressors, while the red arrows signify bad stressors. Imagine accumulating all of your stressors for a week or a month. The higher your levels of stress, the harder it is on your body.

Internal stressors

Internal stressors come from within the body and are most often the *reaction* to external stressors. For example, if you're repeatedly exposed to toxic chemicals, cancer or other diseases may develop. Even if the toxic chemicals are removed, cancer will continue to stress the body systems. If you're in an unhappy relationship, an external situation, you'll experience a chronic stress response *within* the body. Chronic stressors cause elevated stress hormones in the body, leading to immune suppression, the inability to heal and eventually to disease.

Stress is perceived or interpreted by key control systems of the body—limbic/emotional, hormonal, visceral, nervous, musculoskeletal and subsystems. The green arrows in Figure 1 represent good stressors that are used by the body to regulate and maintain optimal bodily function. The bad or excessive stressors (red arrows) can throw the body out of

balance. The nervous system plays an important role here. All the stressors are funneled together and processed by the nervous system to create an overall stress picture in the body. As shown in Figure 1, you'll stay in the Green Zone (in homeostasis, or balance) if the total stress picture is favorable for your body. When in this zone, response to external stressors such as exercise is favorable. The ability to bounce back from potentially damaging stressors is also much improved.

If for any reason the sum of all the stressors places too great a demand on your body, you'll begin to fall out of balance and move into the Yellow Zone. If you don't make the necessary changes to reduce the primary stress or stressors, your body begins to break down and you progressively move into the Red Zone. Your ability to cope with external stressors such as exercise is progressively diminished, as is your ability to tolerate internal stressors, such as disease. The further you get into the Red Zone, the

11

more easily disease will be able to take hold. This is where the saying "stress kills" comes from.

Nerves of Steel

There are many sayings that link stress and your nerves together: *My nerves are frayed. You're getting on my nerves! My nerves can't handle this!* As indicated above, the nervous system plays an important role in evaluating and processing stress in the body. A brief explanation of how the nervous system works will help clarify how stress affects your body.

The nervous system is a combination of two systems that work together. The *peripheral* nervous system controls conscious movement and the *central* nervous system, which contains the *autonomic* nervous system, controls those actions in the body that you don't normally regulate through conscious thought, such as digesting and eliminating food, releasing hormones, sweating and the regulating of blood flow to different muscles and organs.

The autonomic nervous system is further split into two branches: the **sympathetic** and the **parasympathetic**. When activated, the sympathetic nervous system (SNS) produces a fight-or-flight response. Whenever threatened, our natural inclination is either "fight" to protect ourselves, or "flight"—to run for our lives. A potentially stressful situation will activate the SNS and prepare your body for fighting or running by producing the following responses, among others, within your body:

- Release of stress hormones that elevate your heart rate and blood pressure.

- Shunting of blood away from your internal organs to the skin and muscles—greatly reducing or stopping all digestive and eliminative processes.

- Increased sweating.

You've probably experienced these responses when suddenly faced with a frightening or challenging situation.

The SNS is often referred to as the *catabolic* (tissue-destructive) system. When your fight-or-flight response is activated, levels of the stress hormone cortisol are elevated. If cortisol levels are above normal, your growth and repair hormones are suppressed. Long-term over-production of cortisol leads to a break down of body tissues and fatigue of the adrenal glands. As the adrenals fatigue, the body is unable to maintain balance between stress and immune hormones, which leads to immune system dysfunction. Many years of chronic stress results in disease and premature death.

> **Sympathetic Nervous System:** Part of the autonomic nervous system, which when activated (often as a response to stress) results in the release of stress hormones, increasing your heart rate and blood pressure while decreasing digestive and repair processes—often referred to as a "fight-or-flight" response.
>
> **Parasympathetic Nervous System:** Part of the autonomic nervous system which supports digestive and repair processes, opposes the effects of the sympathetic nervous system.

When repeatedly stressed, you're continually mobilizing your energy reserves for immediate use. At the same time, the parasympathetic nervous system (PNS) is suppressed. The PNS stimulates digestion, metabolism and the release of tissue building hormones (DHEA, growth hormone, testosterone, estrogen and others). If the PNS is constantly shut down, you'll be unable to effectively digest foods and repair your body. This over–stimulation of the SNS is a common cause of many chronic fatigue states and chronic disease processes, not to mention emotional imbalances and distress.

How the Nervous System Responds to a Typical Day

Figure 2 demonstrates how autonomic nervous system responses vary over the course of the day. The blue dotted line shows an optimal response—someone with an ANS that can cope with the stress created in an average day. This person has control over lifestyle factors such as diet, scheduling and finances and can keep their SNS and PNS balanced. The dashed black line in the center of the green arrow represents the division between SNS and PNS dominance; both

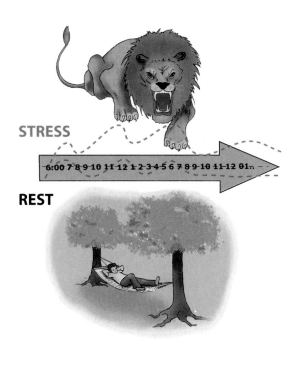

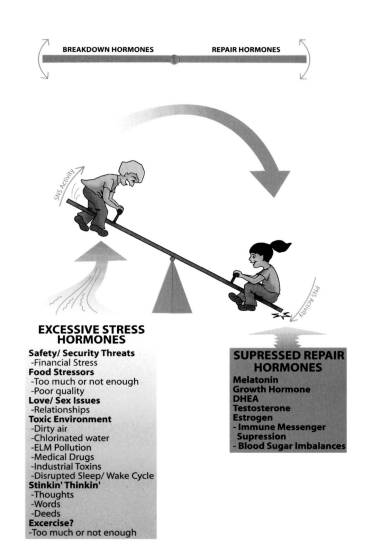

Figure 2: An optimal (blue line) and over-stressed (red line) response of the autonomic nervous system throughout the day. The optimal response represents a balance between the two parts of the nervous system, while the over-stressed response signifies a person whose body is working on high-stress mode for the entire day, limiting digestive and repair processes from taking place.

Figure 3: The Stress/Recovery Teeter-Totter. The more stress your body is under, the more stress hormones it will produce. When your body is overburdened from making stress hormones, it is not able to produce adequate levels of repair hormones to keep your body healthy.

branches of the ANS are always working, it's just a matter of which branch exerts the greatest influence over your physiology at any given time.

The red dotted line shows the response to the typical day depicted at the beginning of this chapter. Waking up tired to an annoying alarm clock immediately activates the SNS, sending you out of the Green Zone. Coffee (an adrenal stressor), along with a diet that does not produce an optimal metabolic response, serves to magnify the response. At this point, you have created a state in your body that is the modern equivalent of running from a hungry lion! Once at work, the lack of sufficient breakfast causes low blood sugar and low energy levels. This kick-starts the SNS again, producing hormones that activate the body's energy stores to make sure there is sufficient fuel to run the brain. This yo-yo syndrome continues, stressing your hormonal system

and keeping you in a fight/flight state all day. In the evening, when you should be winding down, you have to drink more coffee just to make it through the chores and to prepare for the next day. So instead of winding down and letting the PNS work as you rest and repair your body, the SNS is once again sending you out of the Green Zone. Digestion and blood sugar levels are disrupted, resulting in additional internal stressors as well as reducing your ability to get a good night's sleep. Once again, you wake up at 3 a.m. due to the "activating effect" of stress hormones, sweating from an increased metabolic rate. You'll become progressively more tired, fatigued

11

and will start suffering from a string of nagging ailments that may seem unrelated.

In contrast, when you eat regularly planned meals that support your metabolic type, and, as you exhibit control over your daily schedule, you're able to keep your ANS functioning within the Green Zone. This means that when a stressor does occur, *you're capable of adapting quickly*. After dinner, your PNS is activated and becomes the dominant branch of the ANS, facilitating digestion, elimination, immune function, growth and repair processes. You get to bed by 10:30 p.m. and enter a proper sleep, growth and repair cycle (Chapter 12).

For the More Technically Minded - Understanding Your Stress Responses

To better understand our response to stress, we must consider how our brains developed. Research by neuroscientist Paul MacLean shows that our brains are actually made up of three brains: the reptilian brain, mammalian brain and the *new* mammalian brain (known as the human brain).[4]

The reptilian and mammalian brains are actually functional units, yet fully integrated within our more modern human brain. The most important feature inherited from the reptilian and mammalian brain is our primary concern for our own safety, followed by our survival instinct to feed or seek sustenance. The reptilian perspective ranks procreation as the lowest concern.

Reptiles have little emotional capacity and live purely upon instinct. If a predator enters their territory they *fight or flight* because they innately know their lives depend upon their reaction. As humans we have a unique capacity to *ignore* our instincts. When stressful situations arise, we often think irrationally. For example, we ignore our primary reptilian instinct to be secure by spending money that we don't have on cars, jewelry and other status symbols. In this case, we're sacrificing financial security for an improved social status—what our mammalian brain thinks of as rank.

Unfortunately, many people will sacrifice their health by ignoring the second most important concern of the reptilian brain—eating good food. They compromise their well being by eating cheap, poor quality foods so they can afford a fancy car to improve their *status*.

Reptiles and mammals engage in sex for purposes of perpetuating their species, but only when they're safe and well fed. Many humans, on the other hand, prioritize sex over health and safety. An overly stressed body will automatically respond by decreasing the sex drive to preserve energy for the first and second reptilian priorities. The amount of Viagra sold today is but one indication that our human brain has distorted our reptilian drive for safety and sustenance, raising our stress levels so high that many can't enjoy a healthy sexual relationship. If you're suffering from a low sex drive, you'll need to get your reptilian priorities of security and sustenance sorted out. The CHEK Points at the end of this chapter will help with the first priority. Chapters 3 and 4 will show you how to get the food and nutrients your body needs.

Ignoring our reptilian and mammalian (old brain) instincts does very little to improve our stress levels! Modern society is driven by new brain desires to look better and have more material goods, often at the expense of physical and mental health, resulting in more stress and disease.

CHEK Points for Managing Stress

1. Identify your primary stressor

Focus on reducing stress in the area that is causing you the most stress. Generally, the reptilian priorities are: Security, Sustenance and Sex. Alleviating the chief stressor in your life often creates a domino effect, wiping out or dramatically reducing other stressors in succession.

2. Make a plan

Make a realistic plan to address your biggest stressor and set a series of achievable short-term goals, allowing you to clearly recognize progress as it's made. Look for current books, videos or audio tapes that address issues related to your key stressor and how to overcome it. A list to get you started is provided in the Resource Section.

Another effective method is to find someone who has already been successful at overcoming the challenge you now face. There is no better teacher than experience.

3. Eat and drink right

Internal stressors only serve to magnify external stressors! Regardless of what your primary stressor may be, if you aren't eating according to your metabolic type (Chapter 3), you will not be able to effectively replace the stress hormones you're using on a daily basis, which only causes more stress to the body.

Once you know your metabolic type, go out of your way to eat as much organic and free-range food as possible (Chapter 4). The more conventionally farmed food you eat, the more toxins you're consuming. These toxic poisons create a significant stress at a metabolic level, and many of them have been linked to mental and emotional dysfunction.

Dehydration is a common cause of internal stress. A reduction of as little as 1% of water content in your central nervous system can cause significant psychological disorders. Reducing your intake of coffee, tea and sodas, plus drinking more high-quality water, is an easy way to start reducing the internal stress on your body.

4. Move and exercise

Regular exercise can be a major tool to reduce stress. When performed correctly for your particular needs, exercise in the correct dose stimulates an *anabolic* (tissue growth and repair) environment. Your exercise program from Section 3 is carefully constructed so as not to overstress your body.

If you scored high on your stress questionnaire, it's very important that you pay close attention to the Energy Balancing Exercises in Chapter 6. These exercises will help stimulate your parasympathetic system, which is important if you're overstressed.

5. Mental exercise

"You're a living magnet and you inevitably attract into your life, the people, circumstances, ideas, and resources in harmony with your dominant thoughts." (Brian Tracy, *The Luck Factor*).[5] Many successful individuals give credit to the power of positive thinking. Try harmonizing your thoughts, words and actions with your goals and you may find that this will help decrease stress. Doing so is a good example of beneficial mental or psychic stress. Make sure you're talking and thinking about what you *do want*, rather than what you don't. There are many excellent resources available that will show you how to apply this technique in your life.

Other effective approaches to reducing stress include meditation and the use of a computer program called Freeze Frame, an emotional management enhancer that helps you access and maintain mental and emotional balance (see Resources page 249). These modalities will help reduce your stress levels by stimulating the parasympathetic system.

Traits and Functionality Associated with the Reptilian Brain

- Regulates breathing, heart beat, digestion, elimination, sleep/wake cycles and temperature
- The four 'F's: fight, flight, feeding and fornicating
- Instinctual
- Ritualistic (performing the same functions at the same time of day, eating the same foods, behaving a given way during different seasons)
- Defining hierarchy within a group and establishing space in the ecological niche

Traits and Functionality Associated with the Mammalian (paleomammalian) Brain

- Increased sense of subordination (rank, power, authority)
- Increased capacity for memory and learning
- Significant expansion of the emotional centers of the brain (playful moods, fright, passion, joy, sadness, females nurse and protect young)

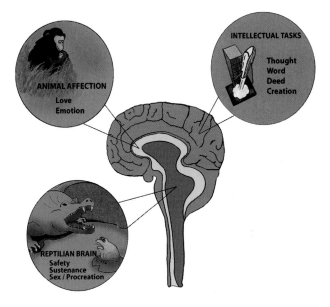

Traits and Functionality Associated with the Human (neomammalian) Brain

- Rational thinking
- Capable of producing symbolic language, enabling intellectual activities such as reading, writing and performing mathematical calculations
- The ability to generate ideas
- The ability to ignore reptilian and mammalian instincts
- Spiritual development

	Old Brain Instincts	New Brain Desires
Safety/Security	Survival Territorial	Financial gain Personal space Material addictions
Feeding	Satiety	Addictive eating Emotional eating
Sex/Appearance	Procreation (only when the above needs are met)	Lust/Desire/Emotional Status driven Procreation

He who is of calm and happy nature will hardly feel the pressure of age, but to him who is of an opposite disposition youth and age are equally a burden.

Plato, *The Republic*

Case History
Jackie Holman, C.H.E.K Practitioner Level 2, Bowling Green, Ohio, client of Paul Chek and Chris Maund, C.H.E.K Certified, C.H.E.K Faculty

After meeting Paul Chek, my life changed forever and I am now much healthier than I could have imagined. My only regret is not having met him earlier and been given the ability to take charge of my health issues sooner.

My name is Jackie Holman, and I am a 41-year-old female C.H.E.K Practitioner Level 2. I have spent the greater part of my life competing in athletics, including basketball at collegiate and professional levels and rugby. After becoming a manager at a World Gym, I immersed myself in body building. I once thought the sport of body building, and body builders themselves, were the ultimate in health and fitness.

One day, a body builder friend recommended the supplement Ripped Fuel™. So, I followed the directions on the back of the bottle: take three capsules, three times a day. I don't drink coffee or any other type of caffeine, so it sent me over the edge. I backed it down to one capsule, first thing in the morning. I performed this ritual for eight years. My rationale for taking Rippled Fuel™ was that I needed the extra energy to get up at 3: 50 a.m each weekday, so I could get my workout in (I weighed 158 lbs, and was able to bench 225 lbs, leg press 1000 lbs, squat 315 lbs and dumbbell press 95 lbs) and start training my first clients at 5: 30 a.m. As my business took off, my days became longer and ended around 6:45 p.m. I needed something to get me through the long day.

While helping my sister on her horse farm, I was bucked off a stubborn horse, landing squarely on my tailbone, displacing and injuring it severely. Since I had no insurance, I tried to rehabilitate myself with body building exercises. This only made things worse. My life was heading in a downward tail spin……but by golly, I looked good, which is the bodybuilder's mentality! Then I started to notice a slight decline in my energy levels and I began putting on a little body fat. My health started to fail. Deep down inside I knew something was wrong.

A few years later, while attending a personal trainer's conference in Chicago, I took a class by Paul Chek. Paul began the class by asking how many of us evaluated our clients before developing their personalized exercise program. In truth, none of us did. Paul challenged the class to identify orthopedic red flags and learn how the body works. A year later, I took the Level 1 of the C.H.E.K Certification course at the Institute in Encinitas, California.

After hearing of my health problems, Paul had me test the function of my adrenal glands. I discovered I was suffering from adrenal exhaustion. I knew I had to make a change in my life, and fast. I was told effective immediately, no more Ripped Fuel™, and I was to get up no earlier than 6 a.m. I quit Ripped Fuel™ cold turkey. At first, I struggled, wanting to take it like a drug addict. But, I was afraid that if I took it just one more day, it would fire up my heart and I would die.

I suffered from low energy, fatigue, lethargy and needed lots of sleep (more than eight hours). I had trouble getting up in the mornings. I started to gain weight and couldn't lose it. I had low blood pressure-heart-rate, menstrual problems-severe cramps, PMS, was very irritable and retained water. I suffered from poor concentration and memory, depression and weakened immune function. I was exhausted and had trouble doing one single exercise.

It's been two long years now and I'm in recovery. I needed to be proactive in my own healthcare. The C.H.E.K Institute was my hospital and the staff, my holistic doctors. If it weren't for the C.H.E.K Institute, I wouldn't be here today. Now, I only eat organic foods. I do not train with machines, but use cable crossovers, Swiss balls, balance boards, medicine balls, free weights and a squat rack. My adrenals are out of the basement. I know I'm not where I need to be yet, but I thank God, I'm not where I used to be. I am a much happier and healthier person. I am enjoying the journey and believe in my heart that the C.H.E.K Institute's practices are the future in health and fitness.

Be proactive and take the time to educate yourself on how to look after your health.

11

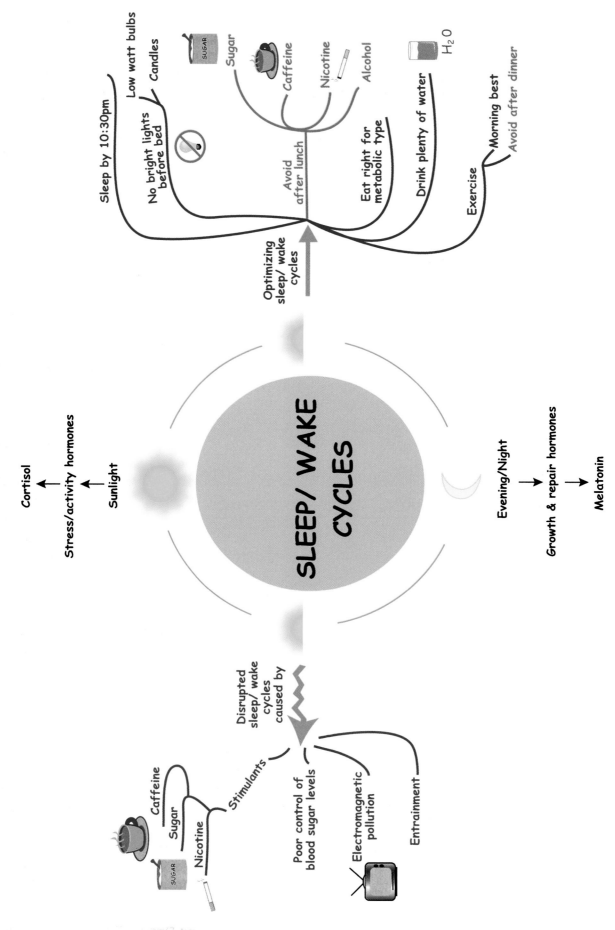

CHAPTER 12

ARE YOU GETTING TO BED ON TIME?

One of the biggest obstacles I face when coaching people to optimal health is getting them to understand the importance of going to bed on time. Today's world of late night TV and bright lights at the touch of a switch make it easy to forget that for thousands of years we lived in sync with the light and dark cycles of day and night. Our physiology is still the same as our ancient sun-driven ancestors – we're simply packaged in fancy clothes, drive cars and use lots of electronic gadgets. Despite the availability of artificial, 24-hour, 365-days-a-year light, we're still tuned to the natural rhythm of daily and seasonal light/dark cycles.

The best way to illustrate my point is to share my own experiences. A few years ago, I began to suffer from a number of nagging ailments such as neck pains, headaches, skin changes, itching, poor recovery from exercise, forgetfulness, dyslexic behavior and was having a hard time focusing at work. I tried several different approaches, and although my health improved, I still noted a general fatigue and lack of focus.

I consulted Dr. William Timmins, a naturopathic physician and founder of BioHealth Diagnostics in San Diego, California, in order to get to the bottom of what prevented me from a full recovery. During our initial consultation, Dr. Timmins asked me to describe my work schedule and a typical day. I explained that for many years I had lectured all over the world, a schedule that had me on airplanes and in many different countries for about six months each year. Most nights I would work until after 1 a.m. Even though I got about seven hours of sleep each night, I usually woke up feeling tired.

Dr. Timmins recognized that the majority of my symptoms were due to **circadian cycle** disruption and sleep deprivation. He convinced me that no matter what else I did, until I got to bed by 10:30 p.m. and got a full eight hours of sleep, I'd be wasting my time and money! While the night owl in me dreaded the thought of changing my schedule so dramatically, I respected his opinion and followed his advice. The changes in my body were dramatic. Within the first week my energy levels and concentration improved and my headaches and neck aches were dramatically reduced. I continue to follow Dr. Timmins' advice to respect my natural sleep/wake cycles and I feel great!

Our Natural Sleep/Wake Cycles

The cycles of light and dark that result from the movements of the sun and planets affect nearly all living creatures. Even though humans had the ability to use fire thousands of years ago, our activity and sleep schedules were still very much in tune with the sun and our environment. To illustrate how influential light is over the physiology of all life in nature, consider that during the solar eclipse on August 11,

> **Circadian Cycle:** A natural physiological cycle of about 24 hours that persists even in the absence of external cues.

1999, birds, horses and many other creatures went to sleep in the middle of the day when the sun was eclipsed.[1]

Whenever light stimulates your skin or eyes, regardless of the source, your brain and hormonal system think it's morning. In response to light, your hormonal system naturally releases cortisol. Cortisol is an activating hormone that is released in response to stress, light being a form of electromagnetic stress (Chapter 11). This activates the body and prepares it for movement, work, combat or whatever may be necessary for survival. We must remember that our physiological systems were well developed long before we even began using fire, so as far as your body is concerned:

Light = Sunshine = Cortisol release = Daytime activities.

As the sun rises, our cortisol levels also rise and peak around 6 - 9 a.m. (Figure 1). They then drop a little but remain high through midday, supporting daily activities. In the afternoon, cortisol levels begin dropping significantly, especially as the sun goes down. Decreasing cortisol levels allow the release of melatonin and increase levels of growth and repair hormones. If we follow our natural sleep/wake cycles, we start winding down as the sun sets and should fall asleep by about 10 p.m. Physical repairs mostly take place when the body is asleep, between about 10 p.m. and 2 a.m. After 2 a.m. the immune/repair energies are more focused on psychogenic (mental) repair, which lasts until we awaken.[2]

Disrupted Sleep/Wake Cycles

Figure 2 shows what happens if cortisol levels are elevated above normal by internal or external stressors (Chapter 11). The continual release of stress hormones may be a great idea for a mountain climber who is climbing hard to avoid a storm and is faced with a climb or freeze situation, but you don't want this response to be an everyday occurrence. Further, a brightly lit house, late night TV and working late into the evening will keep the levels of stress hormones high past sundown. Fluorescent lights, TV and computer screens flicker on and off between 60 and 120 cycles per second, which your brain interprets as morning sunlight. Since cortisol can take hours to clear from your blood stream, this will also prevent the normal release of melatonin and other growth/immune hormones, cutting into your immune system's valuable repair time.[3]

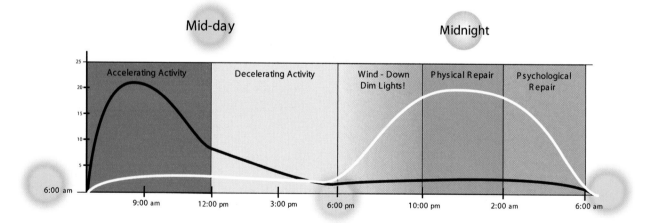

Figure 1: Natural sleep/wake cycle.
Many of our hormones are produced in tune with the cycle of the sun. Stress/activating hormones (black line) are produced as the sun rises and peak around mid-morning. As the day progresses, the levels of stress hormones decrease. The body then begins to increase production of growth and repair hormones (white line) as the sun goes down. Our bodies are designed to wind down from sunset until about 10 p.m. when sleep and physical repair should begin. Psychogenic repair takes place predominantly from about 2 to 6 a.m.

If you go to bed after midnight you've already missed over two hours of your physical repair cycle, which, as I said above, should start around 10 p.m. People working the graveyard shift or parents getting up in the middle of the night regularly have their psychogenic repair cycle disrupted. Such people commonly have a laundry list of nagging musculoskeletal injuries, an increased incidence of headaches, a sagging personality and even neurological disorders.

A disrupted sleep/wake cycle can also result in *adrenal fatigue*. The adrenal glands are located atop the kidneys and produce hormones called glucocorticoids, of which cortisol is one. Chronic exposure to stress and light at night requires the adrenals to produce more cortisol than is normal. Excessive production of cortisol leads to adrenal fatigue, which presents itself in any number of ways, including chronic fatigue syndrome, viral infections, bacterial and fungal infections and headaches. In order to overcome adrenal fatigue, it's very important to respect your natural circadian rhythm and allow your adrenals to rest.

Factors That Can Disrupt Your Sleep/Wake Cycles

1. Stimulants

What do you do for a pick-me-up when you're tired? Most people reach for something sweet, drink a beverage containing caffeine or smoke a cigarette. Some will have coffee with sugar added—while they smoke! Caffeine, sugar and tobacco are all stimulants, which excite your sympathetic nervous system (your fight or flight response, Chapter 11). This triggers the release of (you guessed it!) cortisol! Remember, cortisol tells your brain that it's time to get up in the morning or that it's time for action!

The most popular form of caffeine is coffee. An eight ounce cup of strong coffee contains about 300 mg of caffeine. Caffeine has a half-life of about six hours. So, if you have coffee at 3 p.m., you'll still have 150 milligrams (mg) of caffeine in your blood stream at 9 p.m. Six hours later, well into the psychogenic repair cycle of immune function, you'll have 75 mg of caffeine stimulating your adrenal glands to produce cortisol. Ideally, you should not drink anything containing caffeine after lunch and throughout the evening.

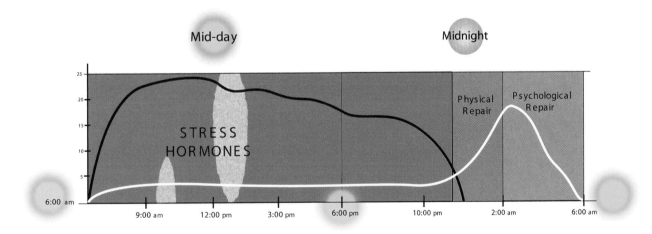

Figure 2: Disrupted sleep/wake cycle.
A typical day for many involves elevated stress levels, resulting in increased levels of stress hormones throughout the day (black line), resulting in decreased levels of growth and repair hormones (white line). Although the healthy body can bounce back from intermittent circadian stresses, chronic (long-term) circadian stress often leads to depressed immunity, illness and chronic fatigue.

One teaspoon of sugar has been shown to suppress your immune system for as long as four hours.[4] When you consider that the average can of soda contains ten teaspoons of sugar, or that the average breakfast cereal is comprised of between 46% and 53% sugar, you can see how easily sugar finds its way into your diet.[5]

A diet that does not match your metabolic type typically results in large fluctuations of blood sugar levels. Blood sugar levels elevate after eating, triggering the release of insulin to break down and store the blood sugar. This often results in an overcompensation response, which in turn leads to a blood sugar low. Unfortunately, your brain considers low blood sugar to be a dire emergency, a major stressor. Stress hormones are released to counterbalance the condition by triggering the liver to release stored glycogen, which elevates blood sugar. Meanwhile, most people feel the effects of low blood sugar, and, before their liver can do its job, they have another sweet snack or caffeine to keep them going. This cycle keeps cortisol levels high, preventing the body from winding down in the evening and getting a good night's sleep.

2. Electromagnetic pollution

Unless you regularly sleep in a cave miles away from human civilization, you'll probably be exposed to low frequency electromagnetic energies. Power lines, electrical circuits in your walls, ceilings and floors and electrical appliances such as electric blankets and TVs all emit such energies. This electromagnetic pollution can disrupt natural sleep/wake cycles.

3. Entrainment

Physiologists and medical doctors have found that you can be entrained, or *synchronized* to a dysfunctional schedule in as little as 7-21 days.[6] This means that if you stay up until midnight for 1-3 weeks in a row, your internal body clock will become trained to wait until midnight to start reducing cortisol output and increasing melatonin production. Just because you didn't start the physical repair on time doesn't mean it's going to get jammed in. Your natural rhythms will automatically begin the psychogenic repair around 2 a.m., thus robbing your body of

two good hours of physical repair. If your body gets used to going to bed late and you then decide to get to bed earlier one night, you'll probably find you have a hard time falling asleep at 10:30 p.m. Now you're faced with the task of entraining your system to release your sleepy-time chemicals early enough so that you can get to sleep on time for a full cycle of physical repair.

For some this is difficult. We live in a world where it's easy to move from one time zone to another with just a few hours of travel. Some people find that their physiological rhythms, including their sleep/wake rhythms, are synchronized to the rise and fall of the sun in the time zone where they were born or brought up. This may be completely different from the place that they currently live. If you're suffering from chronic conditions or pain, and if you have difficulty adjusting to the natural sleep/wake cycle of the place where you live, you may have to return to the time zone where you were born and spent your early years to get better.

CHEK Points for Optimizing Your Sleep/Wake Cycles

1. Get to **sleep** by 10:30 p.m. If you need time to wind down before you sleep, make the appropriate adjustments. Getting in bed at 10:00 p.m. and reading until 11:00 p.m. defeats the purpose!

2. Minimize your exposure to bright lights, particularly fluorescent lights, for at least two hours before going to bed. If you don't have dimmer switches, try lighting your house with candles or lamps with low wattage light bulbs.

3. Sleep in a room that is completely dark.

4. Avoid the consumption of stimulants (caffeine, sugar and nicotine) after lunch. If you're unable to sleep well, be particularly mindful with desserts—especially ones that contain alcohol, sugar and/or caffeine.

5. Eat right for your metabolic type, particularly at dinner. Though we commonly eat sweets or desserts in the evening, doing so will often disrupt the sleep cycle.

6. Drink plenty of water. Our bodies have very little water reserve, and once dehydrated, the body

responds as though it's experiencing stress. Remember, if your body is stressed it produces stress hormones, which are awakening hormones.

7. Exercise! If you aren't following a regular exercise program, implement the plan outlined for you in Section 3. Some type of exercise or physical activity during the day will generally help you to sleep better at night. However, be aware of the time of day and the intensity of your training. You may find that sleep patterns are disrupted if you exercise after dinner, particularly if the exercise is intense. Intense exercise or cardiovascular exercise, particularly when performed for longer than 30 minutes, can increase cortisol levels, making it hard to get to sleep.

8. Try unplugging all electrical appliances in your bedroom, including clocks, TVs and lights. If your sleep quality improves, rearrange your bedroom so that all electrical devices are as far from your bed as possible. Also, don't use an electric blanket. For more information see *Sleep, Biological Rhythms & Electromagnetic Fields* by Chris Maund at www.chekinstitute.com.[7]

9. If you've tried the above CHEK Points and still have trouble getting a good night's sleep, consider consulting a naturopathic physician or a CHEK Nutrition and Lifestyle Coach. When your body has too many unfriendly bacteria, is host to parasites, or is harboring excess toxic waste, your adrenal glands will be under constant stress. This situation will commonly exhaust your adrenal glands, which is likely to disrupt your sleep patterns. Take measures to detoxify your system (Cleansing your colon, liver/gallbladder may be useful). Consult a qualified practitioner to learn more.

Case History
Hank, a professional racquetball player in his 40s, a client of Chris Maund, C.H.E.K Certified, C.H.E.K Faculty, San Diego, CA

Hank was experiencing several nagging injuries which were affecting his match play. He began a corrective exercise program, started getting massage work on a regular basis and also addressed nutritional issues. These steps helped his condition, but, while he was feeling better, he still felt weak at times and was not recovering from injuries as quickly as he would have liked.

It was at this point that Chris noted his sleeping habits. Hank's schedule was quite hectic, and he did not follow a regular routine whatsoever. Many nights he would not eat dinner until 9 p.m. or later and often did not get to bed until 2 a.m., sometimes getting only 5-6 hours of sleep. Other days, he would sleep late and get 10-14 hours of sleep, but still felt tired. Most of Hank's workouts were late at night, between 10 p.m. and 12 a.m.

When Hank changed his sleeping habits and started getting to bed between 10-11 p.m. every night and waking up between 6-7:30 a.m., he noticed a significant improvement in how his body felt and in how he played. He tried to get his training sessions in by 8 p.m. at the latest. If he couldn't train by that time, he would not train at all that day. During this time, Hank increased the number of days he rested from his training and increased the time he spent stretching. He also kept a log of when and how much he was sleeping. This helped him monitor exactly how much sleep he was getting. Along with going to bed by 11 p.m. every night, he also tried to get about 8 hours of sleep each night and a total of 56 hours of sleep each week. While this was a significant lifestyle change for Hank, the results were well worth the effort.

12

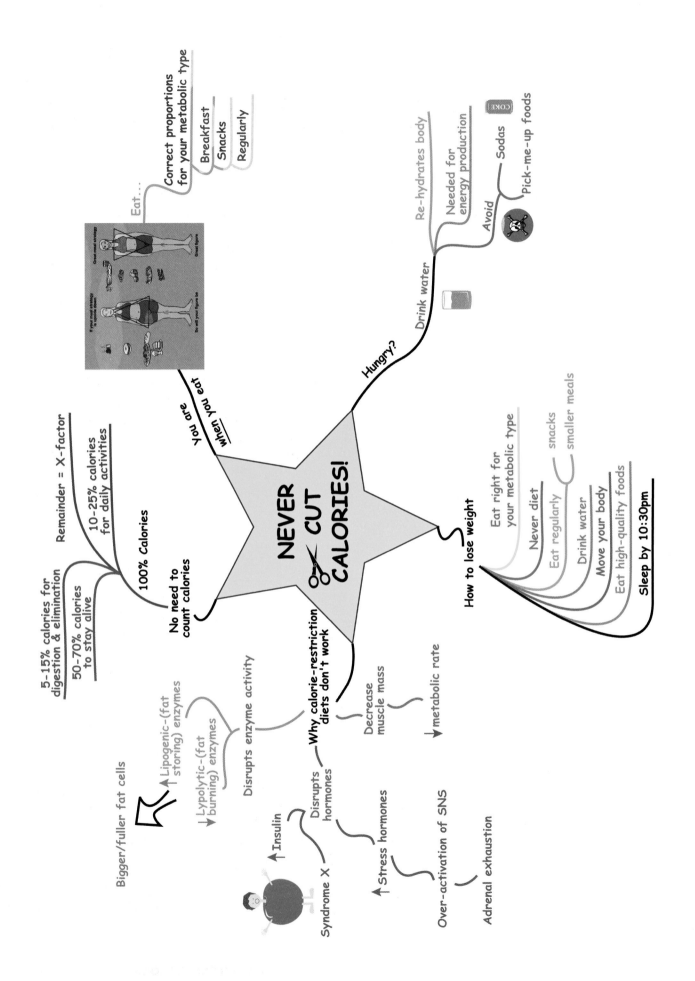

NEVER ~~CUT~~ CALORIES!

You are _when_ you eat

Eat…
- **Correct proportions for your metabolic type**
  - Breakfast
  - Snacks
  - Regularly

No need to count calories

100% Calories
- 50-70% calories to stay alive
- 5-15% calories for digestion & elimination
- 10-25% calories for daily activities
- Remainder = X-factor

Hungry?

Drink water
- Re-hydrates body
- Needed for energy production

Avoid
- Sodas
- Pick-me-up foods

COKE

Why calorie-restriction diets don't work

- Decrease muscle mass
- ↓ metabolic rate
- Disrupts enzyme activity
  - ↑ Lipogenic-(fat storing) enzymes
  - ↓ Lypolytic-(fat burning) enzymes
  - Bigger/fuller fat cells
- Disrupts hormones
  - Syndrome X
  - ↑ Insulin
  - ↑ Stress hormones
    - Over-activation of SNS
    - Adrenal exhaustion

How to lose weight

- Eat right for your metabolic type
- Never diet
- Eat regularly
  - snacks
  - smaller meals
- Drink water
- Move your body
- Eat high-quality foods
- Sleep by 10:30pm

Chapter 13

NEVER CUT CALORIES

Allow me to clearly state my position before we go much further: **Calorie-restricted diets don't work if you want to permanently lose weight!** If you want to lose weight, you're not alone. According to Dr. Jaap Seidell of the International Obesity Task Force, incidence of obesity is on the rise throughout the world, making it one of the fastest developing public health concerns. The World Health Organization (WHO) has described obesity as a "worldwide epidemic." It's estimated that nearly 250 million people worldwide are obese, which is about 7% of the adult population.[1]

Obesity is particularly prevalent in the U.S., where over one third of the adult population is obese, and one in seven children and adolescents are obese.

An incredible 60% of the American population is overweight. Though obesity rates in other countries are lower than in the U.S., the rate of increase in the U.K. and several other countries signals an alarming trend with serious consequences.[2]

You've probably tried some sort of diet—most likely a calorie-restricting plan. There are currently about 2,000 diet books to choose from, each claiming miraculous results. Why, then, is obesity becoming an epidemic? Is it because people have no self-control and simply eat too much? Not likely. It isn't how much you eat, it's what and when you eat. Here's the good news: You don't have to starve or punish yourself with hours in the gym to lose weight. However, you do need to learn how to eat right in order to bring your body back into balance so that it will function at an optimal level.

The beginning of dieting in America

Food shortages were a concern during World War I (WWI), the depression and then again during World War II (WWII). As part of the U.S. WWI strategy, the government created the Food Administration (FA). The FA told Americans to cut down on consumption of flour, meat, butter and sugar, claiming these items were needed to feed the soldiers.

As a means of saving the meat, butter, wheat and sugar for men, women were taught to cut back -- in other words, to diet! In order to satisfy hunger, women learned to fill up on grains, legumes and vegetables. Not surprisingly, by replacing vital nutrients such as meat and butter with carbohydrates (which are rapidly converted to sugar and stored as fat in the body) many women became bigger in spite of so-called food shortages.

During the Roaring 20s, food was once again plentiful. Although men generally rebounded from their war efforts by eating their way into corpulence, the dainty proportions and avoidance of meat and butter continued to be ladylike. Not surprisingly, the slogan: *You can never be too rich or too thin* is a by-product of this era. When the portly look, once associated with wealth in the 19th century, fell by the wayside, dieting became a man's business, too.

During the Depression, the country experienced a surplus of wheat. The government began purchasing the excess to support the farming industry. When reports of malnutrition streamed in from across the country, bread lines sprang up, infuriating farmers who feared that people would learn to live on government handouts. In the meantime,

13

the government continued to purchase surplus grain and meats from farmers to compensate for the public's diminished purchasing power, which was at an all time low.

While the U.S. was knee deep in bread and wheat, newspapers and magazines commonly featured pictures of food either being stored or destroyed alongside people waiting in bread lines.[4] Although people were supposedly starving and meat was considered a rare commodity, the government's farm subsidies produced a stockpile of meat, so much that at one time the government slaughtered six million pigs and dumped them into the Mississippi River, buried them or carted them to dumps to prevent them from coming to market. This manipulation of the food supply was driven by farming lobbyists who wanted to protect farmers from dropping food prices, which in their minds was sure to happen if Uncle Sam started giving away meat.

Paradoxically, while hunger and malnutrition were at their highest in the history of the U.S., women, particularly college girls who had learned to eat like ladies during WWI, were now determined to become thin and attempted one crash diet after another. Some amusing names of such diets were: *The Hollywood 18-day Diet, The Mayo Diet and The United Fruit Company's "Reducing Diet."* By 1933, physicians were tasked with getting the ladies to eat and the men to eat less.

With some of the wiser independent health experts of the day indicting over-consumption of bread and sugar as the source of gluttony, General Mills took a stand to protect their cash cow. General Mills, the food processing company that funded the first nutrition schools in the U.S., created the infamous Betty Crocker. This fictional personality would make her way into almost every magazine, newspaper and media source of the day, espousing the benefits of sugar and white bread. Welch's, along with other juice manufacturers, jumped on the media bandwagon, claiming that their products yielded "quick energy" yet were "never fattening."

Welch's went so far as to say that its predigested grape sugar actually "burned up ugly fat."

By the time the U.S. entered WWII, the American food-processing industry was well underway, with 98% of all bread consumed in the country being white bread, void of nutritional value. The per capita consumption of white flour had risen to an astounding 200 pounds per year. Certainly, it's no wonder that 40-50% of recruits in the U.S. and the U.K. were considered unfit for military service, commonly due to malnutrition and inadequate physical readiness. This led to the government dictum for millers to enrich flour with vitamins in hopes of pepping up the soldiers. Not surprisingly, Mayo Clinic physician Russell Wilder calculated that most of the calories in the American diet were coming from refined sugar and processed, hydrogenated fats, which are void of vitamins.[4]

During WWII, as during the Depression, there was a perceived shortage of meat, yet American cattle ranges were home to more cattle than ever. Again, the government destroyed meat it could not store. In 1942, the average civilian male ate 125 pounds of meat, while the average soldier was allotted 360 pounds annually. Coerced by magazines and trendsetters, women were to eat dainty portions to be lady like. The women were to save meat ("the manly food") for men working in, and for, the war effort. The fear of food shortages was a blessing in disguise for the food processing industry, which successfully marketed canned and packaged foods to women. Due to the extended shelf life of these packaged foods, women were shopping as little as 1-2 times a month instead of several times a week as they had done previously. Further, the meatless consciousness opened the door to soy-based meat substitutes and a host of other food substitutes that were far cheaper than actual whole foods, while allowing longer shelf life and higher profits.

For a detailed history of eating in America, see Harvey Levenstein's books, *Revolution at the Table* and *Paradox of Plenty*.[3, 4]

What Diets Do to Your Body

Calorie-restricting diets don't work in the long run because they disrupt important hormones and enzymes. Skipping just one meal, or eating too many carbohydrates for your metabolic type, can result in changes that make it more difficult for the body to lose fat. Initially, the response to a skipped meal is an elevation of stress hormones (Chapter 11). The body then responds to the stress signal by releasing stored glycogen from the liver into the blood to raise your blood sugar. After all, your body thinks you're in a life-threatening situation. Repeated bouts of stress result in a yo-yoing between high and low blood sugar, creating yet another major stressor on the body. An over-stressed body will not function at an optimal level. For many, this is not the ideal state for losing weight.

If you eat too many carbohydrates, your body must release insulin to lower blood-sugar levels. Skipping meals or not eating enough of the right foods also keeps insulin levels high because the body thinks you're in a famine, and it's forced to store energy whenever it's supplied. If you're active, insulin will store sugar in the muscles. But if your muscles are not being used, or if the muscle cells are full, your extra calories will wind up in the fat cells. Exercising muscles keeps them sensitive to insulin, since an active muscle wants to take in sugar for energy. Inactive muscles become insulin resistant and shuttle more and more calories to fat cells. A diet calling for a high consumption of carbohydrates beyond ideal for your metabolic type will also make you progressively insulin resistant.

Accumulating fat in the middle of your body is an indication that you've become insulin resistant. The medical name for this is Syndrome-X. Again, accumulating unwanted fat around your midsection and Syndrome-X are usually the result of dieting, yo-yo dieting, consuming too many carbohydrates for your metabolic type and lack of exercise. Once the fat cells in your midsection are full, the fat accumulation extends to other areas of the body and you become progressively more obese. Because muscles and fat cells become progressively less sensitive to

insulin, blood sugar levels rise higher, forcing the pancreas to overwork in an attempt to lower blood sugar levels. Eventually, you'll become a Type II diabetic!

Any time you miss a meal—yes, just one meal—your body increases the release of lipogenic (fat storing) enzymes. When these lipogenic enzymes increase, the enzymes you really need, the lipolytic or fat burning enzymes, are decreased.[5] This effect is much more pronounced in women than in men.

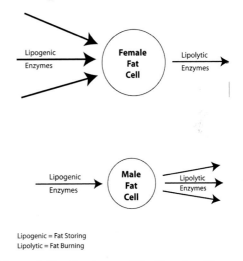

Lipogenic = Fat Storing
Lipolytic = Fat Burning

Figure 1: Fat Storing and Fat Burning Hormones[5]

The entire process of dieting, constantly being in a flight/fight state with elevated sympathetic nervous system activity, and eating incorrectly will leave you tired. Thanks to junk food manufacturers and the media, most people don't understand that they're gaining weight because they're eating incorrectly, not because they're eating too much. Improper eating habits always result in the inability to replace the vital nutrients that keep body systems running correctly and provide additional energy to spend living, not just surviving. Inevitably, people use tea, coffee, soda, sweets and other pick-me-up drinks to compensate for the energy deficit. You must understand that any such stimulant only activates the SNS, releases more stress hormones and eventually requires more and more of the stimulant to get the desired effect. After a while, adrenal glands become exhausted, resulting in a number of symptoms (Chapter 12), all of which are part of the chronic fatigue symptom profile.

If you've lost weight on a diet, you more than likely lost significant amounts of muscle. Remember, muscles burn energy. If you decrease muscle mass, your metabolic rate will be lower—you won't burn as much energy. This increases your chances of gaining back the weight you lost. Then the yo-yo diet syndrome begins, which is even more stressful than a one-time diet. Each time you start and stop a diet, you significantly increase the difficulty of restoring your physiology to normal.

Don't worry about counting calories

Today, magazines, sports stores and specialty shops offer a wide variety of calorie-counting gadgets. You can strap one onto your wrist or ankle, go for a walk, a bike ride or pound the Stair Master for thirty minutes and decide how big a piece of pie you deserve for dessert. Well, there are some serious flaws in this approach!

When trying to determine how many calories to consume each day, many fail to calculate how many calories it takes to meet the demands of just being alive. A whopping 50-70% of all the calories you consume are used to generate the heat and life energy to keep your cells turned on—not cleaning the house or shooting a few hoops, just alive. Another 5-15% of your caloric intake is needed for digestion and elimination. You also need to consider your daily activities and how your individual body functions—this is referred to as the X-Factor.[6, 7]

> **X-Factor:** A variable that can either increase or decrease daily energy expenditure (how many calories you burn) based on several genetic, hormonal and environmental factors. Fidgeting would fall into this X-Factor category.

We don't all lead the same life, nor do we interpret stressors or environment in the same way. If you eat according to your metabolic type (Chapter 3), you'll convert food into energy more efficiently. This means you'll expend or dissipate more of the energy you take on board, leaving less to store as fat. If you follow fad diets and/or eat incorrectly for your metabolic type, your blood sugar balance is disrupted, energy production is inefficient and your cells must

slow down because your meal is causing stress on your body instead of aiding in smooth operations. There will also be more waste material left behind from eating incorrectly, which is often toxic to the body and may get stored in the fat cells to protect the liver while it catches up.

Each of us responds to stressors differently. The X-Factor for determining caloric expense includes such stressors as job and relationship challenges and responding to weather changes. We also display various levels of spontaneous activity, such as fidgeting. As depicted in Figure 2, there are a number of factors that must be considered just to meet the requirements of running your body and keeping it healthy. Be aware that any time you try to run your body without adequate fuel, the right mix of fuel, or on poor quality fuel, you drastically increase your chances of slowing your metabolism and becoming fat.

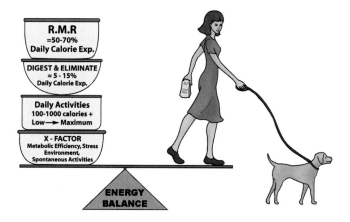

Figure 2: Your body requires different amounts of fuel based on a variety of factors. When you do not provide your body with adequate fuel, the right mix of fuel, or poor quality fuel, you drastically increase your chances of slowing your metabolism and becoming fat.

You Are <u>When</u> You Eat

Few people understand the link between when they eat and their health, let alone their body shape. Starting your day off with a small meal (coffee and toast or a pop-tart), followed by a snack for lunch (bagel), only to come home intensely hungry and pig out will make your body look like your meal proportions (Figure 3).

13

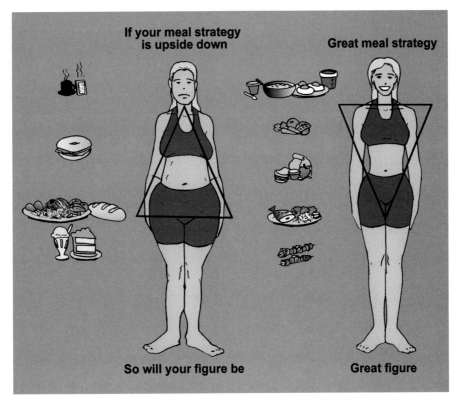

Figure 3: You Are When You Eat

As described in the Chapters 11 and 12, cortisol is an activating hormone. Cortisol levels are highest between 6 a.m. and 9 a.m., which means your metabolism is stimulated and your cells are anxious for you to eat after having fasted all night. For most, particularly women wanting to restore or elevate their metabolic rate, breakfast should be the largest meal of the day, comprising as much as 25% of your daily calories.[8] If you're a carb type, you may do well on smaller breakfasts, making you the only exception to the rule. Carb type or not, all breakfast meals must contain proteins, carbohydrates and fats in the correct ratio for your metabolic type.

Eating a full breakfast will provide you with both staying power and energy. In my experience, people who eat a proper breakfast feel better and are more likely to be physically active during the day. Eating snacks between meals will constantly reassure your body that energy and nutrition are on board, which often results in an elevated metabolism. The body's metabolism is also elevated by eating, simply because the process of digestion, utilization and elimination of food is at work for the body.

When you eat regularly and snack as needed, your metabolic rate will achieve it's genetic set point and you'll achieve your genetic shape. If you don't like the way you look, but are not overweight, consider consulting a C.H.E.K Practitioner to coach you toward shaping a new you (see Resources).

Are You Hungry All the Time?

If you find you're constantly hungry and have gained weight from eating too much, you may not be hungry—you may be thirsty. In his excellent book, *Your Body's Many Cries For Water*, Dr. Batmanghelidj explains that hunger pangs are frequently a symptom of dehydration.[9] I've found this to be true with my clients and in my own experience. If I feel hungry long before I would normally eat, I drink a couple cups of water and hunger pangs usually subside. Until you get in the habit of drinking water regularly throughout the day, it's easy to get dehydrated without realizing it.

Drinking water also gives you energy. Water is a key catalyst in digestion, enzymatic actions and energy production throughout the body. When you drink

13

adequately for your bodily needs, you're less likely to consume soda and pick-me-up foods that generally throw your blood sugar levels off and cause stress on the body.

CHEK Points for Losing Weight

1. Eat right for your metabolic type and **never diet!**

2. Eat regularly to satisfy hunger. Consume slightly smaller main meals and include snacks to elevate your metabolic rate.

3. Eat high-quality food (Chapter 4).

4. Drink plenty of water. Ideally, you should drink half your body weight in ounces of water per day (Body weight (in kg) x 0.033 = how much water you should drink in liters).

5. Move your body. If you don't like a structured exercise program, simply remain active. Park your car at the far end of the parking lot, take the stairs and walk as often as you can.

6. Go to sleep by 10:30 p.m. Disrupting your sleep/wake cycles equals more stress on your body and increases your chances of gaining weight because of hormonal imbalances.

7. Burn your diet books!

Case History

Gwen Miller, C.H.E.K Practitioner Level 1, client of Megan Valente, C.H.E.K Practitioner Level 2, CHEK NLC Level 3, San Francisco/Santa Rosa, CA

When I first met Megan Valente, I was an overweight, unhealthy 39-year-old woman. I had not exercised or followed a healthy lifestyle for over a decade, and two pregnancies in two years had left me de-conditioned, stretched-out and discouraged about ever getting back into shape again. My body fat was almost 38%, and I weighed almost 200 pounds. In addition, I had very poor posture, what I now know as "upper cross syndrome," with extreme forward-head posture, rounded shoulders and chronic low back/sciatic pain. My balance was extremely poor; in fact, I have five scars, three of which required emergency room stitches to repair, as results of falls.

The first thing Megan did was teach me some simple exercises using a Swiss ball as an unstable environment. She explained that, according to the CHEK Principles, I had postural muscle imbalances, that my stabilizers were not firing properly, and for these reasons she was NOT going to put me on machines, and, further, that my transversus abdominis (which I had never heard of!) was "turned off." Megan worked with me, using a Swiss ball and a blood pressure cuff, to train my stabilizers and core musculature to work

again. She began to increase the complexity of the exercises and decrease the base of support as I progressed. For example, to train the internal and external oblique musculature she introduced me to exercises such as the cable wood chop, increasing the level of difficulty by combining the wood chop motion with a weight shift. As my condition improved, she introduced complex exercises such as the single arm row with a weight shift, and then, when I mastered that, she put me on a balance board to perform the exercise!

Megan always kept my program interesting and challenging by following the CHEK Protocol. Within three months, I had lost about 15 pounds of scale weight and my body fat was down to 27%, a decrease of over 10%! Then I discovered that I was pregnant with my third child. What a blow—just when I was getting back into shape again! Now I see that pregnancy as a blessing, but, unfortunately, my attitude was lacking then. Megan encouraged me to continue working with her during my pregnancy and studied program modifications for me that kept me in shape so that at least we didn't lose ground. I trained under Megan until my seventh month, when, at the advice

---

of my doctor, I stopped training due to severe sciatic pain.

The pregnancy and delivery were my healthiest. I birthed my third son completely drug-free, after having had all the drugs and epidurals available for the first two deliveries. Of course, I returned to training under Megan as soon as I could. Within two weeks I was easing back into cardio, and we were training in a month. That third pregnancy left me with a slight weight gain, and I topped the scales at 210 pounds. Within three months, I had shed 20 pounds with exercise alone, and then my weight loss plateaued. My balance and coordination had improved, my body fat was around 25%, I no longer bruised and damaged the left side of my body on a regular basis, but something was still missing. What could it be?

The answer was nutrition. Megan returned from a week-long C.H.E.K Certification Program and gave me about a gazillion pages to fill out—questionnaires regarding my lifestyle and dietary habits, from what I ate for breakfast to how my sex drive was, and everything in between. She also had me read *The Metabolic Typing Diet* (Wolcott and Fahey) and take the self-test to help determine which foods I should eat. We began to look at possible food intolerances, and she instructed me to cut out wheat for two weeks, then dairy, and to "drink only water." Well, I protested. I liked my bread, I was a big milk-drinker from childhood on, I wasn't giving up my coffee, and I had alcohol every day. So Megan loaned me the

Flatten Your Abs Forever video [Editor's note: this video is available from the C.H.E.K Institute] and lights started coming on. Things started making sense. I cut out the dairy first, and replaced that glass of milk I had every meal with two glasses of water. The weight began to come off. Four pounds in a week, I believe it was. Then I cut out the wheat. More weight came off. Then I cut out the alcohol. More weight melted off. Mind you, at this point, I was still exercising, but probably less. I was certainly doing less cardio and about the same amount of resistance/stabilization training, but the main thing that changed was nutrition. No one had ever looked at my nutritional habits before, and it was a huge missing piece.

As I sit here typing this testimonial, I am 60 pounds smaller. I am still a work-in progress, but aren't we all? If I can shed 60 pounds through lifestyle changes and keep it off, as a 42 year-old mother of three, I know it is possible for others to accomplish similar feats.

In fact, I am now committed to helping others the way Megan helped me. I want to help others find the happiness and satisfaction that I have found through functional strength and nutrition, as Megan taught me and as Paul Chek taught her. I am now a Certified Fitness Trainer, and my mentor, Megan, who has become a dear friend over the past three years, is now also a colleague! I am following in her footsteps, studying the CHEK methods and have become a C.H.E.K Practitioner myself.

You must begin to think of yourself as becoming the person you want to be.

David Viscott

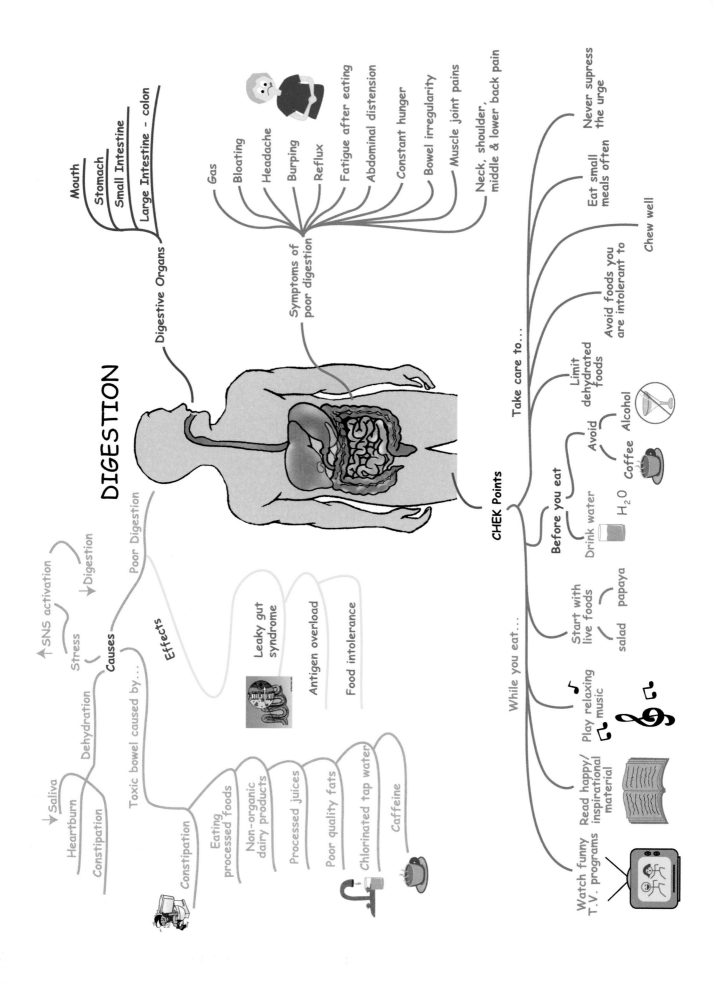

DIGESTION

Digestive Organs
- **Mouth**
- **Stomach**
- Small Intestine
- Large Intestine – colon

Symptoms of poor digestion
- Gas
- Bloating
- Headache
- Burping
- Reflux
- Fatigue after eating
- Abdominal distension
- Constant hunger
- Bowel irregularity
- Muscle joint pains
- Neck, shoulder, middle & lower back pain

Causes
- ↑SNS activation → ↓Digestion
- Stress
- Poor Digestion
- Dehydration
- ↓Saliva
- Heartburn
- Constipation
- Toxic bowel caused by...
  - Constipation
  - Eating processed foods
  - Non-organic dairy products
  - Processed juices
  - Poor quality fats
  - Chlorinated tap water
  - Caffeine

Effects
- Leaky gut syndrome
- Antigen overload
- Food intolerance

CHEK Points

Take care to...
- Never supress the urge
- Eat small meals often
- Chew well
- Avoid foods you are intolerant to
- Limit dehydrated foods

Before you eat
- Avoid
  - Coffee
  - Alcohol
- Drink water
  - H₂O

While you eat...
- Start with live foods
  - salad
  - papaya
- Play relaxing music
- Read happy/inspirational material
- Watch funny T.V. programs

Chapter 14

IS YOUR DIGESTIVE SYSTEM HEALTHY?

In addition to regular exercise, a commitment to good health includes eating responsibly and choosing the right foods. An improper diet can ruin a good digestive system. But perhaps you're eating quality foods in accordance with your metabolic type and still not feeling your best. In order for a new eating plan to be effective, you must make sure your digestive system is fully functional. There's a direct relationship between the health of your digestive system and your overall look, feel and physical performance. In this chapter, we'll discuss:

• The organs in the digestive system and the importance of keeping them healthy

• Common causes of poor digestion

• Healthy options for digestive distress

• The importance of removing unnecessary stressors from your life and diet

• The importance in restoring proper support to the digestive organs

Your Digestive System

Mouth: The digestive process begins in the mouth. For optimal conversion of food to energy, elimination and prevention of unwanted fungi and parasite infestation, food should be chewed until liquefied. While chewing, enzymes from saliva mix with food to breakdown carbohydrates. Proper chewing prepares food for digestion.

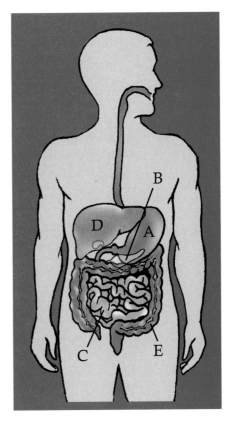

Figure 1: The Organs of Digestion.
A. Stomach B. Pancreas C. Small Intestine D. Liver E. Colon

Chewing too quickly and swallowing prematurely leave food particles too large for stomach acids to break down and kill the parasites and fungi hiding inside. Once unfriendly parasites reach the more alkaline (less acidic) small intestine, they can burrow in to lay eggs. Large food particles also make it difficult for the small intestine to absorb food molecules and extract nutrients. If fungi enter your body through your mouth and survive the stomach, they often begin debilitating the immune system.

Stomach: Food enters the stomach and mixes with additional enzymes and HCL (hydrochloric acid). HCL, produced by special cells in the stomach wall, breaks proteins down into amino acids for absorption in the small intestine. It also kills unfriendly bacteria, germs, fungi and parasites. The ability to properly digest food in the stomach is dependent upon having adequate production of HCL and digestive enzymes.

Nearly all food is absorbed in the small intestine though some, such as alcohol and refined sugars, are absorbed through the stomach.

Small Intestine (SI): The SI is roughly 25 feet long (6-7 m). Each section is lined with special receptor sites that absorb particular foods. Digestive enzymes from the pancreas and bile from the liver are released into the SI to aid in the digestion of foods. Once receptors have digested food, it's sent through the portal vein to the liver for processing. From there, it's delivered to the cells of your body via the bloodstream to be converted into energy and to rebuild or repair cells. Unwanted or indigestible food particles are sent to the colon for final processing before leaving the body.

Large Intestine (Colon): The colon is five to six feet long (1.5 m) and about three inches in diameter. The colon acts as a specialized organ for producing certain vitamins and for recycling useful water for the body.

There are trillions of bacteria inside a healthy colon, some of them friendly, some not. The optimal ratio is 85% friendly to 15% unfriendly. Many people today have closer to 85% unfriendly and only 15% friendly. Friendly bacteria initially come from mother's milk, making yet another argument for the benefits of breast-feeding.

Friendly bacteria produce vitamins B1, B2, B3, B5, B6, B12, A and K. They also produce a lactic acid by-product that helps stimulate peristalsis (movement) of the colon. This prevents constipation and makes the environment unfavorable for unfriendly bacteria.

Consuming poor quality food, especially processed foods, can create an alkaline environment in the colon that supports an overgrowth of unfriendly bacteria. Peristalsis is disrupted, leading to constipation and an even more favorable environment for the unfriendly bacteria and parasites. *A backed-up colon is a toxic colon.*

When the body is dehydrated, the colon squeezes as much water from feces as possible. This results in both constipation and the absorption of toxic fluids into the bloodstream.

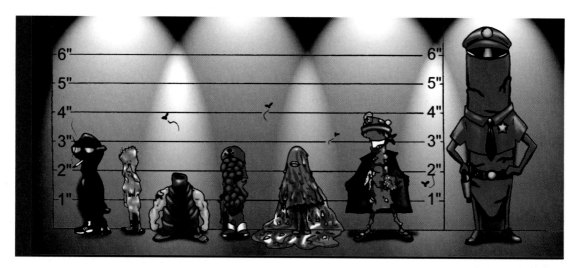

Figure 2: The Poopie Policeman and Poopie Line-up (from right to left: the Flasher, Diarrhella, Pellet Man, the Bodybuilder, Olympic Swimmer, Mr. Sinker 'n' Stinker)

The Poopie Line-up and Poopie Policeman

I developed the Poopie Line-up and Poopie Policeman to teach clients, and their children, how to recognize symptoms of dehydration, poor digestion and toxicity. Ancient physicians relied primarily on physical and emotional symptoms, along with the feces and urine of their patients, to make a diagnosis. They'd smell the feces, examine it, and break it open in search of undigested food particles, worms, blood, mucus, tissue particles and any other indicator of internal imbalance. Ancient physicians actually tasted urine for excess sugar and the level of acidity. While your doctor isn't likely to grovel around in your stool or taste your urine, there is a lot you can learn about your digestion through self-examination.

The Poopie Policeman represents a healthy bowel movement. For a bowel movement to qualify as a "Poopie Policeman," it must:

• Be well shaped and consistent in contour

• Pass easily and pleasurably

• Be light brown in color

• Smell natural, almost earthy - not foul

• Float, yet doesn't require multiple attempts to flush

Familiarity with the following bowel bandits will help diagnose an irregular or dysfunctional digestive/elimination system.

The Flasher: The Flasher gives you a peek at the undigested food particles in the stool. It's *not* normal to see food particles in your stool, as it's a sign of food intolerance or an inflammatory disorder of the digestive system.

Diarrhella: "Diarrhella's" crime is one of passion. It's the body's desperate attempt at detoxification. Even if you're constipated and dehydrated, your body will scavenge extra water to remove toxins from your body. If you fluctuate between constipation and diarrhea once a month or more within a one-year period, it's time to re-evaluate your diet.

Pellet Man: Pellet poops resemble rabbit or sheep manure, and may indicate altered states between peristalsis of the colon and dehydration.

The Bodybuilder: Bodybuilder poops are often larger in diameter than a Poopie Policeman and are hard to pass. Such bowel movements sometimes come from eating too many dehydrated and processed foods, especially protein bars and shakes.

Olympic Swimmer: Lighter in color than the Poopie Policeman due to the high content of undigested fat, I call them Olympic Swimmers because they're difficult to flush. The Olympic Swimmer may indicate a deficiency in bile, which breaks down fats.

Mr. Sinker 'n' Stinker: This mean little bowel bandit often appears after being exposed to processed foods, a toxic environment and/or medical drugs—particularly after undergoing a surgical procedure where general anesthesia was used. Mr. Sinker 'n' Stinker is one of the meanest little fellas you'll ever encounter in the bathroom. If he's yours, he's very hard to get rid of and if he's not, his smell is enough to make your hair stand on end! If Mr. Sinker 'n' Stinker comes to call, take steps to detoxify your body.

Common Causes of Poor Digestion

Symptoms of Digestive Dysfunction	
• Gas	• Fatigue after eating
• Bloating	• Abdominal distension
• Headache	• Constant hunger
• Burping	• Bowel irregularity
• Reflux	• Muscle and joint aches
• Neck, shoulder, middle and lower back pain	

1. Dehydration

For normal physiological and digestive processes to occur, you must consume adequate amounts of water. I recommend at least half your body weight (in pounds) in ounces of water per day. (Body weight (in kg) x 0.033 = how much water to drink in liters)

A dry mouth is an indication that you're dehydrated and digestion will be effected. The first physical act of digestion, chewing food, begins in the mouth and requires the production of saliva. Saliva contains digestive enzymes that begin the breakdown of foods, especially carbohydrates. If you're dehydrated and cannot adequately produce saliva, foods won't be properly prepared for further digestion in the stomach and intestines.

Once dehydrated, the body will scavenge water from vital organs, such as the central nervous system. But the body will first draw water from the mucus membrane in the stomach, and the small and large intestines (organs that play a key role in the digestive process).

As food enters the stomach, hydrochloric acid (HCL) is released to break down proteins. Dehydration robs moisture from the mucus membrane in the stomach, leaving it unprotected from HCL—which is acidic enough to burn a hole through carpet and most certainly capable of causing ulcers. Pain associated with this process commonly causes reflex inhibition of the abdominal muscles, causing susceptibility to injury during physical exertion due to inefficient spine stabilization.

Antacids are a common treatment for indigestion and heartburn, though there are unwanted consequences. Antacids contain high levels of aluminum, which is toxic and suspected to be a cause of Alzheimer's disease.[1] Consuming antacids also inhibits optimal breakdown of proteins before they enter the SI. Aside from water, most of your body is comprised of proteins and fats. If proteins, necessary for repairing cells, are not properly broken down, they're less likely to be absorbed. The body will then begin to break down its own proteins from muscle. Heartburn is a sign of dehydration and should not be treated as an isolated condition.

In addition to drinking at least one half your body weight in ounces (or body weight (in kg) x 0.033 in liters) each day, I recommend 16 ounces (1/2 liter) about 15 minutes before each meal to ensure proper hydration. Adding a pinch of sea salt to each liter bottle of water will increase absorption of water as well as aid in HCL production.

When the mucus membrane of the colon is dehydrated, the *goblet cells* are unable to do their job of providing the necessary amount of lubricating mucus. This makes bowel movements hard to pass and leads to constipation. This is compounded by the fact that one of the primary jobs of the colon is to recycle water from feces, as needed. Dehydration on any level will, therefore, result in the colon *squeezing* more fluid from your feces. This water reducing mechanism was surely necessary during our developmental years as hunter-gatherers while on long hunts or trekking in nomadic conditions where water may not have been available. But today, *there is no excuse for not consuming recommended quantities of water.*

Symptoms of toxicity include:

- Fatigue
- Headaches
- Low back pain
- Asthma
- Nervousness
- Arthritis
- Neck pain
- Cardiac irregularities
- Gastrointestinal upset
- Acne, rash or other skin problems
- Pain between the shoulder blades
- Pain in upper right abdominal region
- Sciatica (pain down the back of the leg)
- Allergies and food intolerance
- Eye, ear, nose and throat problems

2. Toxic bowel

Another cause of poor digestion is a toxic bowel. This often results from constipation and/or an inferior diet of processed foods.

If you experience any symptoms of toxicity (see box), consider changing your diet (review Chapters 3 and 4). The most common culprits that lead to a toxic state are:

- Processed foods
- Pasteurized dairy products
- Processed juices
- Dehydrogenated fats

- Tap water
- Caffeine
- Drug use (recreational and medical drugs)

Constipation

There are conflicting definitions of constipation. I tell clients they should feel a sense of complete evacuation after a bowel movement and that they should be moving about 12 inches of feces per day (this can be as one 12 inch bowel movement, two 6 inch, three 4 inch, etc.).

A body that is continually constipated will become toxic. If food remains in the garbage for several days, it rots and smells foul. Imagine this process occurring inside your warm, wet intestines! When undigested foods remain for more than 24 hours, bacteria that would otherwise remain dormant and be expelled along with other waste matter may become active. This bacteria feeds on undigested remains and produces toxic waste, creating an alkaline environment. This alkaline state inhibits peristalsis.

> **Peristalsis:** Rhythmic waves of contraction of the digestive muscle that pushes food along the colon and triggers bowel movement.

Toxins from these unfriendly critters can seep through a dehydrated mucus membrane. This puts a tremendous load on the liver and kidneys as they strive to keep these toxins out of the blood. The liver then works day and night to neutralize toxic seepage, all the while searching for water to put back into the system for myriad water-dependent physiological functions.

You may be wondering how you can eat three or more meals each day and not be eliminating much. The answer is water composes 70-90% of foods. One of the colon's roles is to extract water from fecal matter for use elsewhere in the body. In a water-deficient person, the colon will squeeze as much water from the feces as possible, leaving the stool compacted in the colon. Thus the saying "You are what you don't excrete."

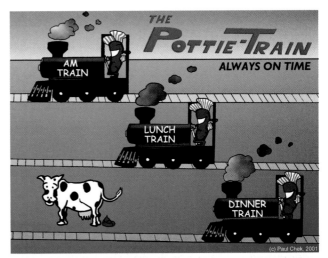

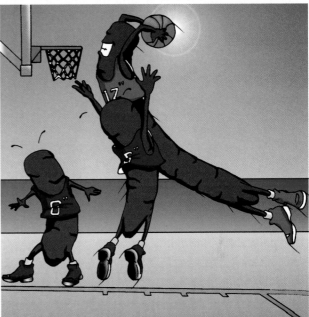

Figure 2: The Pottie Train and Basketball Player Poops. A reminder that a sign of a healthy digestive system is having either a healthy bowel movement after each meal, or excreting at least 12 inches of poop each day.

Processed foods

Today, many foods are so highly processed that the receptors in the SI and the antibodies of the immune system do not recognize them as foods. Processed foods will disrupt proper function within the digestive system.

While many are oblivious to the source of their excessively loose or irregular stools, the problem is literally *right under their nose!* In other words, most people are consuming processed foods that contain a disturbing number of chemical additives, preservatives and colorings, not to mention stabilizers and emulsifiers. There are over 4,000 chemicals used in food processing, a great number of which are recently invented concoctions.[2] Our immune system sees these nasty chemicals as invaders. When the immune system reacts to these chemicals, it works with the body via the intestinal tract to dilute and remove them, thus the appearance of Diarrhella.

If processed foods are not flushed from the body by the immune system's reaction, they may then cause constipation. The chemicals and sugar in processed foods often cause a stress response in the body (increased sympathetic stimulation, Chapter 11). With increased sympathetic action, processes such as digestion and elimination are slowed. This results in decreased peristalsis, which, as indicated earlier, leads to constipation and a toxic colon.

Aside from being potentially toxic and carcinogenic, many of these food-processing chemicals are irritants to the gastrointestinal system. You may say, "Yeah, but I don't often eat those kinds of chemicals," but you probably do. The U.S. Food and Drug Administration (FDA) does not require manufacturers to include additives on the labels of foods that are considered exempt from labeling, such as ketchup and mayonnaise. The package need only say, "artificially flavored," "artificially sweetened," or "contains artificial coloring." The average person consumes about 150 pounds in dry weight of these chemicals each year.[3]

Dairy

Non-organic dairy products contain residual amounts of hormones, antibiotics and pesticides from feed ingested by the animals we eat. Many dairy products today are also colored with dyes. Non-organic butters and cheeses often contain yellow dye #6, which nearly all of my clients who have taken a food additive test discover they are allergic to.

To make matters worse, milk is so badly damaged by pasteurization and homogenization that it is no longer a food. The heat of pasteurization kills the lactase enzymes that naturally break down lactose in milk. During the 1940s, Dr. Francis Marion Pottenger, Jr., performed extensive studies on the effects of processed milk on the health of cats and humans. His study, Pottenger's Cats,[4] revealed that when cats were fed any form of processed milk, they quickly developed significant health problems. By the fourth generation, the cats were unable to reproduce. Not only did Dr. Pottenger see very similar symptoms in his patients who consumed cooked milk products, he continued his study by raising Dwarf beans in the soil from under the pens of the cats fed different foods in his study. This soil was fertilized by the droppings from the cats. The Dwarf beans grown in the soil from under the cages that housed cats fed processed milk products grew crooked and were malformed. On the other hand, the Dwarf beans grown in the soil from under the cages of cats fed only raw milk products and raw foods were not only extremely healthy, these Dwarf beans grew to be six feet tall in some instances! If you consume dairy products, make sure that they're organic and preferably raw.[4]

Processed juices

Processed juices suffer the same fate as processed milk. Natural enzymes, sensitive to temperatures above 108°F (42°C), are killed during pasteurization. These enzymes, like those in raw milk, aid in digestion, making the nutrients more available to your body as an energy source. Cooking the juice, which is necessary for shelf-life, also damages most of the vitamins and other sources of micronutrients that naturally occur in fresh fruits, vegetables and freshly squeezed juices.

Once the nutrients are destroyed, you're essentially left with sugar water that is commonly enriched with synthetic vitamins. Without proper nutrients, your body has to draw from other resources to run the metabolic pathways to digest the juice and detoxify the waste products. When you drink large quantities of processed juices, you set yourself up for indigestion. When deficient in natural enzymes, the body is unable to properly digest sugars. This provides a tasty treat for unfriendly bacteria, parasites and yeast to feed on. These unwanted creatures also have to poop. Their excrement is highly toxic and not only stresses your liver and kidneys but also your immune system.

Fats

As discussed in Chapters 3 and 4, fats are an essential part of a healthy diet. How much fat you should consume depends upon your metabolic type. Also be aware of the quality of the fats you eat.

Far too many dehydrogenated, or partially dehydrogenated fats, most often found in processed foods and foods from fast-food restaurants, are consumed today. When damaged from the heat of processing, the structure of these "bad" fats actually resembles plastic more than fat. Therefore, they're very hard, if not impossible, to digest. Whenever you eat more fat than your system can handle, you'll produce excessive bile to break it down. The excess bile production stimulates peristalsis of the intestinal tract and can cause "Diarrhella." Diarrhea due to excessive fat is evident when you see an oily film in the toilet after a bowel movement.

Tap water

The *Healthy Water* report by Dr. Martin Fox stated that "over 2100 organic and inorganic drinking water contaminants have been identified in the U.S. drinking water supply since 1974. Out of these 2100, 190 of the contaminants have confirmed adverse health effects..."[5]

While tap water is convenient, it's not a good idea to drink it in most cities. Many public water supplies have chlorine added to kill bacteria. Unfortunately, chlorine kills all bacteria that are not immune to it. This includes good bacteria in your gut as well as the bad bacteria in the water. Many notice a big improvement in their bowel habits after drinking water from a high quality filter system that removes chlorine, or by switching to top quality bottled water such as Evian, Vittel, Trinity, Fiji or Eternal Springs.

Caffeine

Caffeine is found in the leaves, seeds or fruits of more than 60 different plants, including coca nuts, mate leaves, guarana and coffee beans. It's commonly found in chocolate and is a flavoring agent in many cola beverages.[6]

Coffee has been used in enemas for almost as long as doctors have been writing about medicine. It does a good job of purging the colon because it's an irritant and stimulates gastric secretion. When coffee comes in contact with the lining of the intestinal tract, peristalsis is stimulated because the body is trying to eliminate it. There's really no point at which coffee stops becoming an irritant to your intestinal tract.

While many enjoy the stimulating effects of caffeine, it's extremely addictive and aside from causing loose stools, it's a diuretic. As discussed above, diarrhea alone will dehydrate you, but toss in a diuretic that also produces loose stools and you're really in trouble. If you have problems with loose stools or diarrhea, try eliminating coffee for 48 hours and see if your bowel habits improve. Note: Replacing coffee with teas like Yerba Mate will minimize caffeine withdrawal while not irritating the digestive tract.

3. Stress

Stress levels in modern society are at an all-time high. In Chapter 11, we discussed the many effects stress has on our bodies. Stress disrupts digestion by activating the sympathetic nervous system (fight-or-flight response), which leads to a decrease in the digestive processes. The sympathetic nervous system's main function is to prepare you to "fight" or "run" for your life. These days, the stress response is activated for a variety of reasons that mostly come down to a primal need for safety.

When you start your day by rushing to prepare for work or school, the digestive system shuts down. This often results in constipation. If you're too busy to stop work for a good meal at midday, stress levels further escalate.

Finally, after battling traffic, you return home for dinner just in time to watch the news, and the process repeats itself. It's easy to get jacked up hearing about the crazy things happening in the world while you chomp away with your head turned to one side, staring in amazement. You get up feeling uncomfortably full, and it's no surprise—*you have eaten three meals today and none of them have come out the back yet. You've created your own traffic jam!*

Over time, digestion becomes progressively challenged. When your body senses that the garbage is not being taken out, it doesn't want more coming in. Soon, you'll have a perpetual sense of fullness, but still feel hungry because your body is lacking nutrients.

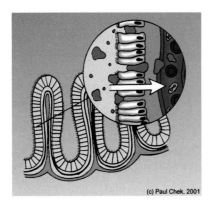

Figure 4: Leaky Gut

Effects of Poor Digestion

Leaky gut syndrome

Food intolerance, as well as all forms of stress, can effect digestion by causing what's referred to as leaky gut syndrome. The leaky gut results in separation of *tight junctions* between the cells of the gut wall (Figure 4). In the leaky gut, undigested or partially digested food particles may cross the gut wall, activating the immune system. The particles that do so become *antigens* (Figure 5A) and invoke a specific immune response when coming in contact with specific cells such as the *ubiquitous mast cells* which line the digestive and eliminative systems. These cells can have as many as 100,000 IgE antibodies attached.[7] When the antibody (Figure 5B) contacts the antigen (undigested food particle), it grabs a hold. When antibodies retain multiple antigens, cross-linking occurs, creating an immune complex (Figure 5C).

Cross-linking of the antigen on the antibodies triggers degranulation of the mast cell, releasing cell mediators such as histamine, which provokes an inflammatory response. This inflammatory response

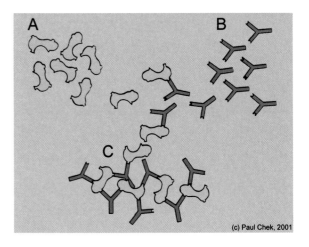

Figure 5
A: Antigens (undigested food particles that cross the gut wall).
B: Antibodies (put out by the immune system grab onto the antigens).
C: Immune Complex (created when antibodies hold onto multiple antigens).

increases permeability of local tissues in an attempt to wash the invader away and to bring more immune cells to the area.

Antibodies cross-link so as to increase the combined size of the particles, making it harder to pass through the gut wall, and so mast cells and phagocytes can recognize them, producing an adequate immune response. Because phagocytes, also known as *big eaters*, do not recognize particles under a specific size, the formation of immune complexes increases particle size so phagocytes can find and eat them. As shown in Figure 6, the phagocyte surrounds and then dissolves the immune complex.

Antigen overload!

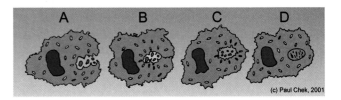

Figure 6: A phagocyte surrounding and dissolving an immune complex. This is an important function, as it prevents food particles from passing through the gut wall into the bloodstream.

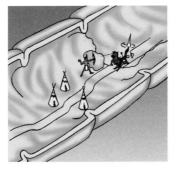

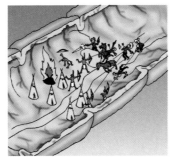

Normally, your first line of defense against antigens is the secretory IgA (sIgA) antibodies found in the mucus membranes lining your digestive and respiratory tracts. The IgA antibodies protect their territory much like the Native American Indians did from cowboys. (Figure 7), As the number of invading cowboys (antigens) try to impose upon the Indians' (sIgA) territory, the Indian adds more warriors. As the number of cowboys invading the Indian village (digestive/intestinal system) increases, the amount of damage done trying to win the war increases; this exemplifies continuance of the offending food(s) or drink(s).

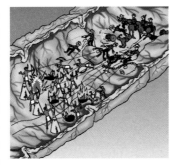

Figure 7: Battle in the Gut

Unfortunately, in this analogy, the cowboys represent food antigens arriving into a leaky gut. While sIgA antibodies are non-inflammatory (they signal for help from other immune cells), their counterparts, IgG, IgM and others, soon come to the rescue and the response they trigger is inflammatory. The immune system's response quickly becomes heated, much like a firefight among battling soldiers. Paradoxically, as described in the book *Enzymes, The Foundation of Life,* by Lopez, Williams and Michlke, when the number of immune complexes entering the blood stream reaches a certain point, the immune antibody system shuts down and a reduction in the activity of macrophages and phagocytes follows.[8] This is one of the reasons people with many kinds of food intolerance and intestinal inflammation suffer from malaise yet can't describe a specific reaction to offending foods.

Immune complexes find their way into joint tissues, organ tissues, nerve tissues and anywhere else accessible via the micro-circulatory system, causing inflammation. *Capillary leakage from inflammation results in fluid retention in subcutaneous tissues, causing the appearance of cellulite!* The result is activation of the *complement system*. The complement system is an enzyme system composed of *killer enzymes*. These enzymes (Figure 8) seek and destroy immune complexes imbedded in tissues. Unfortunately, they aren't specific to the immune complex; they also attack the tissues they're imbedded in. The result is identical to an autoimmune disorder.

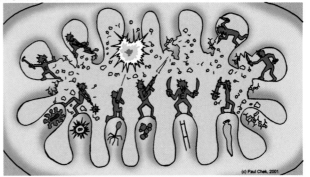

Figure 8: Killer Enzymes

Prolonged activation of the complement system will produce chronic inflammation, which means *chronic pain.* Unfortunately, it's common to treat chronic inflammatory pain, as described above, by prescribing anti-inflammatory drugs or cortisone. However, cortisone is an *immune suppressant,* and anti-inflammatory drugs often produce *gastrointestinal inflammation as a side effect. Further inflammation increases leaky gut which, in turn, produces additional symptoms!*

Prolonged inflammation further immobilizes the immune system while the complement system does its destructive handiwork. Painkillers and anti-inflammatory medication, so often used, allow the patient to ignore the ongoing degradation of tissues. Eventually, cancer, autoimmune disorders and any number of diseases will present themselves. If a natural, functional alternative is not soon applied, it's simply a matter of time before disease appears. The *symptoms are the body's cry for help!*

Current research on the use of enzyme therapies shows that the correctly prescribed type and dose of enzymes will act to break down immune complexes into smaller clusters. For unknown reasons, when the enzymes reduce the number and size of immune complexes in the blood and tissues, the antibody system is triggered back into action. (See Resources section for enzyme recommendations.)

If the complement system or antibody-mediated systems continue to attack at the expense of surrounding intestinal tissues, the gut becomes progressively worse. As intestinal wall leakage continues, more food antigens, chemicals, food additives, etc. make it into the portal vein and find their way to the liver. As you can see in Figure 9, up until about one hundred years ago, the liver dealt only with organic substances that it recognized. Today, the liver is overwhelmed in many cases with the sheer number of food particles, synthetic and organic chemicals it must process. Brostoff states that, **"Someone who is eating an average diet and drinking unfiltered tap water is likely to ingest and be exposed to at least 200 different synthetic chemicals and chemical cocktails every day."** [3] (Realize this is not inclusive of the huge number of *organic* chemicals present in our foods.)

When the liver cannot process food antigens and immune complexes, some of these particles pass into general circulation. Current food intolerance theories suggest that when the immune system becomes overworked it will prioritize resources to handle the most threatening issue at hand. In the meantime, antigens and immune complexes pass into areas of microcirculation, particularly around joint tissues, where they settle. Later, often at night when the immune system becomes more active, antibodies will attack the antigens in the joint tissues. If the number of immune complexes in the blood and tissues rises past the point at which the antibody system "gives up," the complement system of *killer enzymes* may be activated.

If the body has become hyper-sensitized, and/or there are diminished levels of sIgA, a nonspecific attack led by IgE, IgG and IgM antibodies may take place at some point in the continuum of antibody/

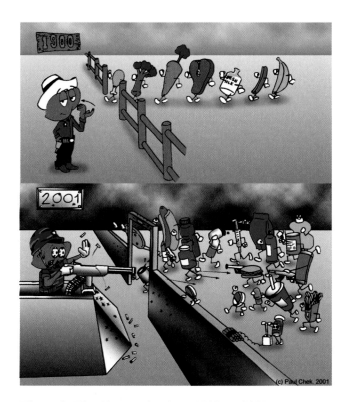

Figure 9: The Liver at the Gate 1900 vs. 2001

complement system activation. This leaves joint tissues inflamed and painful. In my experience, many patients seeking assistance from orthopedic doctors, therapists or chiropractors for unresolved chronic musculoskeletal pain are likely expressing the symptoms of food intolerance and/or chemical sensitivity concomitant with gastrointestinal disorders.

Food intolerance and your stubborn paunch belly!

As you can see in Figure 10, when pain impulses come from the small intestine, bowel or any organ of digestion, there may be some level of inhibition (weakness) and possibly pain in the corresponding region of the abdominal wall. It is important to remember food allergies and intolerance commonly causes inflammation in the gut. The greater the level of inflammation in your digestive system, the greater the likelihood that your abdominal muscles *will not* respond to exercise.

Visit any gym and you'll find scores of people who train regularly to shape their bodies only to have distended and often comparatively unattractive torsos. The exerciser or non-exerciser who has not

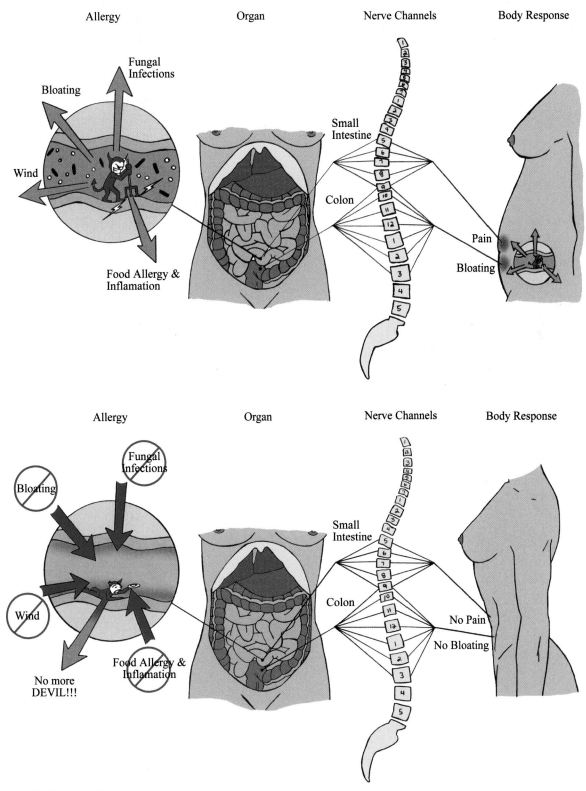

Figure 10: Devil in the Gut.

Pain or inflammation of the digestive organs will reflex to the abdominals, leaving these important stabilizer muscles weak or disabled. No matter how hard you train your abs in such a state, you will not achieve the flat tummy you most likely desire. Once such digestive issues are addressed, you will look and feel better.

addressed food intolerance is likely to exhibit the dreaded paunch belly and commonly suffer from a host of gastrointestinal or digestive disorders. This is why so many people consume a small fortune in expensive vitamins, sports supplements and organic foods yet continue to struggle with their health! *Just because you put it in your mouth doesn't mean it actually makes it so far as to benefit your body.*

Masking messages from your body and the Bowel Bandits with anti-inflammatory and pain medication is also a great concern. When you use any form of drug that repeatedly elevates cortisol levels, you suppress the immune system with a resultant decrease in the immunoglobulin secretory IgA, which is the first line of immune defense throughout all the mucus-lined passages of your body. This includes everything from mouth and nose to anus! Suppressing your front line immune defenses leaves the door wide open for opportunistic organisms to embed themselves in the crypts or folds of your intestinal tract. Here, unfriendly bacteria and parasites have a feast on the food your inflamed gut is unable to digest. You soon begin to accumulate an increasing number of the food allergy and intolerance symptoms listed in this chapter. In the wrong hands, you will also acquire a laundry list of drugs to take every day. *I actually had a client taking 16 different prescription drugs at once, and not one single doctor or therapist had EVER addressed the basics of health and digestion with her!*

Taking Action Against Food Allergy and Intolerance

Blood tests

There are a number of companies that conduct blood testing to determine food allergy and food intolerance. The C.H.E.K Institute has had the most reliable clinical results from Biohealth Diagnostics of San Diego, California (see Resources). While a large number of medical doctors and chiropractors perform food allergy and intolerance testing, you can go directly to an independent testing lab such as Great Smokies (see Resources). Consulting a health care professional does have its benefits, though, as there is a fair amount of patient education and additional dietary management involved.

Elimination and rotation diets

The least expensive way to begin clearing yourself of food allergies and intolerance is by going on either an elimination or rotation diet. An elimination diet calls for the exclusion of suspected problem foods for 8-12 weeks. Questionable foods should then be reintroduced one at a time. If side effects develop from eating the recently reintroduced food, you're probably still intolerant to that particular food and should avoid eating it.

A rotation diet requires that you don't eat foods from the same genetic family more than once every four days. For example, if you eat lamb on Monday, you would not eat it again until Friday. See Appendix page 236 for a sample rotation diet plan.

CHEK Points on Digestion

Now that you have a good understanding of how the Bowel Bandits make their way into your life and how easily digestion can become disrupted, here are a few tips on how to avoid them and how to improve digestion:

1. Never watch the news while you eat! In fact, never watch anything on TV while you eat unless you're sure it's going to be funny or make you feel good. Avoid watching sporting events while you eat, especially if you have an emotional attachment to the outcome. The excitement of watching your favorite team will likely cause that fight-or-flight response which shuts down digestion—especially if they lose!

2. Don't read technical or stressful material while you eat. Reading the newspaper is just like watching the news and will yield the same effect. In fact, if you ate the newspaper, your digestion would probably be better than if you read it while you ate! If you wish to read, read something that makes you happy, something inspirational or something spiritually stimulating.

   If you have poor eyesight, wear glasses or contacts—it's not a good idea to read at all while you eat because the eyes require a lot of energy to run and can drain energy needed for digestion.

3. Play relaxing music. Either classical music or music with a one second beat (such as that from the Baroque period of classical music), or new age

music that has no discernible beat (you can't hum to it), is relaxing to the body and will stimulate the parasympathetic nervous system.

Research from Johns Hopkins University has revealed that rock music causes people to eat faster and to consume larger portions, while classical music—especially slow string music—causes the opposite effect.[9]

4. Drink two glasses of clean, chlorine-free water 15 minutes before each meal.

Always avoid drinking alcohol before meals. When alcohol of *any form* enters your digestive system in the absence *of proteins and fats, it irritates the gut and can lead to leaky gut syndrome,* setting you up for food intolerance and a host of other problems. Also avoid drinking coffee or other stimulants before eating. These drinks cause the activation of your sympathetic nervous system, which in turn shuts down digestion. If that isn't bad enough, a release of insulin from the pancreas and liberation of blood sugar from the liver results. Therefore, anything you eat is likely to be shuttled into *fat cells, which means you'll probably end up wearing it!*

5. Limit use of dehydrated foods and re-hydrate nuts, seeds and dried foods such as fruit, grains and legumes by soaking them for 12- 24 hours before eating.[10] It's also a good idea to flash boil dried fruits once re-hydrated to minimize your chances of parasite infestation.

Dehydrated foods quite often get stuck to the colon wall, where they draw moisture out of the colon. In addition to causing pain, this can lead to problems, particularly in those with diverticulitis, a disease where the colon develops little balloon-like pockets. These pockets often develop from having to force out Bodybuilders, Pellet Poops and Sinkers 'n' Stinkers!

My good friend and associate David Webster, author of *Achieve Maximum Health*, has seen nuts, grains, popcorn, seeds and just about every form of dried food you can think of come out the tail pipe while administering a high colonic.[11] Interestingly, many of his clients had not eaten some of what he was seeing come out of their colons for as long as seven years!

6. Avoid foods that you're intolerant or allergic to.

7. Chew your food until liquefied.

8. Eat smaller meals more often. A number of nutritional experts today suggest that the body can only break down a given amount of protein at any one sitting. They feel that eating smaller portions and dining five or six times a day makes for much better digestion and absorption. Personally, I feel there may be variances among people as to how much protein they can digest, just as there are tremendous differences in the amount of alcohol one can tolerate.

Hypoglycemia is also a growing concern. The onset of hypoglycemia is largely due to the over-consumption of simple carbohydrates in drinks and foods, as well as the consumption of drinks laced with caffeine and similar stimulants. Those with poor blood sugar handling capacity almost always find their concentration and overall level of well being improved when eating more frequent, smaller meals. It's important to remember that all small meals should be correctly proportioned for your metabolic type, as outlined in Chapter 3.

9. Never suppress the urge. You want to have the Poopie Policemen on the job, but you don't ever want to stop a Poopie Policeman from reaching his destination. According to Dr. Tom Benteen, you can entrain (change the timing of, or teach) any physiological system in as little as 7-21 days.[12] This means that if you suppress the urge to defecate each day for as little as a week to three weeks, you can cause a permanent traffic jam in your intestinal tract. This is sure to disrupt digestion, inhibit absorption of nutrients and increase your chances of toxicity through the bowel.

10. Whenever possible, start your meal with raw (live) foods. All raw foods, such as fresh ingredients from a salad, contain enzymes that are beneficial to digestion. Pineapple and Papaya contain enzymes powerful enough to assist in the digestion of meats and are often very tasty in salads.

Case History:

Ru-tee, CHEK NLC Level 2, C.H.E.K Practitioner Level 1 and Certified Health Excel Intermediate Metabolic Typing Advisor, client of Paul Chek

To most of my friends and those that knew me, I was a fit, energetic person with a successful personal training business. They weren't alone – Adidas thought that my image was so good they asked me to be the face of their brand for three years. The truth was that every day was a struggle for me, and it had been that way for a number of years. General lethargy and tiredness upon waking, depression, panic attacks, eczema, rashes, chronic fatigue, abdominal discomfort and bloating, fluid retention, rapid weight gain, strange spacey feelings, excessive thirst, blood sugar level problems (feeling really weak if I didn't eat every two hours), massive appetite – to name but a few of my symptoms – were common ailments which, because of my job, I had become very adept at disguising.

My doctor, I felt, might have thought that I was a hypochondriac. My low energy, he suggested, was due probably to my work as a trainer, and, since I looked as fit as I did, he also suggested that maybe I should cut down on my training. The truth was, I had stopped training myself altogether. Exercise made me feel worse and I gained weight the harder I trained! I improved my diet, cut down on fat and ate fresh vegetables and complex carbohydrates – but these simply made me feel worse! I was sure I was ill and demanded that my doctor take me seriously. I had blood tests, glucose tests, mineral and vitamin tests, and more. All my tests came back as normal – therefore how could there be anything wrong with me?

In the meantime I was getting worse. During photo-shoots I would have to hold my distended pot-belly in for hours at a time. Anytime I relaxed it, people thought I was playing about sticking it out for fun. It was so uncomfortable.

My doctor, who wasn't sure what was wrong with me, but was supportive, referred me to a neurological specialist and a top nutritionist for help—again no improvement, just worsening of my symptoms. It was difficult for these specialists to take me seriously—on the outside I looked great to them and all the tests were negative, so how could there be anything wrong (apart from in my head!).

When I attended a Paul Chek seminar, guess who he decided to pick to demonstrate one of the exercises? Yep, me (and my belly). After completing the exercise (rather well, I thought – with my belly pulled in nice and tight) he asked the audience, "What do you notice about Ru-tee?" No reply. "Well, Ru-tee has an abdominal wall that isn't functioning properly. Look at her lower abdominals; they are not recruiting at all. She definitely has some major digestive issues that need looking in to." This was great news – something was wrong with me! This gave me the confidence to investigate further.

I found out about an environmental hospital that recognized the symptoms I presented. After two weeks of tests, I was diagnosed as suffering from glandular fever, numerous food intolerances and chronic fatigue. A strict rotation diet, desensitizing injections and a truckload of vitamins were prescribed. I followed it religiously and got worse!! It took me weeks to recover from the tests, and I was being told a different thing each time I visited. To make matters worse, I couldn't face taking injections for the rest of my life!

It had cost me £6000 to get to this point, and not one practitioner had been able to explain what was causing the symptoms and how they could be treated effectively. All they wanted to do was treat the symptoms and not find out the cause. Time went on and so did the injections, but I wasn't really feeling any better. I was getting quite panicky about the whole situation, and my stomach, no matter what I ate, was getting bigger and more painful by the day. By this time, I needed a snooze every afternoon just to function, had really bad night sweats, fuzzy head, restless and achy legs, couldn't concentrate and my energy was permanently low.

I had arranged to meet a friend for supper and I really didn't want to go, but I did. And I'm really glad I did. Guess who was there having supper! Paul Chek! I sat down and poured my heart out to him. He was great. He said, "Right, Ru-tee we need to get you straightened out right away."

He took me on as client in September, 2001, and established that I was a fast oxidizer (protein type) —so all the carbohydrates that I had been recommend to eat were wrong for me and were contributing to my feeling worse and to my blood sugar problems. I also had parasites, fungal infections and adrenal fatigue. He put me on a manageable 4-day rotation diet to give my system a break, told me to cut out gluten as I had an intolerance to this, prescribed supplements, Bach flower remedies and organic food. I went on a supplementation program to kill the parasites. He explained that if I started to feel worse, that was good as, my system was starting to detox. Most importantly of all, he told it to me straight—my system was not working correctly and it would take time to heal. He also told me that I needed to cut down on my work and go to bed earlier, try and reduce all the extra stresses in my life, take up Qigong and deep breathing exercises, and also he told me a selection of books that he wanted me to read. If I didn't do something about it now I would probably end up having to stop work in the near future. He was like a breath of fresh air. It is so much easier to make changes when you understand what is going on.

Well, I took his advice and did have some bad moments, but I started to improve significantly. My energy level was higher and I felt things were moving forward. However, at Christmas I went to Jamaica with my fiancé. After two weeks of poor food and a long flight home, my system crashed. All my symptoms (and more) returned and I couldn't work for another five weeks.

Paul was amazing and so caring and understanding. I regularly called him (sometimes in tears). He always had the time to talk to me and coached me on what was happening and what to do (even though he was in the States and I was in England). It made a huge difference to know why I was feeling like this and how to treat it. I gradually started to get back on my feet again and worked closely with a colleague of Paul's here in the UK.

A year on and I'm better than I have been for 12 years. I have made lifestyle as well as nutrition changes, as my case has been quite complicated. I still have a little way to go, but I have my life back, together with a better understanding of how my body works and what it needs to function correctly. In a way, I am glad that this happened to me because I have learned so much and now will be able to help others.

One thing's for sure. Paul really did change my life! Thank you so much, Paul, for making me strong and supporting and guiding me through every step. You are truly an inspiration.

Please understand my friend, that where you find yourself tomorrow is a function of the positive decisions and actions you take today.

Akin A. Awolaja, Educator of *Wise Living*

When Einstein Was My Doctor

Dear Dr. Einstein,

I am writing to follow-up with you, as you requested. It has now been just over six months since I saw you. The education you gave me the day you filled in for my doctor has not only transformed my life, it has transformed my entire family and my family life! The first thing I did after seeing you was purchase the book you recommended, *How To Eat, Move and Be Healthy!* by Paul Chek.

I took the book home and followed the four-step program. Not surprisingly, I scored very high in the Stress, You Are What You Eat and Sleep/Wake Cycle questionnaires. As I read the respective chapters, I could hear your voice in my head telling me many of the same things Paul Chek recommended I do to balance my body systems and build my vitality.

While I had not been taking time to exercise before seeing you, I began with Paul Chek's "No Exercise Exercise" program and incorporated one exercise from zone 3 and another from zone 4. I also forced myself out of bed at 6 am to begin my zone exercises, which ended up helping me get to sleep earlier at night. This really helped me get back on a normal sleep/wake cycle.

Just one month after I saw you, I went back to my doctor for my regularly scheduled follow-up visit. Needless to say, he was very impressed with the initial changes in my blood pressure and cholesterol levels. You should have seen his reaction when he saw your notes in my chart telling me to increase my fat and protein intake! He said he's never seen such an approach before, but, couldn't deny the results. My triglyceride levels were in the healthy range after only one month of eating right for my metabolic type, consuming high quality meats and fats and organic produce as both you and the *How To Eat, Move and Be Healthy!* book suggested.

I returned to my doctor for another follow-up visit three months after seeing you and he was amazed to see my cholesterol levels and blood pressure had normalized! At this point, I had lost 14 pounds, and what really perplexed my doctor, was that I was eating *more calories and more fat than ever!* He said *"only Dr. Einstein could have solved your case with such simplicity!"*

After three months, I was feeling so great, I decided to get a gym membership again, and, to make it even better, the whole family joined. My wife and kids were so amazed at the transformation they saw in my body and energy levels, they too, completed the questionnaires in the *How To Eat, Move and Be Healthy!* book and followed the program.

Dr. Einstein, I can't thank you enough. I feel so fortunate to have had you as my doctor. In just one visit, you educated me and made suggestions that have changed my life – *my whole family's life!* Dr. Einstein, today, I'm off all medical drugs and am excited to tell you I look and feel as good as I did when I was in college. While I wish everyone in the world could have you as their doctor, I know that would certainly take the fun out of your retirement, so, I've done the next best thing – I've told all my friends and family to do what you told me to do – follow the four-step plan in Paul Chek's book, *How To Eat, Move and Be Healthy!*.

Thank you Dr. Einstein. You have changed my life forever!

Sincerely,

Truman Vital

Now, good digestion
wait on appetite,
And health on both!

William Shakespeare, *Macbeth*

There is a time
for many words,
and there is also a
time for sleep.

Homer, *The Odyssey*

Appendix

Diet Plan # 1
Recommended Foods Chart

PROTEINS

MEAT/FOWL — light meats	SEAFOOD — light fish	DAIRY — non/low fat
chicken breast	catfish	cheese
Cornish game hen	cod	cottage cheese
turkey breast	flounder	kefir
pork, lean	haddock	milk
ham	halibut	yogurt
Only occasional lean red meat or restrict entirely	perch	eggs
	scrod	**LEGUMES** — use sparingly
	sole	*high starch:* dried beans
	trout	lentils
	tuna, white	*low starch:* tempeh
	turbot	tofu
		NUTS — sparingly

CARBOHYDRATES

GRAIN — whole grains only	VEGETABLE — high starch	VEGETABLE — moderate starch	VEGETABLE — low starch	FRUIT — all are okay
corn	potato	beet	beet green	apple
couscous	pumpkin	corn	broccoli	apricot
kamut	rutabaga	eggplant	brussels sprout	berry
kasha	sweet potato	jicama	cabbage	cherry
millet	yam	okra	chard	citrus
oat		parsnip	collard	grape
quinoa		radish	cucumber	melon
rice		spaghetti squash	garlic	peach
rye		summer squash	kale	pear
spelt		yellow squash	leafy greens	pineapple
triticale		turnip	onion	plum
wheat		zucchini	parsley	tomato
high starch: amaranth			peppers	tropical
barley			scallion	**LEGUMES** — *high starch:* dried beans
brown rice			sprouts	dried peas
buckwheat			tomato	lentils
			watercress	

OILS / FATS

NUT/SEED — use sparingly	OIL/FAT — use sparingly
walnut	butter
pumpkin	cream
peanut	ghee
sunflower	*oils:*
sesame	almond oil
almond	flax oil
cashew	olive oil
Brazil	peanut oil
filbert	sesame oil
pecan	sunflower oil
chestnut	walnut oil
pistachio	
coconut	
hickory	
macadamia	

Note: nuts are listed from highest to lowest protein content.

Note: High starch foods are high glycemic foods (converts quickly to sugar) and thus are your caution foods if you have blood sugar problems.

Every meal should contain a protein from these sources

Copyright © Healthexcel, 1987

Diet Plan # 2
Recommended Foods Chart

PROTEINS

MEAT/FOWL	SEAFOOD	DAIRY
high purine	*high purine*	*whole fat*
organ meats	anchovy	*low purine*
pate	caviar	cheese
beef liver	herring	cottage cheese
chicken liver	mussel	cream
medium purine	sardine	eggs
beef	*medium purine*	kefir
bacon	abalone	milk
chicken*	clam	yogurt
duck	crab	**LEGUMES**
fowl	crayfish	*low purine*
goose	lobster	tempeh
kidney	mackerel	tofu
lamb	octopus	*medium purine*
pork chop	oyster	beans, dried
spare rib	salmon	lentils
turkey*	scallop	**NUTS**
veal	shrimp	*all are okay*
wild game	snail	
*dark meat is best	squid	
	tuna, dark	

*Every meal should contain a protein from these sources, but dairy, legumes or nuts are **not** a substitute for meats at main meals*

CARBOHYDRATES

GRAIN	VEGETABLE	FRUIT
whole grains only	*non-starch*	avocado
high starch	asparagus	olive
amaranth	beans, fresh	*not fully ripe -*
barley	cauliflower	apple (some)
brown rice	celery	pear (some)
buckwheat	mushroom	*high starch*
corn	spinach	banana
couscous	*high starch*	
kamut	artichoke	
kasha	carrot	
millet	pea	
oat	potatoes, fried in butter only	
quinoa	squash, winter	
rye	**LEGUMES**	
spelt	*non-starch*	
triticale	tempeh	
sprouted grain bread is the only bread allowed	tofu	
	high starch	
	beans, dried	
	peas, dried	
	lentils	

*Sprouted grain breads such as Ezekiel or Manna breads

OILS / FATS

NUT/SEED	OIL/FAT
all are okay	*all are okay*
walnut	butter
pumpkin	cream
peanut	ghee
sunflower	*oils:*
sesame	almond oil
almond	flax oil
cashew	olive oil
Brazil	peanut oil
filbert	sesame oil
pecan	sunflower oil
chestnut	walnut oil
pistachio	
coconut	
hickory	
macadamia	

*Note: nuts are listed from highest to lowest protein content.

Note: High starch foods are high glycemic foods (converts quickly to sugar) and thus are your caution foods.

Copyright © Healthexcel, 1987

Using a Rotation Diet

A rotation diet is an easy, and inexpensive, approach to identifying food intolerances, avoiding symptoms of food intolerance and detoxifying your body, especially your digestive system. It is also a healthy and effective way to lose weight.

The diet plan given here is a four-day rotation. Notice that there are different foods for each day and that no foods are listed on more than one day. A rotation diet is based on taxonomy. Just as there are many species of animals, there are also many species of plants. Foods that are closely related (in the same family) are grouped together in the diet plan because they share similar protein structures and are thus treated similarly by the digestive system. Not all same day foods are in the same family. Each day includes a few different families of plants and animals/fish.

To follow the rotation diet, eat only the foods listed on that particular day. You may have those foods as many times as you like on that particular day, but then you should not consume any of those foods again for the following three days. For example, if you start with day one on Monday, you will not eat any of the day one foods again until Friday. The only exceptions are oils which may be consumed more frequently.

You may start each day at dinner. In this case, you would eat day one foods for dinner (on Monday, for example) and then for breakfast and lunch the following day. You would then switch to day two foods for dinner on Tuesday. This makes it easier if you like to have leftovers for lunch.

If you have a hard time committing to the four-day rotation, start with a "training" rotation diet. Write down everything you eat and drink (excluding water) each day. Do not eat any of the foods you eat on one day for three days following. For example, do not eat the foods you eat on Monday again until Friday. This approach doesn't require rotating by taxonomy or genetic grouping, but still ensures that you are getting adequate variety in your diet. As you get used to eating a variety of foods, start following the rotation plan provided. You may also start with just rotating your protein sources. These are the foods that people often have problems with, so you will likely feel better by rotating them.

Do you need to follow this plan forever? It is ideal to strictly follow a rotation diet for at least three to six months to achieve the maximum benefit. At this point, you will most likely find that you will naturally rotate the foods you are eating. Many people find it easy to continue with a rotation as it makes cooking easy. Again, it is always a good idea to rotate protein sources, especially seafood, to limit your exposure to potential allergens and toxins. With produce and grains, you may decide not to follow the diet plan presented here, but, as long as you cycle a variety of different foods, you will basically accomplish the same thing.

If your total score from your Nutrition and Lifestyle questionnaires was over 260, you should follow the rotation diet plan on the following pages, which is based on taxonomy. This will minimize the load on your immune system which will help reduce your total score and improve your vitality.

Day 1

Carbohydrates

Banana
Currant
Gooseberry
Grapes
Guava
Kiwi
Litchi
Mango
Papaya
Paw Paw
Artichoke
Bell Peppers (Capsicum)
Carrot[1]
Celery[1]
Chicory
Eggplant
Fennel
Lettuce (all types)
Parsley[1]
Parsnip[1]
Tomato
White Potato
Yuca

Protein

Anchovy
Beef
Buffalo
Cheese (cow, sheep or goat)
Codfish
Eel
Herring
Lamb
Liver
Sturgeon
Tarpon
Veal

[1] These items are all from the same family. If you wish to switch the spices to another day, make sure to switch the entire family. Salts and most oils do not need to be rotated.

Miscellaneous

Allspice
Caraway
Cayenne Pepper
Chili Pepper
Clove
Coffee
Coriander[1]
Milk (cow, sheep or goat)
Cumin[1]
Dill
Hops
Fennel[1]
Honey
Macadamia Nuts
Mint
Paprika
Pistachio
Safflower Oil
Sunflower Oil
Tapioca

Day 2

Carbohydrates

Millet
Oats
Rye
Wheat
Barley
Apple
Avocado
Berries (all)
Dates
Figs
Persimmon
Pear
Pomegranate
Cabbage
Cauliflower
Collard Greens
Broccoli
Brussel Sprouts
Kale
Mushrooms
Mustard Greens
Radish
Turnip
Watercress

Protein

Chicken
Duck
Eggs
Goose
Ostrich
Prairie Chicken
Turkey
Tuna
Quail

[2] These items are all from the same family. If you wish to switch the spices to another day, make sure to switch the entire family. Salts and most oils do not need to be rotated.

Miscellaneous

Bakers Yeast
Basil[2]
Bay Leaves
Brewers Yeast
Cane Sugar
Cardamon
Cinnamon
Coconut
Ginger
Hazelnuts
Lavender[2]
Malt
Molasses
Nutmeg
Oregano[2]
Poppyseeds
Rosemary[2]
Sage[2]
Spearmint[2]
Thyme[2]
Tumeric

Day 3

Carbohydrates

Apricot
Blackberries
Boysenberries
Cherries
Loganberries
Nectarine
Peach
Plum
Pineapple
Raspberries
Strawberries
Alfalfa Sprouts
Asparagus
Beans (all)
Chives
Corn
Garlic
Jicama
Leek
Onion
Peas
Sweet Potato
Yams

Protein

Chick Pea
Flounder
Halibut
Kidney Beans
Lentil Beans
Lima Beans
Mung Beans
Navy Beans
Pinto Beans
Pork
Rabbit
Shark
Swordfish
Sole
Soybean
Venison (Deer)

Miscellaneous

Almonds
Brazil Nuts
Carob
Licorice
Peanuts
Pepper (Black and White)
Vanilla
Yerba Mate

Day 4

Carbohydrates

Buckwheat
Rice[3]
Cantaloupe
Casaba
Grapefruit
Honeydew
Kumquat
Lemon
Lime
Orange
Tangelo
Tangerine
Watermelon
Beets
Chard
Cucumber
Okra
Olive
Pumpkin
Rhubarb
Sorrel
Spinach
Squash (all)

Protein

Albalone
Bass
Clam
Crab
Grouper
Lobster
Mackerel
Mussel
Oyster
Salmon
Scallop
Shrimp
Snail
Snapper
Squid
Trout

Miscellaneous

Beet Sugar
Chamomile
Cocoa
Maple Syrup
Pecans
Sesame
Tea
Walnut

[3] You may switch rice to day one.

More on Parasites

If you scored high on the fungus and parasite questionnaire, regardless of your other scores, it is imperative that you read, and strictly adhere to, the advice in ALL the sections listed on your questionnaire score sheet. Always remember to start your study and corrective efforts from the left of your scoring sheet to maximize your time and results. The first issue to address is your diet, so begin by reading Chapters 3 and 4 and then progress to Chapters 11 through 14. If following the advice given here for three months has not notably reduced your parasite score, you will need to seek assistance from a physician trained in the treatment of parasitic organisms.

It is very important to take my advice here *seriously*. When your internal environment shifts to the point that it becomes favorable for fungi and parasites, they will flourish. They can then change your internal ecosystem with the release of their own chemical mediators. The changes these parasitic organisms make in your body include altering your pH levels, releasing immune modulating chemicals so your immune system doesn't recognize them, and eating your food and nutrients before you can! Parasitic organisms also release chemical mediators to trick you into craving sweets—which is the food of choice for most parasites! *When your parasite score is high, you are at war with the bugs – so don't feed the enemy!*

While there are *many* approaches and philosophies for addressing parasite problems, one thing I've learned through clinical experience is that where there are fungi, there are usually other parasites, or soon will be (and vice-versa). The fungi release toxins called *mycotoxins.* Mycotoxins are so powerful that they are used in germ warfare! Some mycotoxins *stun* your immune system, while others alter the release of, and timing of, key immune regulators and messengers so that the fungi become invisible to the immune system. When this happens, should you either keep eating poor quality and/or sweet foods,

you are very likely to feed other parasitic organisms, encouraging their proliferation. I have also heard of many cases in which people were treated for parasites with powerful drugs and felt better while taking the drugs, only to have the symptoms return even stronger after the medication was finished. If this occurs, it is most likely because:

1. The client has a fungal infection modulating the immune system and in the absence of the parasite the drug has just killed, there is now much less competition for food and space for the fungi.

2. The drugs targeted only one of potentially several parasites inhabiting the body, again reducing competition for other parasites.

3. The client was not educated as to the diet and lifestyle modifications that *must* take place to restore the internal ecosystem and immune system to a level of vitality that protects against parasites.

You *must address fungi first to successfully rid yourself of parasites for the long run.* While you may not know if you currently have an active fungal infection, current research presented in *The Fungal Link* by Doug Kaufmann, showed that about 90% of the American population has a fungal infection today. Indications that you do have or are likely to have a fungal infection include recent or current challenges with: dandruff, jock itch, athletes foot, vaginal yeast infection or toenail fungus, or if you have completed a course of antibiotics at any time in your life without re-colonizing the gut with either a human grade probiotic supplement or by regularly consuming raw goats milk or yogurt (raw cows milk or yogurt is helpful but goats milk products are more compatible with the human gut) for about three months.

What do I do?

The first step in any parasite evacuation program is to starve the fungi! There are few reliable tests to indicate the presence of fungi so the best thing to do is put yourself on an antifungal diet preventatively. If you notice a reduction in any symptoms or an improvement in energy levels, sleep quality, mental clarity, or a reduction in anxiety, you have successfully reduced your fungi population. Keep going! A basic antifungal diet consists of the following:

1. Eliminate all simple sugars (even if it's organic)

2. Eliminate all fruit (even organic and dried fruits) with the exceptions of green apples (without the skin) and fresh berries (monitor your symptoms with berries as some people don't respond well to them due to higher than optimal sugar content; this is the best way to satisfy a massive sweet craving if you must).

3. Eliminate all below-ground vegetables with the exception of carrots. You may drink a cup or two of carrot juice with raw garlic, raw ginger or apple cider vinegar each day because these items are strongly antifungal.

4. Do not eat meats that are commercially farmed if at all possible because they feed the animals poor quality grains to fatten them, leaving myco-toxins in the meat, which further weakens your immune system.

5. Eat a diet primarily of high-quality meats and above-ground vegetables, proportioned for your metabolic type.

6. Cook with coconut oil and happily consume high quality saturated animal fats, as they support the immune system! You may also find it useful to freeze cod liver oil capsules and take 2-3 grams first thing in the morning on an empty stomach.

7. Follow the principles of rotation dieting presented on page 236.

8. Consume raw goats milk or yogurt or use a high quality human grade probiotic supplement for a minimum of two months.

While this is a basic outline, I STRONGLY suggest you study *The Fungal Link* by Doug Kaufmann, which is available on-line at www.chekinstitute.com. Most antifungal diets must be followed for a minimum of six months to have a lasting effect and you must be very careful not to start eating junk again as soon as you start feeling good because the parasites are quietly waiting for you to make that mistake!

Due to the complexity of testing for and treating parasites, if following the advice here doesn't lower your scores into the low zone, I strongly suggest you visit the How To Eat, Move and Be Healthy! website (www.eatmoveandbehealthy.com) to view our list of suggested resources and preferred physicians that are experts at eliminating parasites.

In conclusion, I can't over-emphasize the importance of strict adherence to the principles in this book and eliminating fungi and parasites! We live in a toxic environment today and have hectic, stressful lives, which lowers immunity. Always remember, you can't get rid of parasites if you don't make your internal environment unfavorable for them! Parasites don't like healthy, vital people--they are Mother Nature's garbage collectors, so if you want to get rid of them, don't feed them by using your stomach as a garbage can!

Notes

Notes

Chapter 1

1. "Study on Overweight Kids." *Jama*. December 12, 2001.

2. Critser, Greg. "A Get Fit Plan for Physical Education." *Los Angeles Times*. Sunday, December 16, 2001.

3. "High-glycemic Index Foods, Hunger and Obesity: Is There a Connection?" *Nutrition Reviews*. Vol. 58, No. 6.

4. Gottlieb, Scott. "U.S. Drug Sales Continue to Rise." BMJ. March 1, 2003. Online: www.bmjjournals.com.

5. Schlosser, Eric. *Fast Food Nation*. Boston: Houghton Mifflin Co., 2001.

6. "Soft Drinks Add to Childhood Obesity." *Alternative Medicine News Letter*. February 16, 2001. Online: www.healthmall.com.

7. Halandane, J.S. *The Sciences and Philosophy*. Hodder and Stoughton, 1928.

8. Balfour, E.B. *The Living Soil and the Haughley Experiment*. London: Faber and Faber, 1975.

Chapter 2

1. www.zonediet.com

2. www.fatfree.com/diets/ornish.html

Chapter 3

1. Williams, Roger. *Biochemical Individuality*. New Canaan, CT: Keats Publishing, 1956.

2. Price, Weston A. *Nutrition and Physical Degeneration*. San Diego, CA: Price-Pottenger Nutrition Foundation, Inc., 1939, 1970, 2000.

3. Fallon, Sally and Enig, Mary. www.pricepottenger.org. Price-Pottenger Foundation website, includes a variety of articles on nutrition.

4. Wolcott, William. *The Metabolic Typing Diet*. New York: Doubleday, 2000.

Chapter 4

1. Worthington, Virginia MS, Sc.D. *Biodynamics* 224, July/August 1999.

2. Heaton, Shane. *Organic Farming, Food Quality and Human Health Report*. British Soil Association, 2001.

3. Clarke, Porter, Quested and Thomas. *Living Organic*. Naperville, IL: SourceBooks, Inc., 2001.

4. Balfour, E.B. *The Haughley Experiment*. London: Faber and Faber LTD, 1975.

5. Barrett, Stephen, M.D. "Organic Foods: Will Certification Protect Consumers?" Online: www.quackwatch.com.

6. White, Alison. "Children, Pesticides and Cancer." *The Ecologist* Vol. 28, No. 2, March/April, 1998.

7. Schafer, Kristin. *Nowhere to Hide: Persistent Toxic Chemicals in the U.S. Food Supply*. San Francisco, CA: Pesticide Action Network, 2001.

8. Solomon, Gina M.D. *Pesticides and Human Health: A Resource for Health Care Professionals*. Physicians for Social Responsibility and Californians for Pesticide Reform, 2000. Available online at: http://www.psrla.org/pesthealth.htm.

9. Curl, Cynthia, et. al. "Organophosphorus pesticide exposure of urban and suburban pre-school children with organic and conventional diets." Journal of the National Institute of Environmental Health Sciences. Online October, 31, 2002: http://dx.doi.org/.

10. Kellas, William and Dworkin, Andrea. *Surviving in a Toxic World*. Olivenhain, CA: Professional Preference, 1996.

11. Farlow, Christina Hoza, D.C. Food *Additives, A Shopper's Guide to What's Safe and What's Not*. Escondido, CA: KISS For Health Publishing, 2001.

12. Schlosser, Eric. *Fast Food Nation*. Boston: Houghton Mifflin Co., 2001.

13. Price, Weston A. *Nutrition and Physical Degeneration*. San Diego, CA: Price-Pottenger Nutrition Foundation, Inc., 1939, 1970, 2000.

14. Fallon, Sally. *Nourishing Traditions*. Washington, DC: New Trends Publishing, Inc., 1999.

15. Pottenger, Francis Marrion. *Pottenger's Cats*. San Diego, CA: Price-Pottenger Nutrition Foundation, Inc., 1983.

16. Weaver, Sean (interview of Arpad Pusztai). "The Political Science of GE Foods." *Organic NZ* Vol. 60, No. 3, May/June 2001.

17. Epstein, Samuel and Hauter, Wenonah. "Hooked on Nuclear Irradiation Too?" *The Ecologist Report*. June 2001.

18. "Nuclear Lunch: The Dangers and Unknowns of Food Irradiation." Online April, 2001: www.mercola.com. Excerpted from the Food & Water report "Meat Monopolies: Dirty Meat and the False Promises of Irradiation" by Susan Meeker-Lowry and Jennifer Ferrara.

19. Epstein, Samual. "Preventing Pathogenic Food Poisoning: Sanitation Not Irradiation." Online: www.mercola.com.

20. Online: www.mercola.com

21. Crowe, Ivan. *The Quest for Food*. United Kingdom: Tempus Publishing, 2000.

22. Institute of Food and Nutrition. *Introductory Course* (audiotape program). Gig Harbor, WA: HealthComm Inc., 1991.

23. Cook, Wendy. *Foodwise: Understanding What We Eat and How It Affects Us: The Story of Human Nutrition*. Clairview Books, 2003.

24. McArdle, Katch and Katch. *Exercise Physiology: Energy, Nutrition and Human Performance*, 3rd ed. Philadelphia: Lea & Febiger, 1991.

25. Cordain, Loren. "Cereal Grains – Humanity's Double Edged Sword." *World Rev Nutr Diet* Vol. 84, 1999.

26. E. Pfieiffer Himself, audiocassette series. Acres U.S.A.

27. Namey, Thomas. (Ed.) Rheumatic Disease Clinics of North America, Vol. 16, Number 4. *Exercise & Arthritis*. November 1990. Philadelphia, PA: W.B. Saunders Company

28. Simontacchi, Carol. *The Crazy Makers*. New York: Jeremy P. Tarcher/Putnam, 2000.

29. Brown, Myrtle, editor. *Present Knowledge in Nutrition*, 6th edition. Washington, D.C.: International Life Sciences Institute, 1990.

30. "Vaccination Statistics," www.mercola.com.

31. Jensen, Bernard and Anderson, Mark. *Empty Harvest*. Garden City Park, NY: Avery Publishing Group Inc., 1989.

32. Cohen, Robert. "The Cream No Longer Rises To the Top." Online: www.notmilk.com.

33. Cohen, Robert. *Milk the Deadly Poison*. Englewood Cliffs, NJ: Argus Publishing, Inc., 1998.

34. Atiq, et al. "Alterations in serum levels of insulin-like growth factors and insulin-like growth-factor-binding proteins in patiens with colorectal cancer." *Int. J. Cancer*, May 15, 1994, 57(4), pp.491-497.

35. Gillespie, J. et al. "Inhibition of pancreatic cancer cell growth in vitro by the tyrphostin group of tyrosine kinase inhibitors." *Br. J. Cancer*, December, 1993, 68(6), pp.1122-1126.

36. Yashiro, T. et al. "Increased activity of insulin-like growth factor-binding protein in human thyroid papillary cancer tissue." *Jpn. J. Cancer. Res.*, January 1994, 85(1), pp. 46-52.

37. Lipski, Elizabeth and Bland, Jefferey. *Digestive Wellness*. Los Angeles: Keats Publishing, 1996, 2000.

38. Getoff, David. Personal communication, San Diego, CA: 2000.

39. Pollan, Michael. "Power Steer." *New York Times*, March 31, 2002.

40. O'Brien, Tim. "Factory Farming and Human Health." *The Ecologist*, June 2001, supplement.

41. "Is Meat From Diseased Animals Safe For Consumption?" Online: www.mercola.com.

42. USDA Sets Rules For Organic Meat, Poultry. Online: www.mercola.com

43. Jensen, Bernard. *Foods That Heal*. Garden City, NY: Avery Publishing Group Inc., 1993.

44. Cockburn, T. Aidan. Infectious Diseases in Ancient Populations. In: *Culture, Disease, and Healing – Studies in Medical Anthorpology by David Landy*. New York: Macmillian Publishing Co. 1977.

45. Epstein, Samuel and Steinman, David. *The Safe Shopper's Bible*. New York: Macmillan, 1995.

46. Wilson, Edward. *The Future of Life*. New York: Vintage Books, 2002.

47. Seafood Watch. Online: www.montereybayaquarium.org.

48. McTaggart, Lynne. *What Doctors Don't Tell You: The truth about the dangers of modern medicine*. London: Thorsons, 1996.

49. Enig, Mary. *Know Your Fats*. Silver Spring, MD: Bethesda Press, 2000.

50. Simopoulos, Artemis and Robinson, Jo. *The Omega Diet*. New York: HarperPerennial, 1999.

51. Fallon and Enig. "The Skinny on Fats." Online: www.westonaprice.org.

52. Getoff, David. *Attaining Optimal Health in the 21st Century*, videocassette series.

53. McArdle, Katch and Katch. *Sports & Exercise Nutrition*. Baltimore, MD: Lippincott, Williams & Wilkins, 1999.

54. Duffy, William. *Sugar Blues*. New York: Warner Books, 1975.

55. "Refined Sugar – The Sweetest Poison of All." Online: www.mercola.com.

56. Blaylock, Russell. *Endotoxins: The Taste That Kills*. Santa Fe, NM: Health Press, 1997.

57. Pooley, Richard, M.D. *Characteristics of a Traditional Diet* (audio taped lecture). Broda O. Barnes, M.D. Research Foundation Inc.

58. Batmanghelidj, F. M.D. *Your Body's Many Cries for Water*. Falls Church, VA: Global Health Solutions, Inc., 1992.

59. Williams, Roger. *Biochemical Individuality*. New Canaan, CT: Keats Publishing, 1956.

60. "Organic Food." Online: www.hypermesis.org.

61. PANNA: Government Agencies Failing to Cut U.S. Pesticide Use. Online: www.panna.org. October 9, 2001.

62. Surfers Against Sewage: "What is the Problem?" Online: www.sas.org.uk.

63. Fox, Martin, M.D. *Healthy Water*. Portsmouth, NH: Healthy Water Research, 1990, 1998. Online: www.healthywater.com.

64. Stitt, Paul. *Beating the Food Giants*. Manitowoc, WI: Natural Press.

65. Rogers, Sherry. *Detoxify or Die*. Prestige Publishers, 2002.

66. Becker, Robert, M.D. *The Body Electric*. New York: Quill, 1985.

67. Kerner, John, M.D. "Effects of Microwave Radiation on Anti-infective Factors in Human Milk." *Pediatrics*. Vol 89, No. 4, April 1992.

68. Omega Nutrition, catalog, 2002.

Resources: General Nutrition
Price-Pottenger Nutrition Foundation Natural Health and Healing Institute
Books, video and audio tapes, membership and services such as articles on nutrition
www.price-pottenger.org

Weston A. Price Foundation
Education, research, activism, resources such as *Shopping Guide* for finding the healthiest foods in supermarkets and health food stores and quarterly newsletter, *Wise Traditions*.
www.westonaprince.org

www.theecologist.com. The website for the British journal, *The Ecologist*, which covers current issues affecting our environment and food supply.

The Raw Gourmet by Nomi Shannon. A raw-foods cookbook.

Organics
Community Alliance with Family Farmers. www.caff.org. Find farm-fresh products in California.

Wild Oats Natural Marketplace, USA. www.wildoats.com

Whole Foods Market, USA and Canada.
www.wholefoods.com

PCC Natural Markets, Washington State
www.pccnaturalmarkets.com

Gold Mine Natural Food Co.
Organic foods, books and household products
(mail-order)
www.goldminenaturalfood.com or 800.475.3663

Sun Organic Farm
Organic foods and drinks (mail-order)
www.sunorganic.com or 888.269.9888

www.oranicconsumers.org. Organic Consumers
Association website, learn more about food safely,
organic agriculture, fair trade and sustainability
with current updates.

The Grain & Salt Society
Celtic Sea Salt, foods, body care products and
books (mail-order)
www.celtic-seasalt.com or 800.867.7258

Omega Nutrition
Organic oils, food, body care and books (mail-order)
www.omeganutrition.com, 800.661.3529

Wheat-free/Gluten-free
Gluten-Free Pantry
Gluten-free products and books (mail-order)
www.glutenfree.com or 800.291.8386

Wheat-free, Worry-free by Danna Korn. Learn
about gluten intolerance and Celiac Disease,
includes several recipes.

www.coeliac.com. A Celiac DIsease and gluten-free resource.

Dairy
www.notmilk.com. A collection of articles by
Robert Cohen (author of *Milk the Deadly Poison*)
on all aspects of milk and the dairy industry.

www.realmilk.com. Information and resources on
raw milk.

White Egret Farms, Texas. Supplier of raw
goats milk products and organic meats.
www.whiteegretfarm.com or 512.276.7408.

Clay
Pascalite, Inc.
Pascalite clay products
303.347.3872

Meats/Fish
www.cambrianmeats.com. Cambrian Farms, New
Zealand offers high-quality beef, lamb, venison,
chicken and pork within New Zealand, also
available at some markets internationally.

Lasater Grasslands Beef. A family-owned farm
in Colorado, grass-fed beef available to order at
www.lasatergrasslandsbeef.com.

Vital Choice Seafood. www.vitalchoice.com.

Supplements
Ultralife: supplements based on Metabolic Typing
800.654.8191 or 618.594.7711

Ortho Molecular: EFA Supplements (Mega
Omega and Scandinavian Fish Oil) and digestive
enzymes (Digestzyme). Available through the
C.H.E.K Institute, 800.552.8789 or 760.477.2620.

Wobenzym®N. Digestive enzymes, available
through the C.H.E.K Institute, 800.552.8789 or
760.477.2620.

Water Filters
Young Living: www.youngliving.com or
800.371.2928

Microwave Ovens
"Microwave Tragedy." Raytown, MO: Acres,
U.S.A. April, 1994. An article on the dangers of
eating food cooked in microwave oven.

Chapter 6
1. Childre and Martin. *The Heartmath Solution*. Sa
   Francisco: Harper Collins, 1999.

2. Oschman, James. *Energy Medicine*. New York:
   Churchill Livingstone, 2000.

3. Fong Ha. *Yiquan and the Nature of Energy*. Berkeley, CA: Summerhouse Publications, 1998.

Chapter 7

1. Richardson, Jull, Hodges and Hides. *Therapeutic Exercise for Spinal Segmental Stabilization in Low Back Pain*. Churchill Livingstone, 1999.

Chapter 8

1. Schmidt, Richard, and Lee, Timothy. *Motor Control and Learning*, 3rd Edition. Champaign, IL: Human Kinetics, 1999.

Equipment Resources
1. C.H.E.K Institute, U.S.A. Swiss balls, medicine balls wobble boards, the Pro Fitter, Bosu and other functional exercise equipment available at www.chekinstiute.com or 800.552.8789. .

2. Fitter International, INC., Canada. Swiss balls, medicine balls wobble boards, the Pro Fitter, Bosu and other functional exercise equipment available atwww.fitter1.com or 800.fitter1.

3. Body Bar. www.bodybars.com.

Chapter 9

1. Mogadam, Michael MD. Radio interview, Don Bodenbach, San Diego, CA.

2. *Drug Facts and Comparisons 2003*. Facts and Comparisons, October 2002.

3. *Mosby's Drug Consult 2001*. Mosby, 2001. www.mosby.com/genrx.

4. Boos, Norbert et al. *Spine*. 20, 1995. Quoted by Serge Gracovetsky in a lecture.

Chapter 11

1. Mogadam, Michael MD. Radio interview, Don Bodenbach, San Diego, CA.

2. MacKinnon. *Advances in Exercise Immunology*. Champaign, IL: Human Kinetics, 1999.

3. Kimbrell, Andrew ed. *Fatal Harvest: The Tragedy of Industrial Agriculture*. Washington: Island Press, 2002.

4. MacLean, Paul. *Man's Triune Mind*. 1972.

5. Tracy, Brian. *The Luck Factor*, an audiocassette program. Niles, IL: Nightingale Conant.

Stress reduction training tool:
Freeze Frame by Heartmath, available through the C.H.E.K Institute at 800.552.8789 or www.chekinstitute.com.

Chapter 12

1. Smolensky, Michael and Lamberg, Lynne. *The Body Clock Guide to Better Health*. New York: Henry Holt and Company, LLC., 2000.

2. *The Guide to Adrenal Health*. San Diego, CA: Bio-Health Diagnostics, Inc., 2002.

3. Sapolsky, Robert. *Why Zebras Don't Get Ulcers*. New York: W.H. Freeman and Company, 1998.

4. Getoff, David. Personal communication, San Diego, CA: 2000.

5. Stitt, Paul. *Beating the Food Giants*. Manitowoc, WI: Natural Press.

6. Benteen, Tom MD. Personal communication, San Diego, CA: 2000.

7. Maund, Chris. "Sleep, Biological Rhythms and Electromagnetic Fields." Online: www.chekinstitute.com.

Chapter 13

1. Seidell, Jaap. World Health Organization Report.

2. Seidell, Jaap. World Health Organization Report.

3. Levenstein, Harvey. *Revolution at the Table*. New York: Oxford University Press, 1988.

4. Levenstein, Harvey. *Paradox of Plenty*. New York: Oxford University Press, 1993.

5. Waterhouse, Debra Ph.D. *Outsmarting the Female Fat Cell*. New York, NY: Warner Books, 1993.

6. Berardi, John. "Massive Eating, Parts I and II." Online: www.johnberardi.com.

7. Berardi, John. "Appetite for Construction." May 4, 2001. Online: www.johnberardi.com.

8. Ross, Julia. *The Diet Cure*. New York: Viking, 1999.

9. Batmanghelidj, F. M.D. *Your Body's Many Cries for Water*. Falls Church, VA: Global Health Solutions, Inc., 1992.

Chapter 14

1. Watson, Brenda. *Renew Your Life*. Clearwater, FL: Renew Life Press, 2002.

2. Farlow, Christina Hoza, D.C. Food *Additives, A Shopper's Guide to What's Safe and What's Not*. Escondido, CA: KISS For Health Publishing, 2001.

3. Brostoff, Jonathan and Gamlin, Linda. *Food Allergies and Food Intolerance*. Rochester, VT: Healing Arts Press, 2000.

4. Pottenger, Francis Marrion. Pottenger's Cats. San Diego, CA: Price-Pottenger Nutrition Foundation, Inc., 1983.

5. Fox, Martin. *Healthy Water*. Portsmouth, NH: Healthy Water Research, 1990, 1998. Online: www.healthywater.com.

6. Antonio, Jose and Stout, Jeffery. *Sports Supplements*. Baltimore, MD: Lippincott, Williams & Wilkins, 2001.

7. Brostoff, Jonathan and Gamlin, Linda. *The Complete Guide to Food Allergy and Intolerance*. New York, NY: Crown Publishers, 1989.

8. Lopez, Williams and Miehlke. *Enzymes, the Foundation of Life*. Charleston, SC: The Neville Press, Inc., 1994.

9. Campbell, Don. *Mozart Effect*. New York: Avon Books, 1997.

10. Jensen, Bernard. Dr. *Jensen's Guide to Better Bowel Care*. New York: Avery Publishing Group, 1999.

11. Webster, David. *Achieve Maximum Health*. Cardiff, CA: Hygeia Publishing, 1995.

12. Benteen, Tom. Personal communications, San Diego, CA, 2000.

Exercise & Health Care Practitoners
C.H.E.K (Corrective High-performance Exercise Kinesiology) Practitioners
www.chekinstitute.com
then click on "Practitioner in Your Area"

CHEK NLCs (Nutrition and Lifestyle Coaches)
www.chekinstitute.com
then click on "Practitioner in Your Area"

Labs
BioHealth Diagnostics
www.biodia.com or 800.570.2000

Great Smokies
www.gsdl.com

For a complete, updated list of resources, please visit:

www.eatmoveandbehealthy.com

Index